Gender, Global Health and Violence

Feminist Studies on Peace, Justice and Violence

Series Editors:

Tiina Vaittinen, Shweta Singh and Catia C. Confortini

This series provides a forum for the expanding feminist scholarship on questions of justice, peace, and violence, beyond the war/peace dichotomy. It integrates and pushes forward existing feminist contributions to the field of peace research, thus reinvigorating the transdisciplinary traditions of both peace research and feminism. We publish monographs and carefully edited volumes that utilise feminist critical methodologies to shed light on gendered and sexualised violence and injustice in different empirical contexts, with the explicit normative aim of finding ways to lessen the violence and increase justice in the world. Feminists with interests in the study of direct violence (e.g. feminist security studies and feminist work on interpersonal violence), structural violence (e.g. racism and anti-racism, migration and mobility, care, and global health), epistemic peace, and justice (e.g. feminist postcolonial/decolonial and indigenous approaches to peacebuilding, intersectional and transnational analyses of justice, activist/scholar methodologies, feminist approaches to mediation, and conflict transformation) will find an intellectual home in a transdisciplinary series with broad normative dimensions – the feminist-informed inquiry into possibilities for a more just and peaceful world.

Titles in the Series

Gender, Global Health and Violence: Feminist Perspectives on Peace and Disease
Edited by Tiina Vaittinen and Catia C. Confortini

Gender, Global Health and Violence

Feminist Perspectives on Peace and Disease

Edited by Tiina Vaittinen and
Catia C. Confortini

ROWMAN &
LITTLEFIELD
———INTERNATIONAL
London • New York

Published by Rowman & Littlefield International Ltd.
6 Tinworth Street, London, SE11 5AL, UK
www.rowmaninternational.com

Rowman & Littlefield International Ltd. is an affiliate of Rowman & Littlefield
4501 Forbes Boulevard, Suite 200, Lanham, Maryland 20706, USA
With additional offices in Boulder, New York, Toronto (Canada), and Plymouth (UK)
www.rowman.com

Selection and editorial matter © 2020 by Tiina Vaittinen and Catia C. Confortini
Copyright in individual chapters is held by the respective chapter authors.

All rights reserved. No part of this book may be reproduced in any form or by any electronic or mechanical means, including information storage and retrieval systems, without written permission from the publisher, except by a reviewer who may quote passages in a review.

British Library Cataloguing in Publication Data
A catalogue record for this book is available from the British Library

ISBN: HB 978-1-78661-116-1
        PB 978-1-78661-117-8

Library of Congress Cataloging-in-Publication Data Available
Library of Congress Control Number: 2019953149

ISBN: 978-1-78661-116-1 (cloth : alk. paper)
ISBN: 978-1-78661-117-8 (pbk. : alk. paper)
ISBN: 978-1-78661-118-5 (electronic)

To our children [and John Lennon too]

Contents

About the Editors ix

Acknowledgements xi

List of Acronyms xv

1 Introduction: Analysing Violences in Gendered Global Health 1
Catia C. Confortini and Tiina Vaittinen

PART I: REVISITING STRUCTURAL VIOLENCE 23

2 Replenishing Bodies and the Political Economy of SRHR in Crises and Emergencies 25
Maria Tanyag

3 Rethinking Global Health Priorities from the Margins: Health Access and Medical Care Claims among Indonesia's *Waria* 47
Néstor Nuño Martínez

4 'I Cannot Know That Now I Have Cancer!': A Structural Violence Perspective on Breast Cancer Detection in Uganda 70
Deborah Ikhile, Linda Gibson and Azrini Wahidin

5 HIV Politics and Structural Violence: Access to Treatment and Knowledge 89
Elina Oinas

PART II: VIOLENCES ENTANGLED — 115

6 Fighting Symbolic Violence through Artistic Encounters: Searching for Feminist Answers to the Question of Life and Death with Dementia — 117
Dragana Lukić and Ann Therese Lotherington

7 ¡Malas Madres, Malas Mujeres, Malas Todas!: The Incarceration of Women for Abortion-Related Crimes in Mexico — 139
Camilla Reuterswärd

8 When Is It Torture? When Is It Rape? Discourses on Wartime Sexual Violence — 159
Élise Féron

PART III: TOWARDS PEACE AND JUSTICE IN GLOBAL HEALTH — 179

9 Therapeutic Justice for Survivors of Human Rights Violations and Wartime Violence — 181
Debra L. DeLaet, Shannon Golden, and Veronica Laveta

10 Domestic Violence and Public Health: Beginning Steps for Creating More Just and Effective Community Responses — 206
Laura Finley

11 Exposed to Violence While Caring: From Caring Self-Protection to Global Health as Conflict Transformation — 227
Tiina Vaittinen

12 Conclusion: Violence and the Paradox of Global Health — 251
Sophie Harman

Index — 267

About the Authors — 283

About the Editors

Catia C. Confortini is Associate Professor in the Peace & Justice Studies Programme at Wellesley College in Massachusetts (US). Her research and publications explore the contributions of women's peace activism to peace studies as an academic field and as a practice, as well as feminist theorising of peace and violence. She is the author of *Intelligent Compassion: Feminist Critical Methodology in the Women's International League for Peace and Freedom* (OUP 2012); co-editor (with Tarja Väyrynen, Élise Féron, Peace Meadie, and Swati Parashar) of *The Handbook of Feminist Peace Research* (forthcoming, Routledge 2020); and co-editor (with Tiina Vaittinen and Shweta Singh) of the book series Feminist Studies on Peace, Justice and Violence (Rowman & Littlefield International). Her current interests lie at the intersection of feminist peace research and global health. As a feminist peace activist, she has served as Vice President of Women's International League for Peace and Freedom (WILPF) from 2015 to 2018.

Shweta Singh is senior Assistant Professor at the Department of International Relations, Faculty of Social Sciences at the South Asian University (a University established by the SAARC nations) in New Delhi. As a feminist scholar from the global south, she has strived to foreground a South Asian voice in the field of feminist International Relations, and critical Peace and Conflict Studies. She has published extensively in the areas of Women, Peace and Security (South Asia), critical peace and conflict studies, peace education and armed conflict in South Asia (like Kashmir and Sri Lanka).

Tiina Vaittinen is Academy of Finland Postdoctoral Research Fellow at Tampere University, Finland. She holds a PhD in Peace and Conflict Research. Drawing broadly on feminist theories of peace, ethics of care, new materialisms, science and technology studies, her work focuses on deconstructing the global politics of care and care needs. She has published in journals such as *International Feminist Journal of Politics*, *Women's Studies International Forum*, *Peacebuilding*, and *Global Society*. Her monograph on the global biopolitical economy of needs will be published in 2020 (Rowman & Littlefield International).

Acknowledgements

This book, like all academic work, has been a team effort that owes gratitude to a large number of people. First, we would like to express our sincere thanks to all the authors, for bearing with the several rounds of revisions and, at times, surely, rather tedious editorial requests, resulting from our aim to produce an internally consistent volume. Thank you all also for the intellectually stimulating discussions we had in Tampere in January 2018, when workshopping through our first drafts at Tampere Peace Research Institute TAPRI, at Tampere University. Thanks also to TAPRI for hosting the workshop at its premises.

This workshop would not have taken place without the financial support of the International Studies Association (ISA) Venture Workshop Grant, or without the practical, always helpful, and friendly guidance from ISA Grant Manager Lembe Tiky. Wellesley College provided financial support for indexing the manuscript. Thank you. We are also most grateful to Kristiina Tuokko and Johanna Laine, of Tampere University Congress Services, especially Johanna for taking care of all practical arrangements from booking the flights to booking restaurants and accommodations, without any additional cost to our project. To all neoliberal universities across the world: professional conference services of this kind are the most efficient use of resources and facilitate enriching experiences for scholars.

While grateful for the chance of workshopping the book in Tampere, we, however, also need to express our sincere apologies for choosing a venue in the global north, which due to its strict visa regime turned out to be inaccessible for some of our potential authors from the global south. This exclusion is yet another manifestation of (gendered) violence, a concrete reminder of the ways in which physical borders matter in the academia, every day. We bear the responsibility for choosing the venue without thinking ahead, and have certainly learned our lesson for future projects.

We also want to thank the anonymous referees who reviewed the original proposal and some chapters of the book, as well as those who refereed the proposal for the series on Feminist Studies on Peace, Justice and Violence. Your comments and suggestions for revisions were most useful. We have tried to integrate them in this final version, while the mistakes, of course, remain ours. At Rowman & Littlefield International, we want to express our heartfelt gratitude to the most amazing Commissioning Editor, Dhara Snowden, who has guided us through the process of both the book and the series launch with enormous friendliness and supportive encouragement. We very much look forward to working with you in years to come. Thanks to our series co-editor Shweta Singh for launching the series with this edited volume. We are so happy that this is just the beginning of our collaboration.

In the ISA Global Health Section, we want to thank Sophie Harman, Adam Kamradt-Scott, João Nunes, and Anne Roemer-Mahler for rooting for us when we first presented the idea of the book to you, sometime in 2016. Without your encouragement, we might not have had the nerve to take on such a transdisciplinary and challenging project. The fabulous feminists of the Feminist Peace Research Network (FPRN) as well as the ISA Feminist Theory and Gender Studies Section have unconditionally cheered us along the way. From FTGS we thank, in particular, Laura Shepherd for believing in the project early on.

As to our own writing, we want to express our gratitude to various colleagues who took the time to read and comment on the draft of the introductory chapter, including Annariina Koivu, who provided much needed feedback and encouragement early on in this project; the FPRN members at a workshop at Lund University in Spring 2017; and the participants at the TASER (Tampere Security Studies) seminar, organised by Rune Saugmann. As an early career scholar employed through external funding, Tiina's work for this book would not have been possible without salary from the Academy of Finland project on Mundane Practices of Peace (project #297053, PI: Tarja Väyrynen) – thank you. Catia received the financial support of Wellesley College for travel to Tampere, Lund, and various ISA meetings, where early drafts of our ideas took shape. She was able to put the final touches to the manuscript face-to-face with Tiina in Tampere thanks to a Fulbright Finland Foundation Scholarship and the generous hospitality of TAPRI and Tampere University. Larry Rosenwald – literary master, polyglot, translator, Trekky – questioned and critiqued, always with both meticulousness and kindness. Cecelia Lynch read through and gave much needed feedback on multiple drafts of our introduction with the patience only an unconditional friendship can give.

It goes without saying that we could not have completed this project without the endless support from our families, but also without one another. Catia, I love co-authoring with you, and love it that this is only the beginning. Tiina, I feel I need to thank ISA-Northeast for the serendipitous moment when we met and hit it off. What a beautiful partnership we have created! At this point, we probably should also thank Skype and Google Docs and Dropbox for not only spying on us and gathering our information for all kinds of dodgy purposes, but making it possible to co-author across the Atlantic Ocean, as if we shared an office each week.

Tampere, Finland, September 9, 2019
Tiina & Catia

Acronyms

AD	Alzheimer's Disease
ADD	Alzheimer's Disease and other Dementias
AIIA	Australian Institute of International Affairs
AIPEN	Australian International Political Economy Network
ART	Antiretroviral Therapy
ASEAN	Association of Southeast Asian Nations
BME	Black Minority Ethnic
BSE	Breast Self-Examination
CBE	Clinical Breast Examination
CEDAW	UN Committee on the Elimination of Discrimination against Women
CEIPAZ	Centro de Educación e Investigación para la Paz
CVT	Center for Victims of Torture
DRC	Democratic Republic of the Congo
FPRN	Feminist Peace Research Network
GBV	Gender-Based Violence
GRO	Grassroot Organisation
IACHR	Inter-American Commission on Human Rights
ICC	International Criminal Court
ICTR	International Criminal Tribunal for Rwanda
ICTY	International Criminal Tribunal for the former Yugoslavia
IDMC	Internal Displacement Monitoring Centre
IPPNW	International Physicians for the Prevention of Nuclear War
IR	International Relations
ISA	International Studies Association

KEBAYA	Keluarga Besar Waria Yogyakarta (Large Waria Family Jogjakarta)
LCSW	Licensed Clinical Social Worker
MAPW	Medical Association for the Prevention of War
MCANW	Medical Campaign against Nuclear Weapons
MDG	Millennium Development Goals
MilDVE	Milwaukee Domestic Violence Experiment
MSF	Médecins Sans Frontières (Doctors Without Borders)
NCD	Non-Communicable Disease
NGO	Non-Governmental Organization
OECD	Organisation for Economic Co-operation and Development
OUR	Observatory on the Universality of Rights
PKBI	Perkumpulan Keluarga Berencana Indonesia (Indonesian Family Planning Association)
SGBV	Sexual and Gender-Based Violence
SIPRI	Stockholm International Peace Research Institute
SRHR	Sexual and Reproductive Health and Rights
SSA	Sub-Saharan African
TAC	Treatment Action Campaign
TAPRI	Tampere Peace Research Institute
UN	United Nations
UNCAT	United Nations Convention against Torture
UNFPA	UN Population Fund
UNGA	UN General Assembly
UNSC	United Nations Security Council
VAWA	Violence against Women Act
VCT	Voluntary Counselling and Testing
WHO	World Health Organization
WPS	Women, Peace and Security

Chapter 1

Introduction: Analysing Violences in Gendered Global Health

Catia C. Confortini and Tiina Vaittinen

Gender has for a long time been a central category of interest in global health discourses, policies, and practices. Global governance institutions, including the United Nations (UN) and the World Health Organization (WHO), however, still understand gender narrowly. They tend to equate gender with women and/or girls, assuming women's relevance to global health primarily as biological reproducers, or adding gender as an afterthought to policies and recommendations designed in 'gender-blind' ways (Harman 2016). As feminist analysis has shown, gender, of course, is not a synonym for women and girls. It is an organising code in society, where things coded as masculine are taken as the norm and therefore centred and prioritised, whereas things coded as feminine are marginalised, made invisible, and deemed as irrelevant (Peterson 2005). When gender as an ordering principle is not understood in global health politics – and public health discourses more generally – it follows that the everyday health needs coded as masculine are normalised, whereas the needs that are understood as feminine are either exceptional or marginalised or both. Furthermore, the health needs that are difficult to code according to this binary order – such as those of sexual minorities and non-binary individuals, or feminised health problems among men – may become silenced altogether. Such silencing and erasure of gendered health needs by the global health agenda shape the lives of intersectionally gendered men and women and non-binary groups of people across the world – often in violent ways. This volume's purpose is to address such violences through a range of empirical case studies and rigorous feminist analysis.

Even though critical literature on Global Health offers useful lessons for looking at the various intersections between violence and health (as we show later in this chapter), these discussions tend to be scattered across different scholarly fields. In this volume, feminists coming from a range of fields – Peace Research, International Relations (IR), Gender Studies, Political Science, Public Health, Sociology, and Medical Anthropology, for instance – bring together these multidisciplinary concerns. In this regard, the edited collection has been a collective research project crossing disciplinary boundaries and discourses, so as to understand gendered violences in global health better. It began at an International Studies Association–funded workshop at Tampere Peace Research Institute (TAPRI) in January 2018, proceeded through several rounds of revisions, editing, and conversations with all the authors, and finds its end – and hopefully new beginnings – here, within the covers of this book.[1]

To create a common language for such a transdisciplinary effort, we have brought together perspectives from two transdisciplinary fields of research that are, or at least ought to be, interested in questions of gender, global health, and violence – namely Global Health and Peace Research. In this introductory chapter, we elaborate upon the benefits of analysing gendered violence in global health at the intersection of these two research fields.

The purpose of the chapter is fourfold. First, reviewing different bodies of literature we pinpoint the connections between Peace Research and Global Health. Second, we elaborate on a number of understandings of violence, and discuss the ways in which they are used as analytical tools in the chapters of this volume. Third, we explain how our approach builds on and yet departs from prevalent IR approaches to global health, which focus on securitisation theories. Finally, we show how critical Global Health literature has addressed gendered violence and injustice from multiple angles, and how these discussions would benefit from the more nuanced conceptualisation of violence that Peace Research can provide. We maintain that, particularly when understood from a feminist angle, the concept of violence in its entire complexity – and beyond the most common articulation of structural violence (e.g. Farmer 2004) – would be an analytically useful tool for global health scholarship, as it seeks to advance the health and wellbeing of populations and societies. These goals, in turn, are central components of the just and peaceful social transformation that Peace Research seeks to attain.

CROSS-POLLINATING PEACE RESEARCH WITH GLOBAL HEALTH

Widening the horizons of what it means to study violence, peace, and justice in the intersectionally gendered every day, this volume shows how bringing feminist Global Health together with feminist discussions of peace and violence can enrich both scholarly traditions. In contemporary Peace Research, there is relatively little engagement with questions of Global Health. We think this is unfortunate, since engaging with the global health scholarship would immensely benefit peace researchers, as they seek to understand violence, conflict, and peace in different empirical contexts. Simultaneously, with its multidimensional understanding of violence, in/justice, and peace, Peace Research has the capacity to provide the analytical tools that would help us to understand better the ethically and politically complex worlds of global health.

In many ways thus, the volume seeks to do the same for the relationship between Global Health and Peace Research that others have sought to do for the relationship between Global Health and IR, where the study of global health has grown rapidly over the past two decades. Sara E. Davies and colleagues, for instance, have shown how the emergent global health scholarship within IR expands our 'understanding of the politics that shape global health practices', while simultaneously allowing for the emergence of different understandings of IR (Davies et al. 2014, 829). Similarly, by bringing in the gendered questions of global health and violence to Peace Research through an interdisciplinary compilation of feminist interventions, we seek to expand peace researchers' disciplinary imaginations. We draw on the work of critical global health scholars in IR (e.g. Howell 2014; Nunes 2014), who have criticised the tendency of IR to analyse global health politics through securitisation theories. We agree that often the state-centric securitisation frame fails to capture the transnational world of Global Health, and particularly, as O'Manique and Fourie (2018) argue, how it shapes, and is shaped by the intersectionally gendered every day. The chapters in this book suggest that a focus on the entanglements of violence/peace is much more suited for these purposes. Through a nuanced analysis of violence, peace, and justice beyond questions of security or even direct violence, we aim to deepen our understanding of the intertwined domains of politics and ethics as they shape Global Health. Furthermore, demanding that both fields take seriously the complexities of gender and sexuality, we believe that feminist perspectives provide the most fruitful tools for Peace Research to engage with Global Health, and vice versa.

This volume is partly motivated by our conviction that Peace Research should go beyond the metaphors about healthy societies and recognise concrete, embodied health as pivotal to the study of peace/violence. In this regard, this volume is part of an emerging movement to make feminist approaches to Peace Research visible, not only as a question of 'women' but as a wider question of the hierarchies between masculinities and femininities (as many of the chapters in this volume also underscore). After all, despite decades of feminist work, the patriarchal hierarchies in Peace Research continue to silence feminist perspectives despite their relevance (McLeod and O'Reilly 2019; Vaittinen 2017, 41–64; Vaittinen et al. 2019; Wibben et al. 2019). Consequently, also feminised questions such as public health, sickness, corporeality, and sexuality have become overshadowed in Peace Research by the more masculine realm of the specific violence of armed conflict and war. Simultaneously, for feminist Peace Research it is crucially important to engage with global health scholarship more directly and explicitly than before. In the following section, we look at the ways in which Peace Research has engaged with health thus far, and elaborates peace researchers' understanding of violence, which we believe would benefit global health scholarship.

Peace Research and Health

Although sometimes understood as a mere sub-field of IR, Peace Research is a transdisciplinary scholarly field of its own (e.g. Galtung 1964; *Journal of Conflict Resolution* 1957; Wibben et al. 2019). As such, it aims at better understanding violence and injustice in different empirical contexts, so that peaceful interventions for a more just world may be made possible. Unlike in most analyses of IR then, or in popular parlance, peace for peace researchers is not about the absence of armed conflict only, but about wider questions of justice globally and transnationally. In Peace Research, the term 'peace' has multiple meanings: *negative peace* refers to the absence of direct, personal violence (Galtung 1969); *positive peace* stands for the absence of *all kinds* of violence, and the presence of social justice (e.g. Confortini 2006; Galtung 1969, 1996; King 1963). Feminist peace researchers have called into question these static definitions, which construct peace negatively as the absence of violence. Feminists also claim that such definitions presuppose an ultimate, fixed vision, thus disregarding how the day-to-day work to build the world we seek also constitutes peace. Jo Vellacott proposes instead the phrase *dynamic peace*, which refers to 'the ongoing process of laying a solid foundation for peaceful relations between people, groups or nations' (Vellacott 2008, 203). Elise Boulding (drawing on Jane Addams 2007) refers to peace as an 'action concept, involving a constant shaping and reshaping of understandings, situations, and behaviors in a constantly changing lifeworld' (Boulding 2000, 1). A post-human account of peace would include the non-human world and the environment (cf. Braidotti 2013, 2017; Boulding 2000; Shiva 1989, 2015).

Interested in the wellbeing of the living in the broadest sense, then, Peace Research bears a lot of resemblance with the study of Global Health, and indeed health metaphors have often been used to describe the nature and aims of the discipline. Peace Research is, for instance, perceived as embracing normative goals akin to those in medicine and public health, with peace researchers portrayed as physicians in a world of violence (Barash 2014; see also Jutila, Pehkonen and Väyrynen 2008). Beyond such metaphors, however, Peace Research rarely tackles questions of health or disease per se. Consequently, there are very few self-identified peace researchers working on global health issues.

When Peace Research engages with health, this takes place mainly in the context of war, humanitarianism, or post-war interventions. The recent literature on 'post-liberal peace', for example, encompasses public health questions implicitly or explicitly within discussions about human security, emancipation, or welfare (e.g. Berents 2015; Beswick and Jackson 2011; Campbell, Chandler and Sabaratnam 2011; McLeod 2015; Richmond 2010, 2011). Furthermore, Peace Research that emphasises the relationship between conflict and development often talks of health in terms of human development, or in relation to trade-offs, for instance, between resources for war and resources for health care (e.g. O'Gorman 2011; Williams and MacGinty 2016).

Similarly, the medical peace movement has for decades fostered a dialogue between medical practice and Peace Research. This movement includes organisations such as International Physicians for the Prevention of Nuclear War (IPPNW), the Medical Campaign against Nuclear Weapons (MCANW), and the Medical Association for the Prevention of War (MAPW). The two last mentioned were merged into Medact in 1992, which today has a broad agenda that incorporates 'the health threats posed by climate change and structural violence as well as violent conflict', while seeking to abolish nuclear arms and 'reduce the power and influence of the global military-industrial complex'. Medact also 'promotes the universal right to health as a platform for peacebuilding and more effective international diplomacy and cooperation' (Medact n.d.).

These examples show that there exist some important forums for the shared interests of Peace Research and Global Health scholars. Yet, we feel that in Peace Research, these forums, and consequently the interest in Global Health, are not particularly well noted. Furthermore, apart from the recently broadened agenda of Medact, in many forums, there still remains an over-emphasis on questions of war, post-war, and humanitarianism in the analysis of questions of health and peace. This focus on *negative* peace overshadows the intersections of global health and different forms of direct and indirect violence in the gendered everyday beyond armed conflict. What is therefore needed, we argue, are joint feminist peace and global health scholars' interventions: while Peace Research has a lot to learn about peace and justice from and in the field of Global Health, it can simultaneously contribute to global health scholarship by providing it with nuanced concepts, empirical data, and methodological tools for analysing violence and its intersections with and in global health. Such interventions would contribute to the existing forums and discussions by expanding and complementing the two fields' agendas. We intend this volume to be the beginning of this mutual engagement.

VIOLENCE(S) IN PEACE RESEARCH

Peace Research is a transdisciplinary field of scholarly work, the purpose of which is to uncover different forms of violence within and across societies, with a normative goal to lessen or eradicate violence and increase justice. As noted earlier, peace in its positive form refers to the absence of violence of all kinds, sometimes articulated as the presence of conditions for the flourishing of human and non-human life (Boulding 2000). Often, if not always, Peace Research begins with the search for violence in particular empirical contexts. Violence, however, takes multiple forms, as does, as we have seen, peace (Galtung 1969, 167; Wibben et al. 2019). The chapters in this volume discuss a wide variety of violences, as they emerge from and entangle with the embodied gendered realities of global health. In this introduction, we would like to draw attention to three forms of violence, namely direct (personal), structural, and epistemic.

Structural violence, as defined by the Norwegian peace researcher Johan Galtung (1969, 171), is harm that is indirectly caused by political and economic structures, rather than an easily identifiable actor directly harming the other (as in the case of personal violence – perhaps the most straightforward and common understanding of violence). As further discussed, this concept of indirect, structural violence is familiar to most scholars of Global Health (see our discussion on Paul Farmer as well as Ikhile, Gibson, and Wahidin's contribution to this volume), and Galtung himself draws on examples from health care. While he defines violence broadly as 'the cause of the difference between the potential and the actual, between what could have been and what is' (Galtung 1969, 168), structural violence manifests itself very evidently in health and life-expectancy differentials. For instance, if a person dies of tuberculosis today, when medicines are available, there is violence involved, since the potential of keeping the person alive is not realised. If the reason for this death is that someone decided to withhold the medication on purpose, the violence is direct – even genocidal, as argued by HIV/AIDS activists in Mbeki's South Africa (see Oinas, this volume) – but if the medication is not available due to poverty, inequity, inequality, structural racism, or other systemic factors, the violence is structural.

Drawing on Galtung, Jai Frithjof Brand-Jacobsen uses the metaphor of an iceberg to explain how direct violence is only the most visible and smallest part of the formation, which is, like structural violence, largely below water (Brand-Jacobsen 2002, 17). Similarly, Lee (2016) emphasises that understanding structural violence in the context of global health is crucially important, because structural violence has often deadly consequences of massive proportions. Drawing on the findings of Gernot Köhler and Norman Alcock (1976) and James Gilligan (1999) among others, Lee argues that up to eighteen million deaths each year are caused by structural violence. This means that global and local socioeconomic inequalities cause several times more 'excess death and disability' than do 'suicide, homicide, and warfare *combined*' (Lee 2016, 110, emphasis in the original). Lee further stresses that structural violence tends to work through both gender and racial disparities. Utilising World Bank data on gender and development, she points out that in low- and middle-income countries, 'women account for an estimated 3.9 million excess deaths each year . . . . About two-fifths are never born due to a preference to sons, a sixth die in early childhood, and over a third die in their reproductive years' (Lee 2016, 112). Simultaneously in higher-income countries, structural racism leads to racialised groups' unequal access to resources, opportunities, and risks, which in turn lead to overrepresentation in prisons, higher risk of unemployment, disparities in access to health care, and lower life expectancies (see also Alexander 2012; Hinton 2016; Jones et al. 2009; Roberts 2012).

In our reading of these concepts, and in the contributions to this volume, direct and structural forms of violence are not mutually exclusive. And it is here where we partially depart from Galtung, who sees structural violence as being without 'an actor that commits the violence' (Galtung 1969, 170). For the authors of this volume, instead, violent structures are continuously (re)produced by identifiable actors and political decisions, including actions by the state, one of whose tasks is the protection of its population from violence (see Reutersward, this volume). As all the chapters in this volume exemplify, usually those suffering from gendered structural violence in health care are victims of multiple intersecting forms of violence.

Neoliberal capitalism in its global and local manifestations (re)produces these violent intersections through the logic of capital (profit) accumulation and economic growth, which underpins the differential access to health care for precarious populations. The structures of global capitalism enable the wellbeing of some bodies and populations at the cost of others' suffering (e.g. Kelly 2015), which makes neoliberal capitalism – and its agents – violent by definition. This violence is particularly evident in the realm of gendered global health (Schrecker and Bambra 2015).

In this volume, the authors flesh out many such violent intersections, while drawing attention to the potential of peaceful transformation. In particular, we invite Global Health scholars to rethink gendered violence beyond structural violence, and here the concept of epistemic violence plays an important role. This form of violence is produced by particular epistemic orders – such as the biomedical discourse in Global Health – where only certain kinds of pain and suffering make sense, and the pain of others is rendered incomprehensible and unspeakable, and thereby potentially untreatable. We borrow the term from postcolonial feminism, and particularly Gayatri Spivak's work on subalternity, to highlight how in mainstream discourses of global health, the feminised and racialised voices of the Other are silenced and muted as voices of the irrational.

In her widely cited essay 'Can the Subaltern Speak?' Spivak (1988) argues that the colonial project continues to (re)constitute the colonial subject as the subaltern Other in global political and economic orders. As the constitutive outside of the predominant episteme, the subaltern cannot speak – in her own voice – without simultaneously being assimilated in the order, and thereby losing one's own history and being. This complete erasure of the subaltern from the episteme is epistemic violence, and it can be confronted and mitigated, by expanding the epistemic order so as to 'grant the subaltern the possibility of logic' (Spivak 2008, 1:02:02). Many of the chapters in this book seek to do exactly that (see, for example, Oinas; Lukić and Lotherington; Féron; Vaittinen).

In bringing together discussions of gendered and sexualised violence in marginalised realms of global health, this volume aims to widen the episteme of global health scholarship. Such a widened field would be better equipped to listen to what those in the margins have to say about their suffering and to respect their knowledge and expertise in matters relating to their health. This is particularly important since epistemic violence – that is, the fundamental incapacity of the marginalised to speak in the language of the oppressive episteme without losing their own voice – often leads to or intersects with other forms of violence too. Indeed, the relationships between different forms of violence are never uncomplicated and, rather, they are full of tensions, which themselves may lead to intersecting cycles of violence. Attempts to eradicate structural or direct violence, for instance, may embody epistemic violence, which makes it impossible for certain forms of violence to be seen and spoken about, thus further reproducing cycles of violence. This is seen, for example, in Féron's chapter, which brings to light how attempts to address sexual violence in conflict end up erasing the voices of male victims of sexual violence. DeLaet, Golden, and Laveta, on the other hand, point to the violence that retributive forms of justice may reproduce when the needs of torture survivors are not put at the centre of post-conflict justice efforts.

Questions of silence and silencing in global health interventions have been taken up strongly in what is now the prevalent IR approach to global health, securitisation theory, as well as its critiques. In the following section, we examine how securitisation can help us understand the relative disregard of global politics for certain diseases, namely those which are not constructed as threats to state security. At the same time, we explicate how our approach distinguishes itself from securitisation by focusing both on the gendered embodied every day and the multidimensional and multi-sited aspects of violence.

Securitised Global Health – and Beyond

While Peace Research seems disinterested in wider global health questions, in the related discipline of IR, global health has gained increasing attention over the past decade. Here, the so-called securitisation theories form a predominant frame of analysis (Nunes 2014). For us, these theories, and especially their critics, provide important openings for thinking about entangled forms of violence in gendered global health.

Securitisation can be defined as 'a political and dialogical process whereby a social problem becomes a security issue and is conceived as an existential threat' (Meger 2016, 19). Critical approaches to Global Health note that the securitisation of global health has resulted in a disproportionate amount of attention and funding for diseases that are constructed as existential threats to the state. Such has been the case, for example, of infectious diseases, which by their nature easily cross borders and can potentially affect populations in the global north (e.g. HIV/AIDS, Ebola, and Zika). To the extent that it emphasises how certain diseases rise to the status of state security threats, thus becoming subjects of global health interventions, while others do not, the securitisation paradigm may help explain the dearth of responses and resources to non-communicable diseases (NCDs). At the same time, by diverting attention to the language of threats – even if critically so – this paradigm offers few tools to analyse how the non-securitised (and thus politically invisible) concerns of NCDs can be best responded at the global level. Furthermore, as noted by João Nunes (2014, 942), securitisation theories tend to portray security merely as a negative logic, as dangerously excessive state governance over life that is to be resisted. In the realm of health in/security, however, government intervention is often a prerequisite for the delivery of healthcare services, a prerequisite that is concealed if concepts such as health and social security are read only in a negative light. What remains 'lacking is an appreciation of the different meanings that "being secure" can have in the case of health' (Nunes 2014, 943). For these reasons, the securitisation paradigm is inadequate for understanding multiple, entangled, and embodied forms of harm in global health, as well as the potential for remediation.

Our critical approach to the use of securitisation theory in global health follows Alison Howell's (2014) work. According to Howell, it is not that global health issues only recently became a matter belonging to the exceptional realm of national security, exiting the 'normal' realm of politics. Rather, since the nineteenth century, medicine and social/national/international security have developed symbiotically, and together they share a common 'strategic logic in defense of the population' (Howell 2014, 962). Medicine and warfare 'share practitioners, resources, techniques, and language' (Howell 2014, 976). Securitisation theory, Howell claims, is fundamentally ahistorical in ignoring this symbiotic relation, but it also posits false dichotomies between the 'normal' realm of politics and the 'exceptional' realm of security. Consequently, securitisation theory ends up constructing harmful distinctions between social and national/international security, and by extension between the domestic and the international.

These dichotomies, we would add, are deeply gendered discursively. Namely, whereas the securitised dilemmas of global health have the power to call for responses at the high-level (masculinised) politics of international diplomacy, the concerns that require approaches of social policy are easily deemed as domestic issues of the (feminised) welfare state. Furthermore, in neoliberal domestic politics throughout the world today, the (masculinised) biomedical discourse of health tends to override the (feminised) politics of social security. Consequently, many concerns that would require the tackling of structural violence by means of social policy are left unattended in the global politics of health. Thus, in terms of policies and practices as well as theoretically, the securitisation of global health may prevent the emergence of approaches that seek to integrate global health *and* social policy with an aim towards a more just and less violent world.[2] For such an approach, we believe, transdisciplinary dialogues between feminist Peace Research and feminist global health scholarship have a lot to offer.

In her criticism of securitisation theory, Howell calls for ridding ourselves of global health security and proposes instead the new field of Global Politics of Medicine, which would allow us to be curious about new questions of ethics beside the economic reductionism of health 'goods' distribution. We respond to Howell's call in this volume by demonstrating how a feminist focus on violence/peace allows for a deeper understanding of embodied forms of harm, ethics, and agency in various gendered realms of global health. Feminist reflections on violence/peace allow us to illuminate the ways in which the politics of medicine must engage with the politics of social care on an equal basis. It is, for instance, possible to study the epistemic violence inherent in 'the global politics of the inequitable *imposition* of medicine and medical authority' (Howell 2014, 984; see also Oinas, this volume) as well as the structural violence of the inequitable distribution of power in global health and global health governance. Simultaneously, by taking seriously the social movements that struggle 'against the potential violences of medicine' (Howell 2014, 987), a feminist focus on peace/violence enables us to locate hidden spaces and agencies of resistance which stand against the gendered securitisation of health.

João Nunes (2014), too, takes a critical stand against the concept of global health security, which he argues focuses excessively on national security and the securitising efforts of the elites, while disregarding the concrete insecurities experienced in individual lives. He does not fully reject the concept of health security, however, but rather reworks it to embrace better the multiple facets of health *in*security, beyond methodological nationalism. Here, Nunes takes the embodied human being as the 'primary referent for thinking about security' (Nunes 2014, 944). Building on the so-called Aberystwyth school of critical security studies (e.g. Ken Booth and Andrew Linklater), Nunes understands insecurity as a defining condition of human life, which he argues should be taken as a starting point in the analysis of health. However, very similar premises undergird feminist theories of vulnerability, care, dependency, and human security (e.g. Robinson 2011), all of which are relevant for this volume. Indeed, like Nunes, this volume seeks to provide analytical insights to embodied health insecurities, and ways to mitigate them. However, while Nunes' account does not attend to the differences that the intersections of gender, sexuality, class, race, and age produce in the field of health in/security, the chapters in this volume take such situated realities of life as their foundation.

In order to rethink global health in/security, Nunes suggests a new theoretical approach that builds on the concept of domination. This approach, he argues, both deepens and broadens the analysis by connecting the individual experience of insecurity with the social meaning-making practices, as well as the structures that form the conditions of possibility for both the experienced in/securities and their interpretation (Nunes 2014, 947–952). He argues that the domination approach helps to comprehend better the multiple faces of insecurity, as they are manifested through different kinds of (direct and indirect) harm, unpredictability, and dimensions of inequality. We are highly sympathetic to Nunes' suggestion of analysing global health in/securities through different dimensions of domination, and in many ways the interventions presented in this volume are complementary to his approach. We believe that the concept of violence provides similar, yet more, nuanced tools of analysis, than does domination. Specifically, our widened focus on messily entangled forms of violences brings to light, first, the agency/power of the victims of violence in addition to domination as power-over (see Allen 2000; Carroll 1972); and, second, the complex *relational* agencies that emerge as 'agential cuts' (Barad 2007) between the allegedly powerful and the powerless, in the practices of global health. This move allows the chapters in this book to disentangle power from violence in productive ways.

In the following section, we argue that, while feminist global health scholarship has highlighted the operation of structural violence in the politics of global health, widening the scope of analysis to include also other forms of indirect violence – such as epistemic – would serve more fruitfully the goals of feminist justice.

GLOBAL HEALTH APPROACHES TO VIOLENCE

Given the role of health care in the promotion of equality and equity across intersectional differences, universally accessible public health is one of the key means in battling violence across the world. This underlines the importance of increased dialogue between Global Health scholars and peace researchers. In some areas of interest, such dialogue already exists, and many scholars and practitioners of medicine see equity in health as central to promoting peace and non-violence in societies. For example, psychiatrist and violence studies specialist Bandy X. Lee has proposed a systematic framework for violence prevention, to be applied especially to global health approaches (e.g. Lee 2015, 2016). She combines 'bio-psycho-social' and 'structural-environmental perspectives on violence', while drawing on a wide range of interdisciplinary literature from psychology to anthropology to political science to economics. Studying the causes and cures of violence in the field of Global Health, Lee also makes use of peace researchers' work on structural violence.

Similarly, the international journal *Medicine, Conflict and Survival* – founded in 1985 as *Medicine and War* – engages with the ethical and political dilemmas that war and social violence generate for public health and medical professionals. In their edited volume, Howard, Sondorp, and ter Veen (2012), in turn, look at the effects of violent conflict on public health, and the multiple facets and challenges of delivering health services during humanitarian crises and post-conflict peacebuilding. This global health scholarship, however, does not describe or analyse health, health policy, or health governance *themselves* as questions of violence. One notable exception is anthropologist and physician Paul Farmer, who argues for an understanding of health inequalities through the lenses of structural violence (Farmer 2004 and 2005; see also Farmer 1992; Rilko-Bauer and Farmer 2016).

Indeed, as Sophie Harman notes in the concluding chapter of this volume, while peace researchers may fail to engage with Global Health, scholars of global health have embraced the concept of structural violence, notably starting with the work of Nancy Scheper-Hughes (1992) and Paul Farmer (1992; 2004; see also, for example, Anderson 2015; Basnyat 2017; Mills 2016). The influence of Farmer's work in particular is evident in some of the chapters of this book. Yet, the volume also goes beyond Farmer-inspired engagement with structural violence in global health.

As critics of Farmer's approach have noted (Baer, Singer and Susser 2013; Dubal 2012; Wacquant 2004), an exclusive focus on structural violence risks de-politicising health interventions by presenting problems as results of abstract systems – as when Galtung elides the agents of structural violence – rather than the sum of political decisions and actions *by someone*.

We recognise the value of seeing systemic oppression as violence, as we note earlier in regard to the heuristic value of Nunes' focus on domination. However, in this volume, we are concerned not only with the violence of structures but also with the potential dilemmas and contradictions that arise when structural violence is understood as the most central or even sole type of indirect violence in global health, rather than in a complex and sometimes contradictory relationship with other forms of violence.

For example, as the book shows, structural violence is often the breeding ground for other types of violence, such as direct violence. Yet, a simple focus on the crude division between structural and direct violence *only* may hinder us from seeing other types of subtle forms of violence in gendered global health, such as epistemic, symbolic, and cultural violence, all of which point to silent processes of exclusion that the concept of structural violence alone fails to capture. Such exclusions can be seen as harming transgender people in Néstor Nuño Martínez's chapter, for instance, domestic violence victims in the chapter authored by Laura Finley, male victims of sexual violence in Élise Féron's contribution, and persons living with dementia in the 'developed' West in Dragana Lukić and Ann Therese Lotherington's as well as Vaittinen's chapters. All these cases involve structural violence, but focusing on structural violence alone risks reproducing the silence about these other types of violences – and when there is silence, violence cannot be addressed for purposes of justice in global health.

What is needed, therefore, is first an articulation of the complex entanglements of different forms of violence in such cases, and second, analytical efforts to disentangle the violences so that solutions to mitigate each form can be found. This volume seeks to showcase such *feminist Peace Research methods*, which use different understandings of violence as analytical tools when examining gendered violence in global health in varied empirical contexts.

In feminist Global Health, there are similar studies that analyse the gendered entanglements of violence in health. These studies, too, operate with concepts of structural or direct violence, shedding light on the complex ways by which violence intertwines with the health needs of embodied individuals in their gendered everyday lives. Emma-Louise Anderson (2015), for instance, relates the gender discrepancies in HIV infection rates in Malawi to structural violence: where responses to the epidemics are framed in the individualistic and technocratic terms of neoliberal approaches to global health and development, they fail to challenge the gendered violences, which are structurally embedded in habits and practices that underpin such differential risks. Neoliberal responses, Anderson claims, also undermine women's various forms of resistance and responses to the structural violence in their lives.

Elizabeth Mills (2016, 87), in turn, examines HIV positive women's and their children's bodies as 'corporeal sites of structural and interpersonal violence', tracing the intersecting pathways through which precarity enters the women's lives. Set in South Africa, where the state infamously failed to provide antiretroviral therapy and drugs to prevent the mother-to-child transmission of the diseases, Mills' ethnography draws attention to complex intersections of violence. Simultaneously, however, her analysis highlights the ways in which these embodied entanglements of violence give rise to resistance and 'constrained agency' in the midst of precarity: for instance, when the women redefine their relationship with the structurally violent state through health activism (see also Oinas, this volume; Nuño, this volume). The value of Mills' analysis is that its intricate ethnographic detail demonstrates the complicated entanglements of gendered violence in global health, while simultaneously challenging the dichotomous 'assumptions of women as either "deserving subjects" or as "autonomous agents"' (Mills 2016, 89).

Indeed, as also this volume seeks to show, the analysis of gender, violence, and global health requires a better recognition of the ways in which different forms of violence get entangled in global health challenges and responses. Furthermore, it requires an understanding of how these violences interlace with differentially gendered and sexualised bodies and lives, which can challenge and shape the violence – thus exercising a form of power – even from the most vulnerable positions. To even begin to analyse such complexities, the invisibility of gender and gendered relations of power in global health governance is to be taken seriously.

Sophie Harman (2011, 2016) has highlighted the 'conspicuous invisibility' of women in this domain, despite women's indispensable care roles in formal and informal health systems (see also Tanyag, this volume), and with the exception of a few women in high-profile institutional positions. This invisibility 'reinforces gendered norms of care and social reproduction' (2016, 524) and 'sidelin[es] gender expertise' (2011, 214) in global health strategies, policies, and practices. Therefore, not only are women invisible, but short-term and long-term responses to disease outbreaks are also not informed by gender analysis. Harman points out that the scope and depth of feminist public health scholarship on HIV/AIDS, for instance, have reflected an increased attention to questions of gender in public health institutions around the disease, but such attention has remained isolated to specific public health sectors. In other words,

> The conspicuous invisibility of women in global health governance confirms what we know about gender assumptions and male bias in international public policy making, but also extends our knowledge to show how women's care roles can be such a conspicuous essential of everyday healthcare yet be willfully invisible from discussion or strategy on global health. (Harman 2016, 527)

Such silences have serious consequences for the wellbeing of women and other gendered subjects, as they reflect in poorer health outcomes and higher mortality rates for those who remain invisible to global health institutions. From a Peace Research perspective, it is worth analysing such invisibility in terms of violence: the silencing of gender as well as sexuality in global health can be seen as epistemic violence.

Feminist Analyses of Violence: Tools for the Future of Global Health

To sum up, this volume starts with the premise that there are so far underexplored, but potentially fruitful synergies between Peace Research and Global Health, not only as academic fields, but also as fields whose practical aims are emancipatory – albeit often articulated differently. We have highlighted the ways in which the chapters use violence as an analytical framework. For sure, all authors place emphasis on different ways to conceptualise violence, but all – implicitly or explicitly – deal with direct, structural, and epistemic violence. Therefore in this chapter, we have devoted some attention to disentangle the messy relationship between these three forms. IR literature on global health, securitisation theories, and especially their critiques are foundational to our discussion, yet we depart from them in important ways. Feminist critical approaches in this literature are the bedrock upon which our analysis stands, since they see gender as a central category of analysis, rather than simply a social arrangement. Our feminist Peace Research approach adds a more nuanced and complex understanding of violence, as an analytical tool with practical utility for our fields as they seek to advance dynamic peace. This fundamental process of societal transformation is central to both Peace Research and Global Health.

The book is divided into three sections: the first one – with chapters written by Maria Tanyag; Néstor Nuño Martínez; Deborah Ikhile, Linda Gibson, and Azrini Wahidin; and Elina Oinas – revisits the question of structural violence. They show how feminist analysis reveals the gendered and embodied forms structural violence can take in contexts of sexual and reproductive health care in crises and emergencies, in the lives of transgender *waria* in Indonesia, for women with breast cancer in Uganda, and in the multidimensional politics of HIV in South Africa. Already this first section leads us to consider not only structural violence, but the ways in which it entwines with and includes also other types of violence. Taking cues from these discussions and foregrounding questions of symbolic, cultural, and epistemic violence, the second section – with chapters authored by Dragana Lukić and Ann Therese Lotherington; Camilla Reuterswärd; and Élise Féron – analyses the complex ways in which different forms of violence entangle in specific contexts of global health. Each case – from the question of life and death when living with dementia in 'western' societies, to the incarceration of women for abortion-related 'crimes' in Mexico, to the violent consequences of silencing wartime sexual violence against men – paints a multidimensional and sometimes messy and contradictory picture of the entanglements. The third section offers examples of ways forward, creative attempts to eliminate or at least ameliorate violence, where spaces of justice are painstakingly carved out in the midst of intertwined gendered violences. Here, the chapters outline the possibilities of feminist justice in different areas. Debra L. DeLaet, Shannon Golden, and Veronica Laveta explicate the benefits of therapeutic justice approaches to post-conflict transitions and human rights violations; Laura Finley proposes a public health model in relation to intimate partner abuse; and Tiina Vaittinen conceptualises feminist global health as 'caring self-protection' and conflict transformation, while drawing on her ethnography of intimate dementia care.

To be clear, we do not intend for the multiple and entangled forms of violence in the book, or our roadmaps to justice, to be a once-and-for-all or static list. Rather, we see the book as a starting point for a more reflexive mode for studying (and doing) global health, also in the difficult sites where global health seems to intertwine with gendered violence. Indeed, Peace Research may have once been fascinated with producing exhaustive typologies and theories of violence with the aim of mapping a route for a peaceful world order (e.g. Galtung 1969). Yet, compiling this volume with authors from different scholarly backgrounds has reminded us about an important feminist lesson of researching peace: namely, typologies of violence – or peace or justice or health – never pre-exist the gendered empirical contexts in which the violences take place and entangle with one another. Therefore, the lessening of violence and the pursuit of justice in practices of global health require situated knowledges and understandings of harm. Furthermore, where old typologies fail to grasp the gendered experiences of violence, novel conceptualisations of violence that derive from the empirically grounded and embodied everyday are required. For this, critical feminist analysis will provide the tools also in the future.

NOTES

1. For the sake of clarity, it should be noted that, throughout the volume, we capitalise initials of academic fields and disciplines (e.g. Global Health scholars). We use lower cases to refer to practices, policy fields, and objects of study (e.g. global health politics).

2. It goes beyond the scope of the present project, but in the transdisciplinary context of this volume, it is indeed worth noting that, for the purposes of more just global health politics, a better integration and increased dialogue between the two scholarly fields of Global Health on one hand and Global Social Policy on the other would be welcome.

REFERENCES

Addams, Jane. 2007. *Newer Ideals of Peace*. Chicago: U. of Illinois Press.
Alexander, Michelle. 2012. *The New Jim Crow: Mass Incarceration in the Age of Color Blindness*. New York: The New Press.
Anderson, Emma Louise. 2015. *Gender, HIV, and Risk: Navigating Structural Violence*. Basingstoke: Palgrave Macmillan.
Baer, Hans A., Merrill Singer and Ida Susser. 2013. *Medical Anthropology and the World System: Critical Perspectives*. 3rd edition. Santa Barbara, CA: Praeger.
Barad, Karen. 2007. *Meeting the Universe Halfway: Quantum Physics and the Entanglement of Matter and Meaning*. Durham, NC: Duke University Press.
Barash, David P. 2014. 'Introduction: Approaches to *Approaches to Peace*'. In *Approaches to Peace: A Reader in Peace Studies*, edited by David P. Barash, 1–4. New York: Oxford University Press.
Basnyat, Iccha. 2017. 'Structural Violence in Health Care: Lived Experience of Street-Based Female Commercial Sex Workers in Kathmandu'. *Qualitative Health Research* 27: 191–203.
Berents, Helen. 2015. 'An Embodied Everyday Peace in the Midst of Violence'. *Peacebuilding* 3, no. 2: 1–14.
Beswick, Danielle and Paul Jackson. 2011. *Conflict, Security and Development: An Introduction*. New York: Routledge.
Boulding, Elise. 2000. *Cultures of Peace: The Hidden Side of History*. Syracuse: Syracuse University Press.
Braidotti, Rosi. 2013. *The Posthuman*. Cambridge, UK and Malden, MA: Polity Press.
Braidotti, Rosi. 2017. 'Posthuman Critical Theory'. *Journal of Posthuman Studies* 1, no. 1: 9–25.
Brand-Jacobsen, Jai Frithjof. 2002. 'Peace: The Goal and the Way'. In *Searching for Peace: The Road to TRANSCEND*, 2nd edition, edited by Johan Galtung, Carl G. Jacobsen and Jai Frithjof Brand-Jacobsen. London and Sterling, VA: PlutoPress.
Campbell, Susanna, Chandler, David and Meera Sabaratnam, eds. (2011). *A Liberal Peace? The Problems and Practices of Peacebuilding*. London: Zed Books.
Carroll, Berenice A. 1972. 'Peace Research: The Cult of Power'. *The Journal of Conflict Resolution* 16, no. 4: 585–616.
Confortini, Catia C. 2006. 'Galtung, Violence, and Gender: The Case for a Peace Studies/Feminism Alliance'. *Peace and Change: A Journal of Peace Research* 31, no. 3: 333–367.

Davies, Sara E., Stefan Elbe, Alison Howell and Colin McInnes. (2014). 'Global Health in International Relations: Editors' Introduction'. *Review of International Studies* 40: 825–834.

DeLaet, Debra L., Shannon Golden and Veronica Laveta. 2019. 'Therapeutic Justice for Survivors of Human Rights Violations and Wartime Violence'. In *Gender, Global Health and Violence: Feminist Perspectives on Peace and Disease*, edited by Tiina Vaittinen and Catia Confortini. London and New York: Rowman & Littlefield.

Dubal, Sam. 2012. Renouncing Paul Famer: A Desperate Plea for Radical Political Medicine. *Being Ethical in an Unethical World*, 12 May 2012. http://samdubal.blogspot.com/2012/05/renouncing-paul-farmer-desperate-plea.html. Accessed 7 September 2019.

Farmer, Paul. 1992. *AIDS and Accusation: Haiti and the Geography of Blame*. Berkeley: University of California Press.

Farmer, Paul. 2004. 'An Anthropology of Structural Violence'. *Current Anthropology* 45: 305–325.

Farmer, Paul. 2005. *Pathologies of Power: Health, Human Rights, and the New War on the Poor*. Berkeley, Los Angeles, London: University of California Press.

Féron, Élise. 2019. 'When Is It Torture? When Is It Rape? Discourses on Wartime Sexual Violence'. In *Gender, Global Health and Violence: Feminist Perspectives on Peace and Disease*, edited by Tiina Vaittinen and Catia Confortini. London and New York: Rowman & Littlefield.

Finley, Laura. 2019. 'Domestic Violence and Public Health: Beginning Steps for Creating More Just and Effective Community Responses'. In *Gender, Global Health and Violence: Feminist Perspectives on Peace and Disease*, edited by Tiina Vaittinen and Catia Confortini. London and New York: Rowman & Littlefield.

Galtung, Johan. 1964. 'An Editorial'. *Journal of Peace Research* 1, no. 1: 1–4.

Galtung, Johan. 1969. 'Violence, Peace and Peace Research'. *Journal of Peace Research* 6: 167–191.

Galtung, Johan. 1996. *Peace by Peaceful Means: Peace and Conflict, Development and Civilization*. Oslo: PRIO.

Gilligan, James. 1999. 'Structural Violence'. In *Violence in the United States: An Encyclopedia*, edited by Ronald Gottesman, 229–233. New York: Charles Scribners and Son.

Harman, Sophie. 2011. 'The Dual Feminisation of HIV/AIDS'. *Globalizations* 8: 213–228.

Harman, Sophie. 2016. 'Ebola, Gender, and Conspicuously Invisible Women in Global Health Governance'. *Third World Quarterly* 37: 524–541.

Harman, Sophie. 2019. 'Violence and the Paradox of Global Health'. In *Gender, Global Health and Violence: Feminist Perspectives on Peace and Disease*, edited by Tiina Vaittinen and Catia Confortini. London and New York: Rowman & Littlefield.

Hinton, Elizabeth. 2016. *From the War on Poverty to the War on Crime: The Making of Mass Incarceration in America*. Cambridge, MA: Harvard University Press.

Howard, Natasha, Egbert Sondorp and Annemarie Ter Veen, eds. 2012. *Conflict and Health*. New York: Open University Press.

Howell, Alison 2014. 'The Global Politics of Medicine: Beyond Global Health, against Securitisation Theory'. *Review of International Studies* 40: 961–987.

Ikhile, Deborah, Gibson Linda and Azrini Wahidin. 2019. '"I Cannot Know That Now I Have Cancer!" A Structural Violence Perspective on Breast Cancer Detection in Uganda'. In *Gender, Global Health and Violence: Feminist Perspectives on Peace and Disease*, edited by Tiina Vaittinen and Catia Confortini. London and New York: Rowman & Littlefield.

Jones, Camara Phyllis, Clara Yvonne Jones, Geraldine S. Perry, Gillian Barclay and Camille Arnel Jones. 2009. 'Addressing the Social Determinants of Children's Health: A Cliff Analogy'. *Journal of Health Care for the Poor and Underserved* 20 (November Supplement): 1–12.

Journal of Conflict Resolution. 1957. 'An Editorial'. *Journal of Conflict Resolution* 1, no. 1: 1–2.

Jutila, Matti, Samu Pehkonen and Tarja Väyrynen (2008). 'Resuscitating a Discipline: An Agenda for Critical Peace Research'. *Millennium* 36, no. 3: 623–640.

Kelly, M. G. E. 2015. *Biopolitical Imperialism*. Alresford: Zero Books.

King, Martin Luther Jr. 1963. *Why We Can't Wait*. New York: Penguin.

Köhler, Gernot and Norman Alcock. 1976. 'An Empirical Table of Structural Violence'. *Journal of Peace Research* 13, no. 4: 343–356.

Lee, Bandy X. 2015. 'Causes and Cures I: Toward a New Definition'. *Aggression and Violent Behaviour* 25, no. 6: 199–203.

Lee, Bandy X. 2016. 'Causes and Cures VII: Structural Violence'. *Aggression and Violent Behaviour* 28: 109–114.

Lukić, Dragana and Ann Therese Lotherington. 2019. 'Fighting Symbolic Violence through Artistic Encounters: Searching for Feminist Answers to the Question of Life and Death with Dementia'. In *Gender, Global Health and Violence: Feminist Perspectives on Peace and Disease*, edited by Tiina Vaittinen and Catia Confortini. London and New York: Rowman & Littlefield.

McLeod, Laura 2015. 'Feminist Approach to Hybridity: Understanding Local and International Interactions in Producing Post-Conflict Gender Security'. *Journal of Intervention and Statebuilding* 9, no. 1: 48–69.

McLeod, Laura and Maria O'Reilly. 2019. 'Critical Peace and Conflict Studies: Feminist Interventions'. *Peacebuilding* 7, no. 2: 127–145.

Medact (n.d.). 'History'. Accessed 3 May 2019. https://www.medact.org/about/history/.

Meger, Sara. 2016. *Rape Loot Pillage: The Political Economy of Sexual Violence in Armed Conflict*. New York: Oxford University Press.

Mills, Elizabeth. 2016. '"When the Skies Fight": HIV, Violence and Pathways to Precarity in South Africa'. *Reproductive Health Matters* 24, no. 47: 85–95.

Nunes, João 2014. 'Questioning Health Security: Insecurity and Domination in World Politics'. *Review of International Studies* 40: 939–960.

Nuño, Néstor M. 2019. 'Rethinking Global Health Priorities from the Margins: Health Access and Medical Care Claims among Indonesia's *Waria*'. In *Gender, Global Health and Violence: Feminist Perspectives on Peace and Disease*, edited by Tiina Vaittinen and Catia Confortini. London and New York: Rowman & Littlefield.

O'Gorman, Eleanor. 2011. *Conflict and Development: Development Matters*. London: Zed Books.
Oinas, Elina. 2019. 'HIV Politics and Structural Violence: Access to Treatment and Knowledge'. In *Gender, Global Health and Violence: Feminist Perspectives on Peace and Disease*, edited by Tiina Vaittinen and Catia Confortini. London and New York: Rowman & Littlefield.
O'Manique, Colleen and Pieter Fourie, eds. 2018. *Global Health and Security: Critical Feminist Perspctives*. New York: Routledge.
Reuterswärd, Camilla. 2019. '¡Malas Madres, Malas Mujeres, Malas Todas! The Incarceration of Women for Abortion-Related Crimes in Mexico'. In *Gender, Global Health and Violence: Feminist Perspectives on Peace and Disease*, edited by Tiina Vaittinen and Catia Confortini. London and New York: Rowman & Littlefield.
Richmond, Oliver. ed. 2010. *Palgrave Advances in Peacebuilding: Critical Developments and Approaches*. Basingstoke: Palgrave Macmillan.
Richmond, Oliver. 2011. *A Post-Liberal Peace*. New York: Routledge.
Rilko-Bauer, Bauer and Paul Farmer. 2016. 'Structural Violence, Poverty, and Social Suffering'. In *The Oxford Handbook of the Social Science of Poverty*, edited by David Brady and Linda M. Burton, 47–74. New York: Oxford University Press.
Roberts, Dorothy. 2012. *Fatal Invention*. New York: New Press.
Robinson, Fiona. 2011. *The Ethics of Care: A Feminist Approach to Human Security*. Philadelphia: Temple University Press.
Scheper-Hughes, Nancy. 1992. *Death without Weeping: The Violence of Everyday Life in Brazil*. Berkeley: University of California Press.
Schrecker, Ted and Clare Bambra 2015. *How Politics Makes Us Sick: Neoliberal Epidemics*. Basingstoke: Palgrave Macmillan.
Shiva, Vandana. 1989. *Staying Alive: Women, Ecology, and Development*. London: Zed Books.
Shiva, Vandana. 2015. *Earth Democracy: Justice, Sustainability, and Peace*. Berkeley, CA: North Atlantic Books.
Spike V. Peterson. 2005. 'How (the Meaning of) Gender Matters in Political Economy'. *New Political Economy* 10, no. 4: 499–521.
Spivak, Gayatri Chakravorty. 1988. 'Can the Subaltern Speak?' In *Marxism and the Interpretation of Culture*, edited by Cary Nelson and Lawrence Grossberg, 271–313. Urbana and Chicago: University of Illinois Press.
Spivak, Gayatri Chakravorty. 2008. 'The Trajectory of the Subaltern in My Work'. University of California Television. Accessed 3 May 2019. https://www.youtube.com/watch?v=2ZHH4ALRFHw.
Tanyag, Maria. 2019. 'Replenishing Bodies and the Political Economy of SRHR in Crisis and Emergencies'. In *Gender, Global Health and Violence: Feminist Perspectives on Peace and Disease*, edited by Tiina Vaittinen and Catia Confortini. London and New York: Rowman & Littlefield.
Vaittinen, Tiina. 2017. *The Global Biopolitical Economy of Needs: Transnational Entanglements between Ageing Finland and the Global Nurse Reserve of the Philippines*. PhD diss. (published). Tampere Peace Research Institute and Tampere University Press: http://urn.fi/URN:ISBN:978-952-03-0505-5. Accessed 7 September 2019.

Vaittinen, Tiina. 2019. 'Exposed to Violence while Caring: From Caring Self-Protection to Global Health as Conflict Transformation'. In *Gender, Global Health and Violence: Feminist Perspectives on Peace and Disease*, edited by Tiina Vaittinen and Catia Confortini. London and New York: Rowman & Littlefield.

Vaittinen, Tiina, Amanda Donahoe, Rahel Kunz, Silja B. Ómarsdóttir and Sanam Roohi. 2019. 'Care as Everyday Peacebuilding'. *Peacebuilding* 7, no. 2: 194–209.

Vellacott, Jo. 2008. 'Dynamic Peace and the Practicalities of Pacifism'. In *Patterns of Conflict, Paths to Peace*, edited by Larry J. Fisk and John L. Schellenberg, 202–205. Toronto: University of Toronto Press.

Wacquant, Loïs. 2004. 'Comments'. *Current Anthropology* 45, no. 3: 322.

Wibben, Annick T. R., Catia C. Confortini, Sanam Roohi, Sarai B. Aharoni, Leena Vastapuu and Tiina Vaittinen. 2019. 'Collective Discussion: Piecing-Up Feminist Peace Research'. *International Political Sociology*, 13: 86–107.

Williams, Andrew and Roger MacGinty. 2016. *Conflict and Development*. 2nd edition. New York: Routledge.

Part I

REVISITING STRUCTURAL VIOLENCE

Chapter 2

Replenishing Bodies and the Political Economy of SRHR in Crises and Emergencies

Maria Tanyag

Sexual and reproductive health 'is a state of physical, emotional, mental, and social wellbeing in relation to all aspects of sexuality and reproduction, not merely the absence of disease, dysfunction, or infirmity' (Starrs et al. 2018). Sexual and Reproductive Health and Rights (SRHR) emphasise a 'human rights discourse around the body and its needs for security, health and pleasure' (Petchesky 2005, 303).[1] SRHR refer to a range of interrelated freedoms and entitlements such as the freedom to make informed decisions regarding one's body without violence or discrimination, and the entitlement to the progressive realisation of full access to health information, facilities, services, and supplies (CEDAW 2013; Starrs et al. 2018). A rights-based approach to sexual and reproductive health has been the product of long, hard-fought, and ongoing political struggles led by women's movements globally especially in the 1990s and beginning with the International Conference on Population and Development in Cairo (see, for example, Correa 1994). It sets responsibilities for state and non-state actors that as duty-bearers they must ensure that policies and programmes are 'equitable, inclusive, non-discriminatory, participatory and evidence-based' (UNGA 2006, 9).

The promotion of SRHR is a distinctly gendered issue. It is integral to the advancement of gender equality, sustainable development, and justice especially in the aftermath of crisis and emergencies (CEDAW 2013; UNGA 2006). Indeed, as the then Special Rapporteur on Health Paul Hunt noted, 'There is no single cause of death and disability for men between the ages of 15 and 44 that is close to the magnitude of maternal death and disability' (UNGA 2006, 5). Evidence show that the health and wellbeing of women and girls are distinctly impacted by both direct and indirect consequences of crises and emergencies (CEDAW 2013; UN Women 2015; Urdal and Che 2013). In some cases, conflicts kill more people long after the fighting has stopped. For instance, a global time-series study by Urdal and Che (2013) on the impact of conflict on fertility and maternal mortality concludes that further research is still needed to understand whether and why there are gendered health consequences in the aftermath of different types of violent conflict and contexts. Among the main reasons for women's distinct vulnerability, especially their heightened risks for maternal deaths, is that in crisis situations such as violent conflicts, there is a complete absence of emergency obstetric care (Urdal and Che 2013, 496). More broadly, women are often left out of global health governance and this exclusion reproduces the 'conspicuous invisibility' of women's health needs, particularly SRHR, across emergency response and in long-term planning of health systems (Davies and Bennett 2016; Harman 2016).

In this chapter, I argue that an invisible cost of crises is in how women and girls bear compounded harms directly through their distinct sexual and reproductive health needs, and indirectly by mitigating rising care demands in their households and communities. It is precisely these compounded harms that reveal why and how women and girls may experience *excess* mortality – that is, mortality beyond what might be expected across a population – during and after crises and emergencies. Through a feminist political economy analysis of SRHR, I demonstrate the continuum of violence between gender-based violence occurring in times of crisis on one hand, and, on the other, the everyday gendered insecurities rooted in structural and symbolic violence embodied by restrictions to SRHR. Consequently, I situate the replenishment of women's health and wellbeing in times of crisis within the ongoing process of reproducing peace and security in the everyday. Within a continuum of peace – which the inverse of a continuum of violence implies – bridging SRHR gaps is a crucial pathway for recasting women's bodily autonomy as an indispensable component to lasting and inclusive development, as well as post-conflict and post-disaster reconstruction.

Drawing on examples from a regional case study of internal displacements in Southeast Asia, I focus on how women and girls experience routine and protracted displacements in a region perennially beset by multiple forms of crisis. The aim of the regional analysis is to sketch out broad similarities in the linkages between different forms of violence and their implications for women's bodily autonomy and wellbeing, rather than offer an in-depth comparative analysis across different displacement contexts. Internal displacements in Southeast Asia represent a compelling case because the region is considered to be among the most 'crisis-prone' regions globally. Conflicts and disasters routinely displace millions of people in the region, and displacement risks are even projected to intensify in the coming years due to the 'multiplier effect' of climate change (Eckstein et al. 2017). Using a regional perspective to SRHR and internal displacements in Southeast Asia, therefore, has relevance for other regional contexts as well as globally, given predictions that multiple and overlapping forms of crisis such as armed conflicts, economic recessions, health pandemics and environmental disasters will lead to an exponential increase in the number of internally displaced persons (Eckstein et al. 2017; IDMC 2018). Moreover, a regional focus engages with and lends further support to current scholarship on the Asia Pacific that calls for regional cooperation in addressing security issues including in the areas of health and gender (Caballero-Anthony 2018; Nair 2015; Veneracion-Rallonza 2016).

The chapter is structured into three main parts. First, I briefly outline the key components of a feminist political economy analysis and how this lens generates a holistic understanding of different forms of gendered violence in crisis and emergencies. Second, I turn to examine examples of restrictions to SRHR in Southeast Asia to further demonstrate the compounded harms women and girls experience in internal displacements, and consequently, what existing interventions have been in place. Third and last, the chapter makes a strong case for greater research and policy attention to eliminating both material and ideological barriers – that is, structural and symbolic violence – that undermine women's and girls' bodily autonomy and wellbeing before, during and after crises. Through the concept of a continuum of peace, the promotion of SRHR is integral to ensuring that broader groups of women and girls equally contribute to and benefit from lasting peace, security and development.

SRHR AND THE ACCUMULATION OF DIFFERENT VIOLENCES

In recent works, I have developed a political economy analysis that builds on the feminist concept of a 'continuum of violence' between violence against women and global violence (Tanyag 2017, 2018a; True and Tanyag 2018). A feminist political economy perspective enables us to map the interdependence between women's bodies and the political economy governing the allocation of resources and people globally with a focus on crisis situations. This approach demonstrates how pre-existing gendered inequalities rooted in the economic devaluing and unequal distribution of unpaid care and domestic work condition both immediate or physical violence in crisis situations, and gradual or indirect harms that undermine the health and wellbeing of women and girls in the crisis aftermath. As Petchesky (1995, 159) argues, realising SRHR for all groups of women and girls requires us to understand the concrete links between macro-level social and economic changes and women's bodily autonomy. The key importance of analysing women's health and wellbeing for peace and conflict research is precisely because this issue allows us to trace the confluence of insecurities rooted in multiple and different political economy processes that operate before, during and after times of crisis. As further elaborated, there are three dimensions to violence revealed by a feminist political economy analysis of SRHR: (1) layers of violence; (2) forms of violence; (3) phases of violence.[2]

Layers of Violence

In the field of IR, feminist scholarship on the continuum of violence has challenged dominant state-centric definitions of peace and security, by highlighting the ways in which gender relations, as well as women's bodies and their labour, are integral to global processes including war and militarism (Cockburn 2004; Enloe 1989). This body of work highlights the multiple *layers* of violence to link the personal with the international. For instance, as Cynthia Cockburn argues, the process of social and cultural differentiation of men and women is an important ordering principle 'that pervades the system of power and is sometimes its very embodiment'. Gender relations are present 'in every site of human interaction from the household to the international arena' and manifest physically through 'how women's and men's bodies are nourished, trained, and deployed, how vulnerable they are to attack, what mobility they have' (Cockburn 2004, 28). Feminists have further pointed out that gender intersects with other hierarchies such as those based on class, racial/ethnic or religious differences. This means gender may not always be the most salient expression of power, but it nevertheless helps us understand how different forms of inequalities, especially at the global level, are gendered.

The ways in which state behaviour and ideology are gendered have implications for women's everyday experiences especially in times of crisis. This is evident in the case of restrictions to SRHR, particularly in the control of biological reproduction, and specifically women's fertility (e.g. Reuterswärd, this volume). Historically, the so-called developed or first world countries have funded population control programmes substantially in the 1970s. The United States especially was the largest provider of population assistance control (Knudsen 2006, 4). The World Bank and USAID withheld loans and aid unless receiving countries enacted national population policies. This foreign policy approach was underpinned by the belief that rapid population growth in 'poorer' regions posed a threat to the growth of developed countries and the global political and economic order where they were, and are, privileged (Petchesky 2003; see, for example, United States National Security Council 1974). The legacy of state-led population control policies still impacts access to SRHR globally in both developed and developing countries, by shaping, for instance, the health-seeking behaviour of minority and indigenous women (Yuval-Davis 1997; see also Reuterswärd, this volume). Relationships between public health practitioners and minority women are at once shaped by global social hierarchies, particularly given long historical and ongoing abuses through population control measures including forced sterilisations (see, for example, Correa 1994). Health service delivery by the state and international organisations cannot be removed from the suspicion they evoke as a form of coercive control exercised by dominant racial, class or ethnic groups over marginalised groups.

More recently, studies have documented transnational coalitions of 'religious extremist' or 'religious fundamentalist' forces mobilising around key UN international conferences and on their own, through forums such as the World Congress of Families backed by the US Christian Right. The backlash against SRHR from this alliance of conservative governments and international and local non-governmental organisations (NGOs) is internationally visible, highly organised and well resourced (OURs 2017; Petchesky 2005; Tanyag 2017). Gender ideologies propagated by the resurgence of patriarchal authority and religious push back against feminist gains generate differing consequences for women's rights (Kandiyoti 2015; Molyneux 2013; Tanyag 2017). In many countries, especially in developing contexts, the policy impacts of religious fundamentalisms that have been observed include 'limited health rights and reduced fulfilment of reproductive rights; less autonomy for women; increased gender-based violence; restrictions on sexual rights; and diminished rights for women in the public sphere' (OURs 2017, 10).

Similarly, the reinstatement of the US Global Gag Rule under the presidency of Donald Trump in 2017 embodies the influence of religious ideology on SRHR at the global level. Formally known as the Mexico City policy, the Gag Rule has been historically backed by conservative Republicans and the US Christian Right. The policy places limits on US funding distribution by excluding overseas NGOs that perform or promote abortion and related services from receiving financial aid. The reinstatement was accompanied by US withdrawal of funding to the UN Population Fund (UNFPA), the leading UN organisation promoting SRHR. Women who are most dependent on the services delivered by such NGOs and the UNFPA are most impacted by the resurgence of US Christian fundamentalism, for it further undermines overall access to health in developing countries and especially those in crisis situations, where service delivery is more likely to already be constrained to begin with. The layering of violence manifests in how *global* ideological contestations reproduce material realities that are enacted through *national* foreign policies and within *individual* experiences of sexuality and reproduction.

Forms of Violence

In addition to layers, violence occurs in different *forms* and a political economy analysis of SRHR demonstrates how physical, symbolic and structural violence compound particularly for women and girls in crisis situations.

Examining how different forms of violence are tied together means making visible how, especially for women and girls, 'violence is not only directly inflicted on an individual's body but also rooted in structures that relegate unequal status and levels of access to resources and decision-making that significantly impact life chances, as well as in the symbolic representations that justify these inequalities as "natural"' (Tanyag 2017, 41; see also Reuterswärd, this volume; Lukić and Lotherington, this volume; Oinas, this volume; Ikhile et al., this volume).

Dominguez and Menjivar (2014) argue that there is a need to go beyond individualised and 'visible' acts of violence to understand women's lives in marginalised communities such as those residing in low-income neighbourhoods in the United States. They build on concepts of structural and symbolic violence to more fully encompass the accumulation of insecurities for low-income women. Structural violence refers to violence that is 'built into the structure and shows up as unequal power and consequently as unequal life chances' (Galtung 1969, 171). Symbolic violence, drawing on the conceptualisation by Bourdieu (2001), refers to the internalisation of oppression, or the normalisation of domination through the complicity of subjugated peoples (Dominguez and Menjivar 2014; cf. Lukić and Lotherington, this volume). Dominguez and Menjivar (2014, 190) demonstrate the intersections of structural and symbolic violence in how victims of domestic and sexual violence tend to blame themselves for what happened to them (cf. Finley, this volume). At the same time, when they are from low-income neighbourhoods and also belong to racial minorities, they do not necessarily seek out support from state welfare systems that are already shaped by racial and class prejudices that target them as a community (cf. Reutersward, this volume). In effect, many women, particularly those in impoverished contexts, are condemned to a 'slow death' through continuing threats of physical violence from abusive partners and the daily suffering from racial discrimination, social and economic isolation, and loss of self-esteem. Similarly, the revelatory impact of attending to multiple forms of violence draws recognition to the 'victimhood' of men who perpetrate domestic violence at the invisible hands of poverty and racial discrimination.

Political economy research on global health has been crucial in highlighting the adverse consequences of neoliberal economic policies to the sustainability of human reproduction. Such policies include fuelling the marketisation of medical research and intellectual property rights on drug patents which tend to erode public health systems (Benatar, Gill and Bakker 2011; Rai, Hoskyns and Thomas 2014). Austerity, structural adjustments and state retrenchment in public service delivery progressively deplete women's health and wellbeing. First, because women are more dependent on welfare support due to their biological and social reproductive roles in their households and communities;

and second, as a result of added stressors and heightened exposure to diseases and illnesses, as they continue to organise care even when health assistance is scarce or undermined (Elson 2012; Mohindra, Labonté and Spitzer 2011).

Sharon Fonn and T. K. Sundari Ravindran (2011), for instance, investigated the economic impacts of different forms of privatisation on SRHR over a thirty-year period. They found that 'privatisation has increased access to some reproductive health services, albeit not comprehensive services.... Improved equity, however, does not appear to have been achieved' under the prevailing macroeconomic environment (Fonn and Ravindran 2011, 22). For example, a key area of inequality is in that the vast majority of births in low-income and rural areas in developing countries were not assisted by a trained attendant, who could then provide the necessary medical emergency care in the event of complications during the birth. Fonn and Ravindran further noted that privatisation appeared to have worked in expanding SRHR coverage, especially in terms of access to contraception, only where investments in the public health sector continued and were even broadened (Fonn and Ravindran 2011; see also Benatar, Gill and Bakker 2011). Weak public health systems mean that when a crisis such as an environmental disaster or a disease outbreak occurs, the delivery of emergency response both by the state and by external actors will likely fail to address or even exacerbate pre-existing gendered inequalities (Davies and Bennett 2016; Harman 2016; Tanyag 2018b). Therefore, privatisation of health care can create compounded structural harms to everyone, and those that tend to suffer the most are women and girls in crisis settings, who require emergency health service.

The structural violence embodied by inequalities in SRHR is mutually reinforced by symbolic violence in the form of gendered ideals that legitimise self-sacrifice among women. Cultural or religious expectations on altruism help normalise the neglect of women's health and wellbeing in the everyday, and more so during times of crisis (Tanyag 2017, 2018a, b). For example, religious fundamentalists and authoritarian leaders alike have emphasised the role of women as symbolic reproducers and, as such, women are seen to play vital roles in the continuation of national identity and traditional values (Tanyag 2017; Yuval-Davis 1997; cf. Reutersward, this volume). Motherhood, therefore, has political significance especially in the context of conflicts where women's fertility is more directly implicated in either the violent erasure of cultural or ethnic identities, as in the use of rape as a form of genocide, or through coercive, post-conflict pronatalism in order to replenish population size (Correa 1994; Yuval-Davis 1997).

Pre-existing inequalities relating to the lower status of women and girls in societies make them vulnerable to negative health outcomes as a result of crisis. Mohindra, Labonté and Spitzer (2011, 276) note that in societies with a cultural norm of son preference, the health needs of men and boys are prioritised at the expense of women and girls. Similar cultural expectations may even intensify in crisis situations when there may be more widespread and routine resource shortages, which then mean chronic neglect of women's and girls' specific needs. Beliefs on the innate altruism or selflessness of women because they are mothers have physical expressions such that it is women, more than men, who are expected to forego their own health to ensure the overall health of the family in times of crisis (Elson 2012; Tanyag 2018b).

Similarly, pre-existing gender discrimination through women's limited access to land and productive resources exposes them to intensified dependence on men in times of crisis, which may lead to even greater restrictions on their ability to control their own lives in the aftermath (UNFPA 2015). In societies where women are unable to acquire property, they have less economic resources at their disposal (compared to men) to bargain for protection and access emergency relief services in internal displacement camps. In turn, women and girls are more likely to be vulnerable to different forms of sexual and gender-based violence (SGBV) through early/forced marriages, trafficking and exploitation (UNFPA 2015). Having an understanding of the different forms of violence and how they layer on to one another provides insights to the promotion of women's wellbeing in comprehensive and integrated ways. These gendered formations and layered experiences are also subject to the temporal dimensions of violence which I examine next.

Phases of Violence

Violence occurs in *phases*: violence directly linked with crises or emergencies, and therefore more immediate or visible, is distinguished from violence that occurs before and after crisis and that is less visible, more structural or 'normalised'. Crisis is increasingly a technique of global governance informed by assumptions around gender, thus affecting men and women in different ways (Elias 2016; Griffin 2015, 50). That is, the use of 'crisis' as a discourse translates into gendered material outcomes, based on how resources are mobilised, when and for what ends. For example, and as further discussed, crisis responses have reflected a 'tyranny of the urgent' such that the restoration of political order and militarised state security are given priority. In situations of protracted or recurrent crisis, where people can be displaced for extended periods, the temporal dimensions between what constitutes a 'crisis' response and long-term development programming are not as clear cut.

Feminist research in IR has shown the continuum of violence during conflict and in peacetime. Scholars have argued that the restoration of formal political and economic order does not always guarantee the end of violence for women and girls (Cockburn 2004; Tanyag 2018a; True and Tanyag 2018;

cf. DeLaet, Golden and Laveta, this volume). Women's health, and particularly SRHR, helps us 'to pay as much attention to what is not swept up in the rhetoric of crisis as to what is included' (Sjoberg, Hudson and Weber 2015, 530). According to the UN special rapporteur on the Right to Health,

> An aspect of this [human rights] obligation is that the right to health is progressively realisable. However, due to the destruction or diversion of resources to military or police needs, conflicts often reduce the availability of resources which may, at times, be detrimental to the right to health. Even where resources are available, states may not be able to make use of them due to the insecurity and poor infrastructure in many conflict environments. Nonetheless, progressive realisation is a specific and continuous state obligation. It does not dilute certain immediate obligations of states, including taking concrete steps towards the full realisation of the right to health to all, without discrimination and regardless of the status of persons as combatants or civilians. (UNGA 2013, 5)

From a human rights perspective, state and non-state actors therefore have the responsibility under international human rights and humanitarian laws to progressively promote the health and wellbeing of all individuals regardless of crisis. Yet, 'rapid responses' to humanitarian crises are aimed at firstly restoring political order and addressing 'immediate' or visible needs (Davies and Bennett 2016; Harman 2016).

Women, girls and sexual minorities are distinctly impacted by the prioritisation that occurs during crises because their experiences are multi-layered and often compounded by different forms of invisible violence. For example, underreporting for a range of sexual and gender-based violence has been documented, and the invisibility of such violence presents distinct challenges for meeting broad SRHR needs in crisis situations (Starrs et al. 2018; Tanyag 2018a; see also Féron, this volume, on underreporting of sexual violence against men in conflicts, and consequences of this for men's SRHR). Abortion-related services are rarely provided in humanitarian crisis settings, which means victims of sexual violence may be forced to carry unwanted pregnancies (Starrs et al. 2018, 2671). SRHR needs of sexual minorities are also unlikely to become easily 'visible' or identified in the aftermath of crisis in societies, where they continue to face stigma and marginalisation (Starrs et al. 2018, 2670; cf. Nuño, this volume).

Women's distinct needs and contributions are made invisible by structural and symbolic violence that take their care labour for granted and the confluence of multiple violences, including the experience of sexual violence, manifests in physical forms through the deterioration of their health and wellbeing. As Harman puts it, 'a central paradox in global health' is that 'women are conspicuous in the delivery of care and thus the delivery of health, but are invisible to the institutions and policies that design and implement global health strategies' (2016, 526). For example, in the aftermath of environmental disasters (Tanyag 2018b), or disease outbreaks (Davies and Bennett 2016; Harman 2016), women face more burdens as they take on intensified care provisioning for their families and communities. This occurs when women are in the frontline of care service delivery, and their bodies more exposed to heavy physical strain and infection risks. Life in displacement camps without access to proper health and sanitation is made even more difficult by harmful cultural norms around women's 'unclean' bodies during menstruation, which results in further restrictions to their mobility. Menstruating while displaced is a gender-specific insecurity that can amount to a loss of human dignity, and can also serve as a barrier to physically accessing relief assistance (UNFPA 2015). The invisibility of women in global health governance, therefore, becomes a cycle because pre-existing and crisis-induced gender inequalities accumulate to further distance displaced women and girls from ever fully participating in political decision-making.

Furthermore, McInnes and Lee (2006, 6) note how the international agenda on 'health [has moved] beyond the social policy and development agenda, into the realms of foreign and security policy'. However, they argue that instead of addressing how foreign and security policies can facilitate or hinder public health, the focus has largely been on how public health comprises a security risk, as in bioterrorism or epidemic infections (2006, 9). Health falls in the 'remit of security inasmuch as it connects with other "hard" threats' (Nunes 2014, 940). While there has been progress in incorporating health in national and global security agendas, including, for example, reproductive health in the global Women, Peace and Security (WPS) agenda, this effort has not been equally focused on, and connected with, the Sustainable Development Goals agenda towards bridging health inequalities that shape daily life. Indeed, among the current implementation weaknesses to the WPS agenda is that it has not fully engaged with other forms of violence, such as the structural and symbolic harms that pre-exist or are further embedded in the aftermath of conflicts. An example is in its tendency to replicate narrow representations of women, such as those relating to individualised victimhood embodied by the disproportionate attention on protecting them from sexual violence (True and Tanyag 2018).

Yet, feminist scholars especially those working on care and political economy have pointed out that human interdependence means that we are all dependent on giving and receiving care before, during and after crises. 'Vulnerability is a fact of all human life' and our human bodies are 'vulnerable to life itself: to aging and decay, and ultimately, to death' (Vaittinen 2015, 103–104). Rethinking security through the lens of women's bodies, and specifically SRHR, reveals the continuum of violence rooted in the non-recognition of the centrality of care for the daily reproduction of human life. Fiona Robinson (2011) articulates a feminist perspective about human security, based on care ethics. More to the point, a feminist political economy perspective to SRHR helps reveal how health, economic and security systems actually reflect which bodies matter and how they are valued in times of crisis and in the everyday.

THE INVISIBLE COST OF CRISIS: GENDER AND INTERNAL DISPLACEMENTS IN SOUTHEAST ASIA

I now turn to the regional case of Southeast Asia to examine empirically SRHR in crises and emergencies.[3] By focusing on this region, I show that the depletion of women's bodies in internal displacements is a *regional* problem for Southeast Asia, and therefore interventions to stem this depletion need to incorporate both national and regional governance structures. In previous works, I have argued that the cost of the economic devaluing of women's social reproductive labour is the depletion of women's bodies manifested at its extreme by maternal deaths (Tanyag 2017, 2018a, b). Building on the concept of depletion by Diane Elson (2012) and Shirin Rai, Catherine Hoskyns and Dania Thomas (2014), I examined how the deterioration of SRHR globally and in post-conflict and post-disaster situations, in particular, constitutes a form of depletion by embodying the 'structural aspects of social reproduction that undermine the sustainability of the everyday lives of women and men in a given social context' (Rai et al. 2014, 89–90). Depletion also highlights the ways in which women's contributions especially in post-crisis recovery are left unreplenished, and this is normalised precisely because of gendered norms around women's altruism (Tanyag 2017, 2018a).

In the analysis for this chapter, I extend my argument through a regional lens on depletion, which consequently allows me to identify a specific mode of replenishing women's bodies through SRHR across the different layers, forms and phases of violence. A regional analysis of Southeast Asia represents a compelling case to begin accounting for the full cost of multiple crises, especially when peacebuilding and disaster or climate-resilience initiatives continue to neglect health inequalities (CEDAW 2013; UNGA 2013). Less developed countries – predominantly low income or lower-middle income – are generally more affected by multiple crises than industrialised countries. And yet, such countries faced with the greatest need for addressing diseases and health emergencies are also those most lacking or ill-equipped to respond (Eckstein et al. 2017; IDMC 2018). One way in which states can strengthen capacities is through regional cooperation and, for Southeast Asia, this is through the Association of Southeast Asian Nations (ASEAN) (Caballero-Anthony 2018). ASEAN as a regional organisation has made significant strides in collectively committing to human security and protection, including the advancement of WPS concerns (Nair 2015; Veneracion-Rallonza 2016).

Mely Caballero-Anthony (2018) argues that regional organisations play a critical role in health and human security governance. Their role, however, must go beyond traditional health security issues such as state cooperation to combat health pandemics and disease surveillance. Increasingly, in the face of multiple crises including climate change–related risks, regional organisations such as ASEAN must mature into institutions that help 'strengthen national public health systems to achieve health security' (Caballero-Anthony 2018, 603). I contribute to this growing focus on regional health governance by proposing that one pathway is in the area of bridging inequalities in SRHR, especially for internally displaced populations in Southeast Asia. As noted earlier, there is growing evidence that the region is among the most crisis-prone regions in the world. Moreover, a majority of countries in Southeast Asia are characterised by state fragility and political instability (OECD 2016).

The region historically has been exposed to escalating climate change–related risks as well as pre-existing geographical impacts of the Pacific Ring of Fire.[4] These factors help explain why one-third of the total global refugees are in the Asia Pacific at an estimated 3.5 million people. This is in addition to the 1.9 million internally displaced and 1.4 million stateless people (UNHCR n.d.). Globally, 45.8 per cent or almost half of the total new disaster-induced displacements occurred in the East Asia Pacific (where Southeast Asia is located) in 2017. This translates to an estimated 8,604,000 people in a year (IDMC 2018, 16). Internal Displacement Monitoring Centre (IDMC) data indicate that disasters caused twice as many new displacements as armed conflicts with the most incidences dominating in two main regions in the world: South and East Asia and the Pacific (IDMC 2016, 14–15).

According to the Global Climate Risk Index, four Southeast Asian countries were included in the ten countries most affected by long-term climate risks from 1997 to 2016 (annual averages), the highest concentration than any other region (Eckstein et al. 2017, 9). The countries were Myanmar, the Philippines, Vietnam and Thailand. In roughly a decade, the Philippines experienced 289 extreme weather events. Hence, the country was also ranked second among the ten countries identified by IDMC as the worst affected by new internal displacements resulting from conflicts and disasters in 2017 (IDMC 2018). For many of these highly affected populations in Southeast Asia, the recovery phase is always cut short by the next crisis or disaster. Frequent or recurrent crises mean that any gains in economic and human development are set back or undermined by new death and destruction. The rebuilding of economies and societies post-crisis are always short-lived and whole communities are unable to fully recover or must contend with current realities of protracted or permanent insecurity.

Complicating the situation of internally displaced populations is how disasters often intersect with protracted conflicts. A severe example is in Myanmar where in 2015 'floods, landslides and the impacts of cyclone Komen displaced more than 1.6 million people . . . in July and August, resulting in the highest [displacement] worldwide in absolute terms and the sixth highest in relative terms' (IDMC 2016, 15). Yet, many parts of the country are also conflict affected such as Kachin and Rakhine states, in addition to an ongoing humanitarian crisis affecting the Rohingya minority ethnic group (see Davies and True 2017; Hutchinson 2018). This is similar to the Philippine context where, despite the signing of a peace agreement between the government and Moro Islamic rebels in Mindanao, many communities still face risks of displacement due to ongoing clan violence which continues to occur sporadically in the southern part of the country (Tanyag 2018a). The area is also constantly experiencing disasters such as drought and flooding.

Severe and recurrent disasters ultimately undermine long-term development and peacebuilding. In 2016, Cambodia was subjected to one of the worst incidences of drought in the region. As an example of a slow onset disaster, droughts in Cambodia distinctly affected the livelihood and wellbeing of rural communities. Risks of wide-scale displacements due to disasters in the country are exacerbated by the structural legacies of violent conflict forty years after the reign of the Khmer Rouge as many remote parts are characterised by high levels of poverty, illiteracy and poor infrastructures in basic delivery of social welfare services (see CARE, People in Need and Save the Children 2016).

CONTINUUM OF PEACE: SECURITY AND REPLENISHING BODIES

What does it mean to build peace in a crisis-prone region? A feminist political economy analysis of SRHR in crises and emergencies helps substantiate the indispensability of replenishing bodies for connecting capacity for crisis response and long-term resilience in the face of future risks. Depletion can be said to be occurring because the demands on care provisioning are intense in Southeast Asia due to multiple displacements and security risks, yet indicators for SRHR are poor. For example, through the concept of layers of violence I argue that restrictions to young women's SRHR in Southeast Asia is a regional issue that reveals recurrent patterns of violence experienced by households and communities similarly situated within countries beset by multiple and intersecting crises. Official data from UNFPA (2018) indicate that, though globally adolescent birth rates are on the decline, this is not the case in Southeast Asia. In fact, among the highest adolescent birth rates in the world are found in Cambodia, Indonesia and the Philippines.[5] Compared to neighbouring Asian countries, young people in Southeast Asia comprise a significant proportion of the population. Most notably, in Cambodia, approximately 60 per cent of the population is under the age of 30. In the Philippines and Indonesia, two of the most populous countries in the region, the figure is at 17 per cent of the population, respectively, which means an estimated sixty million youth from two countries alone. Regionally, young people are most in need of comprehensive SRHR, because adolescence is a stage in one's human development where knowledge on sexuality and reproductive decision-making can significantly impact one's life course. For girls, early pregnancy can mean foregoing access to education. However, in crises and emergencies, young women's bodily autonomy and wellbeing are undermined even more because 'decreased protection mechanisms, along with increased instability and pressure on families to cope, can all be drivers of child marriage and early union and, therefore, increased rates of adolescent pregnancy' (UNFPA 2018). Individual-level impacts of restrictions to SRHR experienced by young people will affect prospects for long-term national and regional security in Southeast Asia, when significant numbers of youth face constrained human development.

Deteriorating SRHR outcomes is the 'canary in the coal mine' for broader *forms* of structural and symbolic violence faced by women and girls including SGBV in crisis settings. For example, 'Myanmar has been regularly reported to the UN for nearly two decades for state-sponsored human rights violations, protracted displacement and use of child soldiers by the Tatmadaw and non-state armed groups' (Davies and True 2017, 7). A continued failure to stem this broad form of violence by state and non-state armed groups in the country has created an environment ripe for impunity among perpetrators of SGBV against ethnic minorities, particularly the Rohingyas. In order to understand current conflicts and displacements within an ethnically diverse region, direct violence needs to be situated within a continuum of structural violence in the form of historical injustices perpetrated by dominant ethnic groups against specific minorities and in terms of lack of access to justice. For instance, having suffered SGBV, many minority women and girls are then forced to deal with its long-term effects while at the same time being denied adequate protection and redress.

Similarly, in Mindanao, the Philippines, the occurrence of conflicts results in low battle-related deaths, but conflict intensity tends to be cyclical and may register peaks and troughs over time. Davies, True and Tanyag (2016) demonstrate how threats of violence erupting in the form of community or clan feuds structure the everyday lives of the Moro minority group especially women and girls. Clan feuds are triggered by competition over resources such as land or political office. These feuds are also largely honour based and violence is perpetrated in the name of protecting clan identity. Yet, as a driver of instability in Mindanao, clan feuds remain 'below the radar' in national and global conflict monitoring, and a primary consequence is that 'if a conflict is too small-scale to be recorded, the SGBV which is linked to it will also go unnoticed' (Davies, True and Tanyag 2016, 465). The invisibility of specific types of conflicts such as clan feuds in the Philippines has knock-on effects for the mobilisation of resources and political attention to address comprehensive insecurities, including the lack of emergency sexual and reproductive health services. The violence is not counted and, therefore, the necessary health services such as clinical management of rape are also far less likely to be made available (UNFPA 2015, 54).

Against this backdrop of a crisis-prone region, progressively bridging sexual and reproductive health gaps by attending to the different *phases* of violence is a crucial link for a continuous chain of protective measures for internally displaced women and girls, who are faced with pre-existing gender discrimination and heightened risks of SGBV in crisis settings. In Asia Pacific, where protracted conflicts and severe environmental disasters routinely intersect, military spending rose by 5.4 per cent in 2015 and by 64 per cent between 2006 and 2015, reaching $436 billion in 2015 (SIPRI 2016). By contrast, global and regional health outcomes remain politically and economically neglected, despite how fundamental health is underpinning the capacities of households and communities to thrive and adapt to multiple crises. Based on a study by WHO on global public health expenditures, 'higher income or higher general government revenue and spending do not necessarily imply higher priority on health' (2018, 20). Moreover, for low-income countries, steady economic growth has not translated to improvements on government spending on health. Rather, government spending registered a decline from 7.9 per cent in 2000 to 6.8 in 2016 (WHO 2018, 22).

Indeed, a permanent 'health crisis' characterised by endemic shortages in supplies and personnel serves as a backdrop to any humanitarian crisis. According to a 2016 review of the progress on health workforce development in Southeast Asia, WHO found that many countries in the region continue to have a density of skilled workforce lower than the recommended threshold of 22.8 health workers (doctors, nurses and midwives) per 10,000 population (WHO 2016). More broadly, progress towards fulfilling SRHR for all 'has been stymied because of weak political commitment, inadequate resources, persistent discrimination against women and girls, and an unwillingness to address issues related to sexuality openly and comprehensively' (Starrs et al. 2018, 2642).

Regional cooperation among Southeast Asian countries can significantly improve the governance of multiple crises that affect them. It can help generate protection mechanisms that are geared towards strengthening public health systems together with the coordination of emergency response including foreign assistance (see also Caballero-Anthony 2018). Framing SRHR as a regional security issue for ASEAN is also relevant because of ongoing ethnic and religious conflicts. Health governance can be an entry-point for security discussions to broaden and encompass social protection and citizenship entitlements that at present reflect which lives and bodies are recognised as more valuable, that is, worthier of replenishment than others. To this end, important gender equality gains are thus necessary to make visible how promoting women's wellbeing is at the core of how peace and security are understood and promoted in Southeast Asia – before, during and after crises. Indeed, ASEAN as a regional organisation has already made positive strides in adopting a normative commitment to human security and protection, including the advancement of WPS concerns (Nair 2015; Veneracion-Rallonza 2016). ASEAN member states have expressed their support for the 2013 UN Declaration of Commitment to End Sexual Violence in Conflict. This commitment needs to be implemented in the context of ensuring comprehensive protection for internally displaced women and girls to include SRHR.

On 9 October 2013, ASEAN member states adopted the Declaration on the elimination of Violence against Women and Elimination of Violence against Children. This ASEAN Declaration is significant because it explicitly references UN Security Council Resolutions 1325, 1820, 1888 and 1889 that collectively comprise the framework for the global WPS agenda. At the same time, it reaffirms ASEAN member states' commitments to other gender equality instruments such as CEDAW and the Beijing Platform for Action, as well as the Millennium Development Goals (MDGs). Through this declaration, ASEAN espouses a conceptual understanding that violence against women occurring in securitised settings of armed conflict (which falls within the ambit of WPS agenda) is also part of a wider issue of gender equality as addressed extensively by the other gender equality instruments such as CEDAW. This framework holds promise for critical interventions that link SRHR in crisis and emergencies with broader health inequalities in the region. State and non-state crisis responders in Southeast Asia have an institutional basis to further strengthen the tacit recognition of a continuum of violence within this ASEAN Declaration to further establish mechanisms and procedures for addressing gendered insecurities post-crisis and in the everyday. Further research thus is needed to track the progress of ASEAN regional cooperation on health and security, particularly by monitoring the implementation of gender frameworks as an example of how a continuum of peace can be enacted across geographic borders.

SRHR IN THE CONTINUUM OF PEACE

This chapter has mapped out the interconnections between different layers, forms, and phases of violence rendered visible by a feminist political economy analysis of SRHR. In so doing, it has also drawn connections for a continuum of peace which situates women's bodily autonomy as central to engendering human security across societal and global levels. As I argue here, and the other chapters in this edited volume show too, promoting health and wellbeing requires not just the absence of direct or physical violence but also the presence of an enabling environment wherein differentially gendered individuals, in this case especially women and girls, can make safe and informed decisions to exercise their bodily autonomy. Importantly, women's health and wellbeing are a prerequisite foundation for building and sustaining peace in the everyday. Importantly, the project of replenishing bodily health and wellbeing is a progressive and continuous goal rooted in human rights obligations. It requires that bodies are valued in both material and ideological terms.

The predicted risks for displacements in Southeast Asia, a crisis-prone region, will intensify in the coming years. National and regional governance structures must be able to rise to the challenge of such a changing environment. The notion of a continuum of peace informs us that preparing for future security risks requires replenishing bodies now. The experiences of internally displaced populations demonstrate the cumulative impacts of different forms of crises and violence. The absence of critical interventions in health and wellbeing, particularly SRHR that can progressively stem the root causes of gender inequality from emergency relief to long-term development assistance, reinforces the entire invisibility of the gendered bodies that end up bearing the brunt of crises. And yet, women are most impacted by different forms, layers and phases of violence. This is evident in that they may be faced with restricted mobility because of their care dependents and/or due to threats of physical violence, which may mean also that they cannot easily access relief assistance or re-enter the formal paid economy. Despite carrying the primary burden of survival for their families and communities, women are most likely to face barriers in the distribution of benefits or rewards during and post-crisis because the 'private sphere' contributions they provide are valued less compared to the productive labour performed predominantly by men in the 'public sphere'.

Especially for women and girls, the cessation of conflicts or disasters does not necessarily spell out the absence of violence. Discrimination and exclusion from health services based on gender, religion and ethnic identity can still constrain their life chances or heighten their mortality in the aftermath. It is not only the violence of conflicts and disasters that distinctly lead to excess mortality among women in the form of maternal deaths. Women's health is constrained by unequal distribution of resources and access to decision-making before, during and after crisis. Analysing the economic and political neglect of SRHR in crises and emergencies helps reveal the range of structural and symbolic conditions that shape the gendered coping mechanisms and full costs borne by households and communities. Consequently, such an analysis makes a case for women's health as a core pathway to peace that includes the availability of comprehensive protection measures before and during crises, while rebuilding post-crisis societies inclusively and equitably.

NOTES

1. These international human rights frameworks include the Convention on the Elimination of all Forms of Discrimination against Women (CEDAW); Declaration on the Elimination of Violence against Women (DEVAW); International Conference on Population and Development (ICPD) Program of Action; Beijing Platform for Action (BfPA); International Covenant on Civil and Political Rights (ICCPR); and International Covenant on Economic, Social and Cultural Rights (ICESCR).
2. These three dimensions are adapted from True and Tanyag (2018) and applied as a framework to the specific case of SRHR.
3. Southeast Asia comprises the following countries: Brunei, Cambodia, Indonesia, Laos, Malaysia, Myanmar (Burma), Philippines, Thailand, Singapore, and Vietnam.
4. The Pacific Ring of Fire refers to the geographical region marked by several sites of seismic activity (National Geographic n.d.).
5. There are no available subnational data on adolescent birth rates in conflict and disaster-affected areas in these countries. A lack of data on health indicators in crisis-prone areas speaks to larger issue of monitoring the consequences to SRHR and whose body is valued within these countries.

REFERENCES

Benatar S., Gill S. and Bakker, I. 2011. 'Global Health and the Global Economic Crisis'. *American Journal of Public Health* 101, no. 4: 646–653.
Bourdieu, Pierre. 2001. *Masculine Domination*. Cambridge: Polity Press.
Caballero-Anthony, Mely. 2018. 'Health and Human Security Challenges in Asia: New Agendas for Strengthening Regional Health Governance'. *Australian Journal of International Affairs* 72, no. 6: 602–616.
CARE, People in Need and Save the Children. 2016. 'Rapid Assessment of the Drought in Koh Kong Province April 2016'. Accessed 8 August 2019. https://reliefweb.int/report/cambodia/cambodia-final-report-rapid-assessment-drought-koh-kong-province-april-2016.

Cockburn, Cynthia. 2004. 'The Continuum of Violence: A Gender Perspective on War and Peace'. In *Sites of Violence*, edited by W. Giles, 24–44. Berkeley: University of California Press.

Confortini, Catia C. and Tiina Vaittinen. 2019. 'Introduction: Analysing Violences in Gendered Global Health' In *Gender, Global Health and Violence: Feminist Perspectives on Peace and Disease*, edited by Tiina Vaittinen and Catia Confortini. London and New York: Rowman & Littlefield.

Correa, Sonia. 1994. *Population and Reproductive Rights: Feminist Perspectives from the South*. London: Zed Books.

Davies, Sara. 2014. 'Healthy Populations, Political Stability, and Regime Type: Southeast Asia as a Case Study'. *Review of International Studies* 40, no. 5: 859–876.

Davies, Sara and Belinda Bennett. 2016. 'A Gendered Human Rights Analysis of Ebola and Zika: Locating Gender in Global Health Emergencies'. *International Affairs* 92, 5: 1041–1060.

Davies, Sara and Jacqui True. 2017. 'The Politics of Counting and Reporting Conflict-Related Sexual and Gender-Based Violence: The Case of Myanmar'. *International Feminist Journal of Politics* 19, no. 1: 4–21.

Davies, Sara, Jacqui True and Maria Tanyag. 2016. 'How Women's Silence Secures the Peace: Analysing Sexual and Gender-Based Violence in a Low-Intensity Conflict'. *Gender and Development* 24, no. 3: 459–473.

DeLaet, Debra L., Golden Shannon and Veronica Laveta. 2019. 'Therapeutic Justice for Survivors of Human Rights Violations and Wartime Violence'. In *Gender, Global Health and Violence: Feminist Perspectives on Peace and Disease*, edited by Tiina Vaittinen and Catia Confortini. London and New York: Rowman & Littlefield.

Dominguez, Silvia and Cecilia Menjivar. 2014. 'Beyond Individual and Visible Acts of Violence: A Framework to Examine the Lives of Women in Low-Income Neighborhoods'. *Women's Studies International Forum* 44: 184–195.

Eckstein, David, Vera Künzel and Laura Schäfer. 2017. *Global Climate Risk Index 2018*. Bonn; Berlin: GermanWatch.

Elias, Juanita. 2016. 'Whose Crisis? Whose Recovery? Lessons Learned (and Not) from the Asian Crisis'. In *Scandalous Economics*, edited by Aida Hozic and Jacqui True, 109–125. Oxford: Oxford University Press.

Elson, Diane. 2012. 'Social Reproduction in the Global Crisis: Rapid Recovery or Long-Lasting Depletion?' In *The Global Crisis and Transformative Social Change*, edited by Peter Utting, Shahra Razavi and Rebecca Varghese Buchholz, 63–80. Basingstoke: Palgrave Macmillan.

Enloe, Cynthia. 1989. *Bananas, Beaches and Bases: Making Feminist Sense of International Politics*. Berkeley, CA; London: University of California Press.

Féron, Élise. 2019. 'When Is It Torture? When Is It Rape? Discourses on Wartime Sexual Violence'. In *Gender, Global Health and Violence: Feminist Perspectives on Peace and Disease*, edited by Tiina Vaittinen and Catia Confortini. London and New York: Rowman & Littlefield.

Finley, Laura. 2019. 'Domestic Violence and Public Health: Beginning Steps for Creating More Just and Effective Community Responses'. In *Gender, Global*

Health and Violence: Feminist Perspectives on Peace and Disease, edited by Tiina Vaittinen and Catia Confortini. London and New York: Rowman & Littlefield.

Fonn, Sharon and Ravindran, T. K. 2011. 'The Macroeconomic Environment and Sexual and Reproductive Health: A Review of Trends over the Last 30 Years'. *Reproductive Health Matters* 19, no. 38: 11–25.

Griffin, Penny. 2015. 'Crisis, Austerity and Gendered Governance: A Feminist Perspective'. *Feminist Review* 109, no. 1: 49–72.

Harman, Sophie. 2016. 'Ebola, Gender and Conspicuously Invisible Women in Global Health Governance'. *Third World Quarterly* 37, no. 3: 524–541.

Hutchinson, Susan. 2018. 'Gendered Insecurity in the Rohingya Crisis'. *Australian Journal of International Affairs* 72, no. 1: 1–9.

Ikhile, Deborah, Linda Gibson and Azrini Wahidin. 2019. ' "I Cannot Know That Now I Have Cancer!" A Structural Violence Perspective on Breast Cancer Detection in Uganda'. In *Gender, Global Health and Violence: Feminist Perspectives on Peace and Disease*, edited by Tiina Vaittinen and Catia Confortini. London and New York: Rowman & Littlefield.

Internal Displacement Monitoring Centre (IDMC). 2016. *Global Report on Internal Displacement*. Geneva: IDMC.

Internal Displacement Monitoring Centre (IDMC). 2018. *Global Report on Internal Displacement*. Geneva: IDMC.

Knudsen, Lara M. 2006. *Reproductive Rights in a Global Context*. 1st ed. Nashville: Vanderbilt University Press.

Lukić, Dragana and Ann Therese Lotherington. 2019. 'Fighting Symbolic Violence through Artistic Encounters: Searching for Feminist Answers to the Question of Life and Death with Dementia'. In *Gender, Global Health and Violence: Feminist Perspectives on Peace and Disease*, edited by Tiina Vaittinen and Catia Confortini. London and New York: Rowman & Littlefield.

McInnes, Colin and Lee Kelley. 2006. 'Health, Security and Foreign Policy'. *Review of International Studies* 32, no. 1: 5–23.

Mohindra, K. S., Labonté, Ronald and Denise Spitzer. 2011. 'The Global Financial Crisis: Whither Women's Health?' *Critical Public Health* 21, no. 3: 273–287.

Nair, Tamara. 2015. 'Women, Peace and Security in the ASEAN: Need for a Distinct Action Plan'. *RSIS Commentary*, 23 December. Accessed 8 August 2019. https://reliefweb.int/report/world/women-peace-and-security-asean-need-distinct-action-plan.

National Geographic, n.d. 'Ring of Fire'. Accessed 12 February 2019. https://www.nationalgeographic.org/encyclopedia/ring-fire/.

Nunes, João. 2014. 'Questioning Health Security: Insecurity and Domination in World Politics'. *Review of International Studies* 40, no. 5: 939–960.

Nuño, Néstor M. 2019. 'Rethinking Global Health Priorities from the Margins: Health Access and Medical Care Claims among Indonesia's *Waria*'. In *Gender, Global Health and Violence: Feminist Perspectives on Peace and Disease*, edited by Tiina Vaittinen and Catia Confortini. London and New York: Rowman & Littlefield.

The Observatory on the Universality of Rights (OURs). 2017. *Rights at Risk: Observatory on the Universality of Rights Trends Report 2017*. Toronto and Mexico City: AWID and OURs. Accessed 7 September 2019. https://www.awid.org/sites/default/files/atoms/files/ours_trends_report_2017_en.pdf.

Oinas, Elina. 2019. 'HIV Politics and Structural Violence: Access to Treatment and Knowledge'. In *Gender, Global Health and Violence: Feminist Perspectives on Peace and Disease*, edited by Tiina Vaittinen and Catia Confortini. London and New York: Rowman & Littlefield.

Organisation for Economic Co-operation and Development (OECD). 2016. *States of Fragility 2016*. Paris: OECD Publishing.

Petchesky, R. 2005. 'Rights of the Body and Perversions of War: Sexual Rights and Wrongs Ten Years past Beijing'. *International Social Science Journal* 57, 184: 301–318.

Rai, Shirin, Catherine Hoskyns and Dania Thomas. 2014. 'Depletion: The Social Cost of Reproduction'. *International Feminist Journal of Politics* 16, no. 1: 86–105.

Reuterswärd, Camilla. 2019. '¡Malas Madres, Malas Mujeres, Malas Todas! The Incarceration of Women for Abortion-Related Crimes in Mexico'. In *Gender, Global Health and Violence: Feminist Perspectives on Peace and Disease*, edited by Tiina Vaittinen and Catia Confortini. London and New York: Rowman & Littlefield.

Robinson, Fiona. 2011. *The Ethics of Care: A Feminist Approach to Human Security*. Temple University Press: Philadelphia.

Sjoberg, Laura, Heidi Hudson and Cynthia Weber. 2015. 'Gender and Crisis in Global Politics: Introduction'. *International Feminist Journal of Politics* 17, no. 4: 529–535.

Stockholm International Peace Research Institute (SIPRI). 'Trends in World Military Expenditure, 2015'. *SIPRI Fact Sheet, April 2016*. Accessed 27 December 2018. https://www.sipri.org/publications/2016/sipri-fact-sheets/trends-world-military-expenditure-2015.

Tanyag, Maria. 2017. 'Invisible Labor, Invisible Bodies: How the Global Political Economy Affects Reproductive Freedom in the Philippines'. *International Feminist Journal of Politics* 19, no. 1: 39–54.

Tanyag, Maria. 2018a. 'Depleting Fragile Bodies: The Political Economy of Sexual and Reproductive Health in Crisis Situations'. *Review of International Studies* 44, no. 4: 654–671.

Tanyag, Maria. 2018b. 'Resilience, Female Altruism, and Bodily Autonomy: Disaster-Induced Displacement in Post-Haiyan Philippines'. *Signs: Journal of Women in Culture and Society* 43, no. 3: 563–585.

True, Jacqui and Maria Tanyag. 2018. 'Violence against Women/Violence in the World: Toward a Feminist Conceptualization of Global Violence'. In *Routledge Handbook on Gender and Security*, edited by Caron Gentry, Laura J. Shepherd and Laura Sjoberg, 15–26. London: Routledge.

UN Committee on the Elimination of Discrimination against Women (CEDAW). 2013. *General Recommendation No. 30 on Women in Conflict Prevention, Conflict and Post-Conflict Situations*, 1 November. CEDAW/C/GC/30. Accessed 7 September 2019. https://www.refworld.org/docid/5268d2064.html.

UN General Assembly (UNGA). 2006. *Report of the Special Rapporteur on the Right of Everyone to the Enjoyment of the Highest Attainable Standard of Physical and Mental Health, 61st Session, 13 September*. A/61/338. https://www.hr-dp.org/files/2015/06/08/GA_Annual_report,_2006.pdf. Accessed 7 September 2019.

UN General Assembly (UNGA). 2013. *Report of the Special Rapporteur on the Right of Everyone to the Enjoyment of the Highest Attainable Standard of Physical and Mental Health*. 68th session, 9 August. A/68/297. https://documents-dds-ny.un.org/doc/UNDOC/GEN/N13/422/97/PDF/N1342297.pdf?OpenElement. Accessed 7 September 2019.

UN Refugee Agency (UNHCR). n.d. *Asia and the Pacific*. Accessed 31 December 2018. http://www.unhcr.org/asia-and-the-pacific.html.

UN Women. 2015. *Preventing Conflict, Transforming Justice, Securing the Peace: A Global Study on the Implementation of United Nations Security Council Resolution 1325*. http://wps.unwomen.org. Accessed 7 September 2019.

UNFPA. 2015. *Shelter from the Storm: State of the World Population 2015*. New York: UNFPA.

UNFPA. 2018. 'Addressing the Patterns of Child Marriage, Early Union and Teen Pregnancy in Southeast Asia: A Matter of Urgency'. 12 April. http://asiapacific.unfpa.org/en/news/addressing-patterns-child-marriage-early-union-and-teen-pregnancy-southeast-asia-matter-urgency. Accessed 7 September 2019.

United States National Security Council. 1974. *National Security Study Memorandum 200*. 24 April. http://nixon.archives.gov/virtuallibrary/documents/nssm/nssm_200.pdf. Accessed 7 September 2019.

Urdal, Henrik and Chi Primus Che. 2013. 'War and Gender Inequalities in Health: The Impact of Armed Conflict on Fertility and Maternal Mortality'. *International Interactions* 39, no. 4: 489–510.

Vaittinen, Tiina. 2015. 'The Power of the Vulnerable Body: A New Political Understanding of Care'. *International Feminist Journal of Politics* 17, no. 1: 100–118.

Veneracion-Rallonza, Ma. Lourdes. 2016. 'Building the Women, Peace and Security Agenda in the ASEAN through Multi-Focal Norm Entrepreneurship'. *Global Responsibility to Protect* 8: 158–179.

World Health Organization (WHO). 2016. *Regional Workshop Summary Report*. Regional workshop to review progress on the decade for strengthening human resources for health in the South East Asia Region 2015–2024. Bangkok, Thailand, 20–22 April. http://apps.who.int/iris/bitstream/10665/249546/1/2016_HRH_flyer.pdf?ua=1. Accessed 7 September 2019.

World Health Organization (WHO). 2018. *Public Spending on Health: A Closer Look at Global Trends*. https://apps.who.int/iris/bitstream/handle/10665/276728/WHO-HIS-HGF-HF-WorkingPaper-18.3-eng.pdf?ua=1. Accessed 7 September 2019.

Yuval-Davis, Nira. 1997. *Gender and Nation*. London: SAGE.

Chapter 3

Rethinking Global Health Priorities from the Margins: Health Access and Medical Care Claims among Indonesia's *Waria*

Néstor Nuño Martínez

Since the 1990s, neoliberal development practices promoted by global financial institutions, such as the International Monetary Fund and the World Bank, have failed to reduce world inequalities. Some of these neoliberal policies and programmes have included the orientation of local economies towards foreign trade and the privatisation of state enterprises based on the premise that private industry is more efficient. This situation has led to a weakening of the political, economic, social, and health conditions in some of the countries that applied these doctrines (Hanlon 1996; Homedes and Ugalde 2005; Oriol 2006; Sanahuja 2007). In parallel to, or perhaps as a consequence of these interventions, there has been a redefinition of health as a central element to development and poverty eradication worldwide (United Nations 2000).

In this context, international health policies, priorities, and interventions have converged into the new multidisciplinary field of Global Health. According to Craig Janes and Kitty Corbett (2009), Global Health seeks to connect the notions of health and wellbeing with global processes and policies (Janes and Corbett 2009). However, global health interventions have been harshly criticised for being decontextualised, unsuited to local realities, and essentially complicit in the pursuit of neoliberal practices and logics (Keshavjee 2015; Ong and Collier 2008). The re-conceptualisation of health as a central element in development has propitiated the participation of pharmaceutical industries, financing organisations, and non-profit foundations in the processes of global health. Appealing to scientific-based evidence and the benefits of health improvements for world markets, new powerful international partnerships, mainly dominated by private actors, have gradually oriented the majority of global health interventions towards pathologies such as HIV and malaria (Nunes 2014; Petryna and Biehl 2013; Pfeiffer and

Nichter 2008). Some authors have associated the guiding principles of global health interventions not only with the intersection of political and economic processes and actors but also with the spread of ideologies of moral responsibility. These ethical approaches highlight the use of moral sentiments (e.g. guilt, blame, and responsibility for the suffering of others) to legitimise discourses and practices focused on vulnerable and defenceless populations (Fassin 2011; Nichter 2008).

The aim of this chapter is to critically investigate the focus of mainstream global health priorities on pathologies such as HIV. Despite the benefits of these interventions for vulnerable populations, their logic and design (mainly based on biomedical paradigms) overshadow different day-to-day health needs. As a consequence, new forms of violence and discrimination emerge, reinforcing the perpetuation of vulnerability for such groups. In this chapter, I analyse these dynamics in the specific case of Indonesia's *waria* living in the city of Jogjakarta, and illuminate the socio-political claims and negotiations that groups who are considered vulnerable enact to reduce health inequalities among their peers.

The term *waria* is the current neologism used to describe the male-to-female transvestite community of Indonesia.[1] *Waria* are people born with male bodies who do not conform to social stereotypes of masculinity and wear women's clothing (Oetomo 2002).[2] Tom Boellstorff defines *waria* as individuals with male bodies and female souls (*jiwa*): they have a masculine body by birth but their god-given destiny (*takdir*) is being *waria*, which implies feminine attitudes and practices. For Boellstorff, being *waria* is not a rational realisation but a social imposition: 'Unlike *gay* men, *waria* never speak of "opening themselves" (*membuka diri*) in terms of revealing who they are; indeed they often discover who they are because others point it out to them' (Boellstorff 2004, 165).

Waria are a social group historically discriminated and excluded in Indonesia because of their gender identity (Boellstorff 2004, 2014; Koeswinarno 2007). They are exposed to direct, social, and, most importantly, structural violence. As discussed in various chapters of the volume (e.g. Confortini and Vaittinen; Oinas; Ikhile, Gibson and Wahidin; Harman), structural violence is defined as an apparatus consisting of social and political structures (e.g. economy and religion) that harm and discriminate against vulnerable populations. Structural violence is inextricably tied to power relations, insofar as it is discursively shaped by – and in turn affects – the power to decide over the distribution of resources in any given context. The development and replication of legitimising social norms make structural violence acceptable and normalised (Dilts et al. 2012). According to Paul Farmer (1996), structural violence is complicated to observe for two main reasons. First, individuals commonly develop an exoticised or indifferent construction of the suffering of others. Second, the dynamics and logics that generate, distribute, and perpetuate structural violence are poorly understood.

Structural violence shapes the position of *waria* in Indonesian society, where they are almost only accepted and respected as sex workers, *ludruk* artists (traditional dances), street musicians, and stylists (Balgos, Gaillard and Sanz 2012). They usually belong to the most marginal social strata and subsist in a context of constant vulnerability, employed in temporary, informal, and precarious jobs without regular income (Hardon and Ilmi 2014; Nuño 2016). In contemporary Indonesia, there are also *waria* who work in television; run small businesses; have university careers; and work as politicians, fashion designers, or teachers (Nuño 2017c).

This chapter examines the multi-faceted and complex interpersonal, socio-economic and structural realities that affect *waria*'s health and wellbeing and the possibilities for epistemic and social justice for these communities. The data used comes from an anthropological study carried out in 2014 in the city of Jogjakarta, where I conducted semi-structured, tape-recorded, or annotated interviews; participant observations; and focus-group discussions. Some of the results presented in this chapter have been previously published in Spanish-language journals (Nuño 2017a, b, c).[3] Participants provided tape-recorded informed consent to participate in the research. All real names have been replaced by pseudonyms to maintain confidentiality for participants and safeguard the integrity of the research process.[4]

The chapter proceeds as follows. First, I explain how neoliberal logics influence global health policies and practices in the empirical context where *waria* live in Jogjakarta. Second, I present the impact of structural violence and HIV stigma on *waria*. Third, I introduce different dimensions that limit the *waria*'s access to public health services. Finally, I describe the processes through which *waria* make socio-political claims and negotiations to reduce health inequalities.

THE NEOLIBERALISATION OF GLOBAL HEALTH

As discussed in the introduction, the growth of global health is inscribed in neoliberal health policies and programmes. Different authors propose that neoliberal health policies are mainly driven by geopolitical and economic objectives rather than principles of health equity and human rights (Castro, and Singer 2004). As a consequence, they reinforce and perpetuate dynamics that promote health inequalities such as the increment in bureaucratic obstacles to health care and the appearance of discriminatory practices against vulnerable populations (Ayala and García 2009; Biehl 2004; Huffman, Veen and

Hennink 2012; Larchanché 2012; Warner and Gabe 2004). It is important to note, however, that neoliberal logics not only undergird global health institutions, but they also model and shape identities based on specific ideas about freedom based on individualism (Keshavjee 2015; Rose 1999).

Michel Foucault's concepts of biopower, biopolitics, and governmentality are helpful in this context. Biopower is theorised as a set of principles and technologies applied on bodies that seek to control and regulate life and maintain security. Practices of self-care and self-control, such as being concerned about maintaining good health, constitute some of the mechanisms through which biopower is exerted. Consequently, biopolitics are the general principles, policies, and strategies that guide biopower actions. They are developed to govern populations and discipline subjects according to discourses, habits, attitudes, and normalising standards. Biopolitics are then applied using governmentality, which is the set of procedures and tactics implemented by disciplines and institutions (e.g. through statistics, anatomy, the education system) to generate, introduce, and reproduce power mechanisms (Foucault 1978). According to Foucault's conception, biopower, biopolitics, and governmentality constitute the ontological foundations of liberalism and individualism, as these principles are intended to define the body as the pillar of growth and development and produce and guarantee the mechanisms for economic neoliberalism (Foucault 2009).

Resilience, in turn, is a technique of governmentality that highlights the principles of adaptation to guarantee security in adverse and vulnerable contexts. Since the 1970s, non-governmental (NGO) and humanitarian organisations have promoted resilience discourses across the Global South, with a consequent spread of neoliberal markets logics, free markets, and the information industry (Ong 2007). Some authors suggest contemporary resilience discourses have progressively become techniques of neoliberal biopolitical governance, where attention turns away from dimensions and structures that perpetuate structural violence and discrimination in societies, and resilience turns into adaptation skills for people who survive under difficult circumstances (Keshavjee 2015; Kleinman and Lock 1997; Lock and Nguyen 2010). While the majority of health-related social movements' claims in the past have focused on economic and social equity or restructuring of institutions, today a number of them are primarily focused on the construction of health as a right and responsibility based on normative standards or shared conditions, but not as a matter of structural change (Fassin 2010). Some examples are organisations of seropositive people in Brazil (Biehl 2004) and South Africa (Fassin 2007) seeking affordable treatments, marginalised social groups in Brazil who want to perform aesthetic operations as subsistence strategies (Edmonds 2007), organisations of people with muscular dystrophy in France (Rabeharisoa 2006), and survivors of the Chernobyl tragedy (Petryna 2002) who use their biological condition to generate public concern. When these movements use resilience logics to improve the health and welfare of certain social groups, they generally do not address structural dimensions in the form of institutional changes, which are intimately related to the non-provision of adequate health care for marginalised populations in general. Some of these structural claims may include the development of alternative health systems based on principles of social justice, protection, and sustainability that guarantee health protection to all in society (van de Pas 2016). Resilience logics also shape the global health interventions that affect the lives of *waria* in Indonesia.

For *waria*, embracing these discourses has its origin in recent sociopolitical changes and in the promotion of different development programmes in Indonesia. For instance, between 2006 and 2010, the NGO *Perkumpulan Keluarga Berencana Indonesia* (Indonesian Family Planning Association – PKBI) conducted a community development programme to train *waria* in topics such as human rights, community participation, and management. Constructed from a scenario where *waria* saw themselves as passive spectators of national policy and programmes, this initiative helped them to become more politically active citizens. This transformation is reflected, for instance, in the change of focus in *waria* groups. While in the past these groups sought to increase their acceptance in the city's neighbourhoods, promote their economic inclusion and independence, and generate support networks, today their priorities are oriented towards political visibility, legal recognition, and social rights (Nuño 2016).

Critical approaches to global health highlight that, instead of empowering vulnerable people, resilience may reinforce the importance of adapting and accommodating populations on the same terms, scopes, and discourses that macro-level structures impose (Joseph 2013). This means, for instance, that vulnerable populations must frame their claims in ways that follow the logics and procedures established by political and legal international schemes (e.g. human rights statutes) instead of fostering their own constructions of justice and equity (Devillard and Baer 2010). While these normatively based claims are useful to somehow reverse concrete and specific situations of inequality and discrimination, further reconsiderations or criticisms of the logics that perpetuate structural violence, unequal power relationships, and discrimination suffered by vulnerable populations rarely appear. Lindroth and Sinevaara-Niskanen (2014), for instance, have argued that demands for resilience among vulnerable populations diffusely reinforce individual aspirations and values that, in the end, adapt and reproduce practices and beliefs according to specific and normative schemes of subordination and violence (Lindroth and Sinevaara-Niskanen 2014).

Throughout this chapter, I use particularly the concept of resilience to present the different causes that promote the emergence of socio-political movements among *waria*. In this case, understanding resilience as a particular technique of neoliberal biopolitical governance is useful to illustrate the logics and dynamics that govern these claims. In the following section, I present the history, implementation, and impact of the most common global health interventions among *waria* – HIV programmes. From the existence of different interpersonal and structural dimensions that these programmes do not address, new forms of discrimination and structural violence towards *waria* emerge.

HIV STIGMA AND STRUCTURAL VIOLENCE AGAINST *WARIA*

Since the first case of HIV appeared in Bali at the end of the 1980s, AIDS has become a public health issue in Indonesia. Cases have increased uncontrollably nationwide (growing from 7195 cases in 2006 to 76,879 in 2011), turning AIDS into the communicable disease with the highest growth rate in the country (United Nations Programme on HIV/AIDS 2012). In light of this worrisome reality, numerous HIV prevention and treatment programmes have emerged. These strategies have been heavily influenced by Western models of HIV prevention as opposed to structural approaches. While Western models are focused on the selection of beneficiary groups based on epidemiological evidence and the development of individual behavioural change strategies, structural approaches seek to transform the environment and conditions in which people live, in order to influence individual and collective behaviours and attitudes (O'Manique 2004; Ramin 2007). In Indonesia, almost all HIV strategies have focused on minority groups (e.g. female sex workers), yet they have not targeted other social groups that interact with them, such as sex work clients (Hammar 2010). Recurrently, organisations such as USAID have categorised *waria* as a population at risk of HIV based on data regarding prevalence and transmission (Joesoef et al. 2003; Morin 2008; Prabawanti et al. 2011).

Situated in the centre of the Island of Java with a population of about 600,000 (Badan Pusat Statistik 2010), the city of Jogjakarta is a vibrant commercial, cultural, and academic metropolis. The city is known for housing a relatively large population of *waria*, between 80 and 300 individuals.[5] For decades, HIV has had a significant impact among *waria* in Jogjakarta. Although there are no official statistics, the aforementioned NGO, PKBI, estimates that 30 per cent of *waria* in Jogjakarta are infected with the virus. Since 1993, when the first case of HIV infection was diagnosed among *waria* in the city, PKBI has mainly focused on HIV prevention. Currently, PKBI promotes four different strategies: monthly meetings to educate *waria* on sexual behaviours, peer education to promote the use of condoms, free Voluntary Counselling and Testing (VCT) for HIV, and a mobile clinic to promote VCT in residential *waria* areas. Facing the increasing incidence of HIV among *waria* and the reluctance of PKBI to provide Antiretroviral Therapy (ART), in 2004, a group of *waria* who had been peer educators with PKBI mobilised and founded the grassroot organisation (GRO) *Keluarga Besar Waria Yogyakarta* (Large *Waria* Family Jogjakarta) – KEBAYA. Today, KEBAYA provides ART and organises support groups for seropositive *waria*.

After years of implementation, the interventions of PKBI and KEBAYA have led to remarkable outcomes. Particularly significant achievements have been greater acceptance and awareness of condom use in sex work areas and the promotion and sustained implementation of mechanisms for free VCT and ART. Although no official statistics are available, *waria* consider the impact of these programmes to be significant. In 2005, at least seven *waria* died in a month; whereas between 2010 and 2012, the population lost 10 *waria* to the disease. According to KEBAYA representatives, there have been no cases of AIDS-related death of *waria* in Jogjakarta since 2012 (Nuño 2017b).

Undoubtedly, these two programmes have improved *waria*'s quality of life. However, this success must be understood in the context of different socio-cultural dimensions that emerge during the implementation of HIV programmes. In the words of Colleen O'Manique (2004), HIV responses cannot be constructed in terms of rational scientism free of interpretations or context. Rather, important political, social, and historical factors must be taken into consideration. Historically there have been two dominant models to define the disease. These models heavily influence, among other aspects, how we construct the disease and conceive of its solution. First, the biomedical (or allopathic) model views AIDS as a pathology resulting from viral infection. In this sense, the disease is only considered within biological limits and is accordingly restricted to biological explanations (Menéndez 1988). In this case, a single strategy to address the disease is based on the knowledge and application of biomedical technologies. The public health model represents the second prevalent way to construct the disease. Here HIV transmission is portrayed as the result of risky behaviours (e.g. sex without condoms). This paradigm primarily focuses on prevention and seeks to modify 'inappropriate' habits and attitudes at the individual level.

These two models are employed in a complementary manner, as PKBI and KEBAYA do in the case of *waria*, and are both focused on addressing the disease from a perspective centred around individuals with specific and measurable behavioural risk factors and biomedical indicators (United Nations 2014; United Nations Programme on HIV/AIDS 2004). Such singular construction of HIV, while abiding by the neoliberal focus on individual resilience, rejects the possible impact that collective, socio-cultural, and structural factors have on the predisposition to the disease, and to its transmission, prevention, and treatment (Castro and Farmer 2005; Farmer 1993, 1996; Nguyen 2010; Singer 1996). In the case of *waria*, the success of HIV campaigns is intimately connected with unequal power relationships and negative beliefs and attitudes about the origins and transmission modes of the disease, and hence structural violence.

For instance, *waria* still mentioned new cases of HIV infection in areas of sex work where there had been campaigns promoting condom use. Despite the awareness of *waria* regarding condom use, clients were still reluctant to use condoms for two principal reasons: first, clients thought that *waria* might suspect they had a sexually transmitted disease and, secondly, clients reported less pleasure during intercourse. For these reasons, regular clients attempted to negotiate condom use and sway *waria* with compelling arguments regarding their responsible nature and 'clean record'. Ultimately, some *waria* conceded to regular clients' wishes in order to keep a consistent and reliable source of income. Some *waria* perceived this practice as safe, believing that regular clients had no other sex partners. However, in practice, oftentimes regular clients also have sex with their spouses and other sex workers, which greatly magnifies the risk of HIV transmission (Gysels, Pool and Bwanika 2001; Thomsen, Stalker and Toroitich-Ruto 2004).

Another form of structural violence that emerges from power relations, social structures, and a complex system of beliefs is the stigma surrounding HIV (cf. Harman; Oinas, this volume). In turn, stigma is strongly influenced and connected to social inequalities, discrimination, physical violence, and poverty (Castro and Farmer 2005). The appearance of the HIV epidemic in Indonesia has led to the emergence of a strong stigma against seropositive individuals in general (Hammar 2010), and *waria* in particular. *Waria* are socially perceived as axiomatic carriers of the disease based on the limited knowledge Indonesian people have regarding HIV/AIDS (Badan Perencanaan Pembangunan Nasional 2012, 69–71; United Nations Programme on HIV/AIDS 2012, 34–35) and the prevalent portrayal of *waria* as sinful and immoral in the eyes of God (Safitri 2013). The combination of these two contextual factors have promoted the belief that AIDS is a divine curse that God sends *waria* as punishment for their gender condition and corrupt sexual behaviour. This reality leads to direct discrimination (e.g. social rejection and public violence) against seropositive *waria*, which also can act as a syndemic factor[6] that perpetuates their poor health and vulnerability (Singer 1996; Singer et al. 2006).

Oftentimes, seropositive *waria* have been forced to abandon their families and towns because the general population is fearful of infection. For this reason, seropositive *waria* often experience immense fear and anxiety in learning their HIV status, and are not likely to disclose their condition to relatives, friends, or neighbours – but rather only to other *waria* who will support them. The overwhelming fear and shame experienced by seropositive *waria* lead them to develop mechanisms to circumvent certain situations, as illustrated in the following interview excerpt: 'My sibling came when I was taking the [HIV] pill and he asked me: "What medicine are you taking?" "It is for tiredness", that is all I said. He asked me again, "why so many?" "Because it is from the doctor, to cure me when I am tired"' (Mkala, interview on April 6, 2014).

Some *waria* in fact do not want to know if they are seropositive in order to avoid having to lie about their status or, alternatively, facing stigma. These fears also generate insecurities about ART. Actually, some *waria* taking ART decide to stop taking the medication, as hiding their condition to relatives and neighbours becomes too much pressure: 'because for me it is just about dying, if I die today, it's because I am starving . . . but if I die tomorrow it's because of AIDS, so it is just the same. The point is being dead' (Tiara, interview on 11 March 2014). Although the stigma surrounding HIV is a pressing issue for *waria*, it is not a priority for PKBI and KEBAYA. The organisations have only addressed the issue with the general population after specific incidences, for example, when HIV stigma generated tensions in the neighbourhoods where *waria* live. In 2004, one of the communal latrines in the neighbourhood of Badram displayed a sign prohibiting *waria* from entering, supposedly to prevent the transmission of HIV. PKBI and the local *waria* group in the area mobilised to inform and educate neighbours about the disease until the sign was finally removed in 2005. The fact that the organisations do not address the problem of HIV stigma in their programmes generates tensions between *waria* and the organisations, sometimes exacerbating the stigma in the wider community:

> When that car [PKBI mobile clinic] comes, people here do not know why. When they see *waria* going into the car, people start asking: 'What are they doing here? Do *waria* have a new disease or something? It is just for *waria*'. I told this to [PKBI member]: 'It is your programme, not mine. My programme is with people here. If you want to do something for *waria*, you can tell me to go to PKBI but do not come here, because people do not know about AIDS'. I am scared, because maybe people can think, 'eh, look at *waria* . . . all of them are infected!' (Malula, interview on 24 April 2014)

The organisations' disinterest in the structural impacts of HIV negatively influences *waria*'s welfare, compounding the dynamics of discrimination and violence against them. Although initiatives to promote condom use are necessary, their exclusive focus on sex workers generate forms of structural violence based on power relationships and economic and social inequalities (Majuelos 2014). The same principle applies to the proliferation of

HIV-stigma. Given that HIV strategies developed by the organisations are primarily focused on individualistic approaches, they have failed to reach their potential due to overshadowing these relational and collective dimensions. Although KEBAYA emerged to improve *waria*'s health and welfare by promoting an intervention that PKBI refused to provide, it gradually ended up sustaining the same principles of mainstream neoliberal HIV programmes. These cases are not an exception, as most HIV interventions worldwide follow the same neoliberal, individualistic, and cost-effective principles (Parker, Easton and Klein 2000; Ramin 2007; Sumartojo 2000). In the next section, I explain how these principles in practice silence the demands, needs, and perceptions of *waria* and reproduce unequal, hierarchic, and discriminatory dynamics.

HEALTH ACCESS AND MEDICAL CARE PROBLEMS AMONG *WARIA*

The opening of Indonesia to global markets has facilitated the promotion of neoliberal ideologies and practices, including the deregulation of state competences and the transfer of part of their management to external organisations (Hadiz and Robison 2005). Prior to 2004, health access in Indonesia operated through direct payments or private health insurances. The Indonesian government launched the first phase of the *Akesin* plan to promote universal health coverage in 2004, and in 2008, this programme evolved towards the current *Jamkesmas*, focusing on low-income populations. In the global neoliberal landscape, the implementation of a national health programme such as the *Jamkesmas* is, however, complicated due to fragmented financing flows among districts and regions (Thabrany 2008). In 2010, about 60 per cent of Indonesians did not have any health coverage and out-of-pocket spending remained high among those covered. In addition, there were significant deficiencies in the quality and availability of *Jamkesmas* coverage, differences in its admission criteria across districts and poor programme knowledge and management. These dimensions resulted in poor coverage, leakage in non-poor populations, diminished resources, and poor accountability and feedback mechanisms (Harimurti et al. 2013). In other words, the *Jamkesmas* can be viewed as another example of an unhealthy health policy given its bureaucratic and management problems, demonstrating how neoliberal schemes operate as an apparatus of structural violence.

Although these violent marginalising practices impact vulnerable populations in general, they specially affect populations who do not meet social gender norms and normative stereotypes, such as *waria*. Gender-non-conforming individuals around the world face barriers for accessing health services as they commonly live in the margins of society and suffer gender discrimination and exclusion (Fraser 2016; Ming, Hadi and Khan 2016; Reisner et al. 2016; Winter et al. 2016). In what follows, I offer some examples of how structural violence is embedded in regulations about healthcare access for *waria*.

One of the main problems *waria* have highlighted during my research is their difficulty in accessing health services, and this is the result of multiple entangled dynamics of marginalisation. To participate in the *Jamkesmas*, it is mandatory to have a valid identification card in the region of residence. However, *waria* who were born outside the Jogjakarta region and moved to escape domestic violence, social discrimination, or ostracism are usually unable to access the programme. In order to obtain an identification card, relatives of displaced *waria* must sign a legal document authorising the change of residence. Families of displaced *waria* commonly refuse to sign the document due to the shame of having a *waria* in the family (Boellstorff 2004). For this reason, there is an indeterminate number of *waria* in the city of Jogjakarta without social, political, or legal recognition. This example represents a fierce exercise of structural violence as *waria* are stripped of their legal status due to norms and policies that do not consider their specific conditions of vulnerability.

Another example relates to the way in which HIV status determines which *waria* have access to adequate health care. While health access and care for seropositive *waria* are guaranteed by PKBI and KEBAYA regardless of possession of an identification card, undocumented non-seropositive *waria* have to pay out-of-pocket for public health services. The price per consultation in a *Puskesmas* (primary care centre) is around 60,000/70,000 IDR (3.78/4.41, euros respectively) and in a hospital about 200,000 IDR (12.61 euros), while private insurance has an approximate cost of 121,000 IDR per month – 7.56 euros. These amounts are prohibitive for *waria* because of their socio-economic status. For example, *waria* who work as street musicians can earn around 200,000 IDR per month. As a consequence, when *waria* need treatment for health issues, they use medical drugs recommended by other *waria* (Hardon and Ilmi 2014; Nuño 2016), rather than go to a *Puskesmas*. While these practices reveal the resilience that helps *waria* to survive social discrimination and structural violence, they bear high risks not only among *waria* but also more widely. For instance, when the recommended drugs are antibiotics, the practice of self-help among the community leads to uncontrolled antibiotic use. This is known to increase anti-microbial resistance, which, in turn, is one of the biggest threats to global public health (Wuijts et al. 2017).

These examples show how in healthcare systems, structural violence is embodied in the norms and rules about which populations are authorised to receive proper health care, and which are excluded and forced to rely on their own 'resilience' because of their socio-economic, religious, or health conditions (Basnyat 2017; Farmer et al. 2006).

SHIFTING THE SITUATION: *WARIA* CLAIMING ACCESS TO HEALTH AND MEDICAL CARE

The structural barriers discussed in the previous section are a consequence of the neoliberal logics that guide HIV interventions and prevent the improvement of all *waria*'s welfare. For years, PKBI and KEBAYA were the only institutions permitted to receive funds, which limited the healthcare options for *waria*. The majority of these funds were destined to HIV programmes and not to other various dimensions that are important for *waria*. Hence, as the following exchange illustrates, some *waria* who had worked for the organisations began to question whether the money was really used to meet all of their necessities.

> I think PKBI has a double moral standard. On the one hand, they help *waria* communities to develop. However, they do not let this happen without their control. Before, PKBI wanted to coordinate *waria* groups that already existed. They asked for funds using our names, which is not really nice . . . . I worked with them for some years and the salary was really low compared to the regular personnel . . . . I tried to talk to them clearly about this but they never listened. You know, the field-staff always does the hard work while they only write the reports. (Interview with Tika, 22 April 2014)

Waria also reported cases where they felt discriminated against and excluded by the organisations. For instance, some *waria* entrepreneurs programmes organised by PKBI and KEBAYA were purposely established only for seropositive *waria*. The organisations justified this criterion by claiming seropositive *waria* needed the money more; however, the decision generated strong critiques and propagated the feeling that the organisations were using *waria* for their own benefit (Nuño 2017b).

In face of these disagreements between *waria*, KEBAYA, and PKBI, some undocumented *waria* formed their own legal organisations. Their main objective was to obtain an administrative status to apply for national and international aid programmes. Nowadays, at least three *waria* groups in Jogjakarta exist as official autonomous institutions that are able to receive funds and negotiate directly with the local government and health authorities:

> We started to claim our rights. We learned the laws and what our constitution says. *Waria* should be included in the state programmes. Therefore, we

demanded and finally the government accepted our claims. In 2008, the government gave the *Jamkesmas* to 65 people, 24 of them were *waria*. It was the first time we achieved something like that. (Interview with Vilma, 10 March 2014)

These *waria* groups provide identity cards to their members and have legal authority to facilitate free healthcare access to undocumented *waria*. *Waria* who receive approval letters signed by the group are thus able to ask for health services at *Puskesmas* centres. The information is then verified with the *waria* group, allowing the *waria* patient to freely access immediate health services, receiving the official *Jamkesmas* cards in about two weeks. Furthermore, some of these *waria* groups are also able to provide free HIV prevention and treatment programmes. The success achieved by these autonomous groups is motivating *waria* from other cities and regions such as Palembang, Medan, and Bali to move to Jogjakarta in order to obtain free medical access and identification cards:

In the last saloon in Jakarta where I was working I was fine and pleased. One day my friend Vilma called me and told me I had to come back to Jogjakarta for my identity card. For the procedures I needed seven days, more or less. However, my boss only gave me two. Then I had two dilemmas, obtaining an identity card or continuing working in a job I loved. Finally, I decided to leave the job and got my identity card. I did not know if I was going to have the opportunity again in my life. (Interview with Sandi, April 4, 2014)

However, the *Jamkesmas* also has its limitations. It only offers hospital, ambulatory, maternal, and preventive health care, and the majority of its beneficiaries only receive basic medical coverage – expensive treatments and therapies are not covered (Harimurti et al. 2013). These regulations pose yet another form of structural violence against vulnerable populations, who are more susceptible to develop co-infections and complicated diseases (Singer et al. 2006). To overcome these limitations, the autonomous *waria* groups began negotiating with local authorities and health personnel. The story of a *waria* from Batam called Shasa provides an example of how the autonomous *waria* groups work to improve *waria*'s health and wellbeing.

At the end of 2012, Shasa started to lose hir[7] vision due to *toxoplasmosis*.[8] Doctors recommended her to move to Jakarta for the treatment; however afterwards (s)he discovered the *Jamkesmas* did not cover it. The price of the medicines for three months was approximately nineteen million IDR (1229.31 euros), a price that Shasa could not afford as (s)he depended on the support from other *waria*. Another *waria* from Jogjakarta then recommended Shasa to move to Jogjakarta to obtain free medical care. (S)he moved to the city and contacted an autonomous *waria* group. They informed Shasa about a state programme to provide free medical care for low-income and disabled people, and began negotiations with the health authorities to provide Shasa access to the programme. The medical doctor suggested an operation instead of the regular treatment, arguing too much time had passed since Shasa's blindness began. After a few weeks had passed and the medical doctor did not approve the intervention nor respond to *waria*'s calls, the *waria* group proposed moving forward and organising meetings with the hospital director and health authorities in order to continue the negotiation. These *waria* described these practices of constant pressure and negotiation as necessary, as medical staff do not commonly make efforts to facilitate treatments to *waria*-patients, and sometimes they outright refuse to help.

These experiences have helped autonomous *waria* groups to establish relationships and networks with other *waria* groups in the country. For them, these exchanges are useful for providing a broader knowledge of their rights as citizens and confronting health vulnerability, as the following exchange illustrates:

> *Mback*: Honestly, Gila is also an activist. (S)he can carry out a programme that we cannot. For this reason, I have learned from hir how to implement it and, in return, I taught hir what we do here.
>
> *Gila*: There is a state programme that says when a patient needs to move to another place for treatment, the government pays for the ticket, companion, and living costs in the new place. I know it works where I live [*Batam*]. (Interview with several *waria*, 3 April 2014)

The emergence of *waria*'s socio-political movements reveals the inadequacy of the Indonesian national health system to serve vulnerable populations. It is also an indication of the diffusion of neoliberal resilience logics among *waria* themselves. As the earlier mentioned cases illustrate, organisations of undocumented *waria* frame the problem of healthcare access as specific to undocumented *waria* in Jogjakarta, not as a general *waria* problem. In turn, only those *waria* who are directly affected by specific policies propose alternatives and solutions. This is one example of how neoliberal resilience logics operate: instead of understanding inequalities as a structural problem that, in one way or another, affects *waria* as a marginalised group, they are individualised based on certain conditions (e.g. documented *versus* undocumented *waria*). These categorisations and differentiations allow some forms of violence to be repudiated while others are normalised and reproduced. Therefore, *waria* cannot be understood as a social group with a collective identity, but as a set of different individuals gathered and organised according to shared conditions and neoliberal aspirations and values (Ong 1995). Their condition as gender-non-conforming subjects living at the margins of society no longer represents an element of unity and solidarity among their peers (Koeswinarno 2007).

The processes of making claims for care described in this chapter then represent some limitations of resilience movements. Despite the fact that undocumented *waria* follow legal and political regulations to make their claims, they find that macro- and micro-level health structures still resist their demands. What explains this conflict is the collective, social, and structural nature of resilience. NGOs usually provide knowledge to vulnerable groups in order to strengthen their individual competences. However, the webs of resilience these groups are able to create are not always enough to promote changes at the structural level (Obrist, Mayumana and Kessy 2010). If the empowerment of marginal groups does not include other social movements and groups, resilience processes are in danger of becoming a permanent and never-ending process of confrontation with single, individualised obstacles (Prozorov 2007, 77).

RESILIENCE VERSUS STRUCTURAL RESPONSES TO HIV

This chapter critically investigates different dimensions of structural violence affecting *waria* (Indonesian male-to-female transvestites) in the city of Jogjakarta. It explores their day-to-day health needs beyond mainstream global health priorities and discusses the impact that neoliberal logics have in the identities of vulnerable populations, in particular as they revolve around the notion of resilience. *Waria* is a social group that has historically been discriminated against and excluded in Indonesia because of its gender identity. As they are categorised as a population at risk for HIV, global health interventions with *waria* have focused on HIV/AIDS prevention and treatment programmes. These interventions have failed to reach their potential due to overshadowing relational and collective dimensions of HIV, such as stigma. In addition, *waria* have had difficulties in accessing and receiving medical care due to the violence embedded in national and international health priorities and processes, and sometimes due to the lack of adequate ID documents. None of the HIV-organisations assisting *waria* have addressed *waria*'s own priorities, as their interventions have followed neoliberal global health logics. For these reasons, groups of undocumented *waria* have formed their own legal organisations in order to obtain access to health care.

The case described in this chapter evidences the inadequacy of the Indonesian state and neoliberal global health schemes to provide health care for vulnerable populations, such as *waria*. In addition, it describes how neoliberal logics model and transform identities based on the principles of individualism and shared conditions, aspirations, and values. Instead of understanding inequalities as a structural problem that equally affect *waria* as a marginalised group, they have created categories based on certain conditions (e.g. documented *versus* undocumented *waria*). These differences have allowed for the normalisation and proliferation of some forms of violence and discrimination, as *waria* organisations make rights-based, rather than solidarity-based, claims. In addition, the claim processes described in this chapter also represent some limitations of resilience movements. Although these movements help undocumented *waria* to improve their health and wellbeing, macro-level health structures are still resistant to accommodating their demands. What explains this problem is the collective, social, and structural nature of resilience. Resilience programmes provide individual competences, but are rarely enough to promote changes at the structural level.

Yet, if the micro- and macro-practices of global health are to genuinely address the plight of marginalised populations, structural responses are required. For instance, as shown in this chapter, the HIV programmes in place tend to emphasise individual resilience in the affected communities. Nevertheless, addressing the structural dimensions of HIV is essential in preventing HIV transmission as well as reducing social, economic, and political inequalities, that is, the structural violence that underlies vulnerability (Sumartojo 2000). HIV interventions that follow structural approaches commonly involve social scientists, medical professionals, seropositive populations, and civil society organisations. These interventions include the implementation of HIV prevention programmes at community and household levels to generate safe environments (Aidala et al. 2005; Argento et al. 2011; Kerrigan et al. 2008) and the development of community strategies involving exclusive use of condoms and condom eroticisation with sex work clients (Philpott, Knerr and Boydell 2006; Sahu et al. 2014). Structural approaches to HIV have demonstrated tremendous success over time in terms of the reduction of HIV incidence and HIV-stigma barriers, as well as the improvement of the social conditions of vulnerable groups (Gupta et al. 2008). These approaches, however, require a global health agenda that goes beyond the resilience of the marginalised.

NOTES

1. Although some scholars define *waria* as transgender, I follow Tom Boellstorff's definition of *waria* (Boellstorff 2004). The concept of transgender emerged in recent decades as a homogenizing category for non-heteronormative identities. However, in my reading, following David Valentine (2007), this definition implies a construction of identities based on political and individualistic approaches that deny socio-cultural, class, or ethnic differences.

2. Historically, different non-heteronormative, socially recognised expressions of gender have existed in Southeast Asia. Some examples are the *kathoey* in Thailand

(Jackson and Sullivan 1999), the *hijras* in India (Nanda 1998), and the *fa'afafine* in Samoa (Besnier 1994). In Indonesia, cases of transgression of masculine/feminine dichotomies such as the *tomboi* and the *bissu* have been documented for centuries (Boellstorff 2005; Peletz 2011). According to Dédé Oetomo (2000, 46–59) and Tom Boellstorff (2004, 159–195), the term *waria* was coined in the late 1970s from the conjunction of the Indonesian words woman (*wanita*) and man (*pria*). *Waria* describe themselves in terms of masculinity and femininity (Oetomo 2000). For Tom Boellstorff, *waria* cannot be defined as third sex/gender because they operate within the orbit of male gender identity and are shaped as feminine males within their society (Boellstorff 2004).

3. All relevant journals have granted permission to reproduce some of the findings.

4. Conducting a research with *waria* had delicate ethical and epistemological dimensions, as also described elsewhere (Taha 2012; Koeswinarno 2007). As a European cisgender male, it was easy for me to get close to *waria* due to a white-male eroticisation *waria* frequently admit (Oetomo 2000). However, my proximity to them also involved delicate moments and evoked feelings of jealousy and discussions among them. At the beginning of my participant observation, in areas that were popular among *waria* sex workers, some *waria* did not understand my role as a researcher, as they were exclusively accustomed to interacting with white males as sex clients. Afterwards, my presence generated disputes because some *waria* thought I unequally dedicated more time to others. I was viewed as exotic, which meant that *waria* wanted to spend as much time with me as possible. In addition, while I organised the focus-group discussions, I was warned about possible problems of bringing together various *waria* communities in the same space for fear that they could end up arguing and fighting. Therefore, in order to soften possible tensions, each focus group included only members of the same *waria* group.

5. According to statistics produced by the PKBI, there are around 100 *waria* in the city. These data contrast significantly with the appraisals of other organisations, such as the NGO *Komunitas AIDS Indonesia* (Indonesian AIDS community), which reports between 80 and 130, and the *waria*-run organisation, *Ikatan Waria Jogjakarta* (*waria* bonds Jogjakarta – IWAYO) which reports 300.

6. I use the notion of syndemic factors to understand the different factors, in this particular case, driving HIV epidemic. The syndemic theory posits the existence of risk factors that interact synergistically to increase vulnerability. For example, co-occurring conditions such as alcohol abuse, clinically significant depression, and violence collectively influence HIV risk behaviours and vice versa.

7. Following the statement made by Boellstorff (2004), I combine the masculine and feminine English pronouns (s)he to name *waria*, as they do not consider themselves neither men nor as women. I use the accusative pronoun 'hir' to refer to the third person singular.

8. Toxoplamosis is an infection produced by the parasite *Toxoplasma gondii*. The contagion can be produced by direct contact with animals or the ingestion of raw or undercooked meat.

REFERENCES

Aidala, A., J. E. Cross, R. Stall and E. Sumartojo. 2005. 'Housing Status and HIV Risk Behaviors: Implications for Prevention and Policy'. *AIDS and Behavior* 9, no. 3: 251–65.

Argento, E., S. Reza-Paul, R. Lorway, J. Jain, M. Bhagya, M. Fathima, S. V. Sreeram, R. S. Hafeezur and J. O'Neil. 2011. 'Confronting Structural Violence in Sex Work: Lessons from a Community-Led HIV Prevention Project in Mysore, India'. *AIDS Care* 23, no. 1: 69–74.

Ayala, Ariadna R. and Sergio García, G. 2009. 'Gestión de cuerpos y actuación de resistencias en una política social. La aplicación de la Renta Mínima de Inserción de la Comunidad de Madrid'. *Revista de Antropología Experimental* 9: 17–36.

Badan Perencanaan Pembangunan Nasional. 2012. *Laporan pencapalian tujuan pembangunan millennium di Indonesia 2011*. Indonesia: BAPPENAS.

Badan Pusat Statistik. 2010. *Daerah Istimewa Yogyakarta Dalam Angka. Subdivision of Regional Balance and Statistical Analysis, Province of Yogyakarta*. Indonesia: Badan Pusat Statistik.

Balgos, B., J. C. Gaillard and K. Sanz. 2012. 'The Warias of Indonesia in Disaster Risk: The Case of the 2010 Mt Merapi Eruption in Indonesia'. *Gender & Development* 2, no. 2: 337–348.

Basnyat, Iccha. 2017. 'Structural Violence in Health Care: Lived Experience of Street-Based Female Commercial Sex Workers in Kathmandu'. *Qualitative Health Research* 27, no. 2: 191–203.

Besnier, Niko. 1994. 'Polynesian Gender Liminality through Time and Space'. In *Third Sex, Third Gender: Beyond Sexual Dimorphism in Culture and History*, edited by G. Herdt, 285–328. New York: Zone Books.

Biehl, Joao. 2004. 'The Activist State: Global Pharmaceuticals, AIDS, and Citizenship in Brazil'. *Social Text 80* 22, no. 3: 105–132.

Boellstorff, Tom. 2004. 'Playing Back the Nation: Waria, Indonesian Transvestites'. *Cultural Anthropology* 19, no. 2: 159–195.

Boellstorff, Tom. 2005. *The Gay Archipelago: Sexuality and Nation in Indonesia*. Princeton: Princeton University Press.

Boellstorff, Tom. 2014. 'Lessons from the Notion of "Moral Terrorism"'. In *Feelings at the Margins: Dealing with Violence, Stigma and Isolation in Indonesia*, edited by T. Stodulka and B. Röttger-Rösssler, 148–158. Chicago: Chicago University Press.

Castro, A. and P. Farmer. 2005. 'El estigma del sida y su evolución social: una visión desde Haití'. *Revista de Antropología Social* 14: 125–144.

Castro, A. and M. Singer. 2004. *Unhealthy Health Policy – a Critical Anthropological Examination*. Maryland: Altamira Press.

Confortini, Catia C. and Tiina Vaittinen. 2019. 'Introduction: Analysing Violences in Gendered Global Health'. In *Gender, Global Health and Violence: Feminist Perspectives on Peace and Disease*, edited by Tiina Vaittinen and Catia Confortini. London and New York: Rowman & Littlefield.

Devillard, M. J. and A. Baer. 2010. 'Antropología y Derechos Humanos: multiculturalismo, retos y resignificaciones'. *Revista de Antropología Social* 19: 25–51.

Dilts, Andrew, Yves Winter, Thomas Biebricher, Eric Vance Johnson, Antonio Y. Vázquez-Arroyo and Joan Cocks. 2012. 'Revisiting Johan Galtung's Concept of Structural Violence'. *New Political Science* 34, no. 2: e191–e227.

Edmonds, A. 2007. '"The Poor Have the Right to Be Beautiful": Cosmetic Surgery in Neoliberal Brazil'. *The Journal of the Royal Anthropological Institute* 13, no. 2: 368–81.

Farmer, Paul. 1993. *AIDS and Accusation: Haiti and the Geography of Blame*. Berkeley: University of California Press.

Farmer, Paul. 1996. 'On Suffering and Structural Violence: A View from Below'. *Daedalus* 125, no. 1: 261–283.

Farmer, Paul E., Bruce Nizeye, Sara Stulac and Salmaan Keshavjee. 2006. 'Structural Violence and Clinical Medicine'. *PLOS Medicine* 3, no. 10: e449.

Fassin, Didier. 2007. *When Bodies Remember: Experiences and Politics of AIDS in South Africa*. Berkeley: University of California Press.

Fassin, Didier. 2010. 'El irresistible ascenso del derecho a la vida. Razón humanitaria y justicia social'. *Revista de Antropología Social* 19: 191–204.

Fassin, Didier. 2011. *Humanitarian Reason: A Moral History of the Present*. Berkeley: University of California Press.

Foucault, Michel. 1978. *The History of Sexuality: An Introduction*. Vol. 1. New York: Random House Inc.

Foucault, Michel. 2009. *Nacimiento de la biopolítica*. Barcelona: Akal.

Fraser, Barbara. 2016. 'Peru's Transgender Community: The Battle for Rights'. *The Lancet* 388, no. 10042: 324–325.

Gupta, G. R., J. O. Parkhurst, J. A. Ogden, P. Aggleton and A. Mahal. 2008. 'Structural Approaches to HIV Prevention'. *Lancet* 372, no. 9640: 764–775.

Gysels, M., R. Pool and K. Bwanika. 2001. 'Truck Drivers, Middlemen and Commercial Sex Workers: AIDS and the Mediation of Sex in South West Uganda'. *AIDS Care* 13, no. 3: 373–385.

Hadiz, Vedi and Richard Robison. 2005. 'Neo-liberal Reforms and Illiberal Consolidations: The Indonesian Paradox'. *The Journal of Development Studies* 41, no. 2: 220–241.

Hammar, L. 2010. *Sin, Sex and Stigma: A Pacific Response to HIV and AIDS*. London: Sean Kingston Publishing.

Hanlon, J. 1996. *Mozambique: Who Calls the Shots?* London: James Currey.

Hardon, A. and N. Ilmi. 2014. 'On Coba and Cocok: Youth-Led Drug-Experimentation in Eastern Indonesia'. *Anthropology & Medicine* 21, no. 2: 217–229.

Harimurti, P., E. Pambudi, A. Pigazzini and A. Tandon. 2013. 'The Nuts and Bolts of Jamkesmas – Indonesia's Government-Financed Health Coverage Program for the Poor and Near-Poor'. In *Universal Health Coverage (UNICO) Studies Series*. Washington, D.C.: The World Bank.

Harman, Sophie. 2019. 'Violence and the Paradox of Global Health'. In *Gender, Global Health and Violence: Feminist Perspectives on Peace and Disease*, edited by Tiina Vaittinen and Catia Confortini. London and New York: Rowman & Littlefield.

Homedes, N. and A. Ugalde. 2005. 'Why Neoliberal Health Reforms Have Failed in Latin America'. *Health Policy* 71, no. 1: 83–96.

Huffman, Samantha A., Jaap Veen and Monique M. Hennink. 2012. 'Exploitation, Vulnerability to Tuberculosis and Access to Treatment among Uzbek Labor Migrants in Kazakhstan'. *Social Science & Medicine* 74: 864–872.

Ikhile, Deborah, Gibson Linda and Azrini Wahidin. 2019. '"I Cannot Know That Now I Have Cancer!" A Structural Violence Perspective on Breast Cancer Detection in Uganda'. In *Gender, Global Health and Violence: Feminist Perspectives on Peace and Disease*, edited by Tiina Vaittinen and Catia Confortini. London and New York: Rowman & Littlefield.

Jackson, P. and G. Sullivan. 1999. 'A Panoply of Roles: Sexual and Gender Diversity in Contemporary Thailand'. In *Lady Boys, Tom Boys, Rent Boys: Male and Female Homosexualities in Contemporary Thailand*, edited by P. Jackson and G. Sullivan, 1–27. New York: Haworth Press.

Janes, Craig R. and Kitty K. Corbett. 2009. 'Anthropology and Global Health'. *Annual Review of Anthropology* 38, no. 1: 167–183.

Joesoef, M. R., M. Gultom, I. D. Irana, J. S. Lewis, J. S. Moran, T. Muhaimin and C. A. Ryan. 2003. 'High Rates of Sexually Transmitted Diseases among Male Transvestites in Jakarta, Indonesia'. *International Journal of STD and AIDS* 14, no. 9: 609–613.

Joseph, Jonathan. 2013. 'Resilience as Embedded Neoliberalism: A Governmentality Approach'. *Resilience* 1, no. 1: 38–52.

Kerrigan, D., P. Telles, H. Torres, C. Overs and C. Castle. 2008. 'Community Development and HIV/STI-Related Vulnerability among Female Sex Workers in Rio de Janeiro, Brazil'. *Health Educ Res* 23, no. 1: 13–45.

Keshavjee, Salmaan. 2015. *Blind Spot. How Neoliberalism Infiltrated Global Health.* California: University of California Press.

Kleinman, Arthur and Margaret Lock. 1997. *Social Suffering*. London: University of California.

Koeswinarno, Oleh. 2007. *Kehidupan Bergama Waria Muslim di Yogyakarta*. Yogyakarta: Universitas Gadjah Mada.

Larchanché, Stéphanie. 2012. 'Intangible Obstacles: Health Implications of Stigmatization, Structural Violence and Fear among Undocumented Immigrants in France'. *Social Science & Medicine* 74: 858–863.

Lindroth, Marjo and Heidi Sinevaara-Niskanen. 2014. 'Adapt or Die? The Biopolitics of Indigeneity – From the Civilising Mission to the Need for Adaptation'. *Global Society* 28, no. 2: 180–194.

Lock, Margaret and Vinh-Kim Nguyen. 2010. *An Anthropology of Biomedicine*. London: Wiley.

Majuelos, F. 2014. 'Trabajadoras sexuales africanas, entre el stigma y la crisis'. *Gazeta de Antropología* 30, no. 2: article 7.

Menéndez, Eduardo, L. 1988. 'Modelo Médico Hegemónico y atención primaria'. II Conferencia de atención primaria, Buenos Aires.

Ming, Long C., Muhammad A. Hadi and Tahir M. Khan. 2016. 'Transgender Health in India and Pakistan'. *The Lancet* 388, no. 10060: 2601–2602.

Morin, J. 2008. '"It's Mutual Attraction": Transvestites and Risk of HIV Transmission in Urban Papua'. In *Making Sense of AIDS: Culture, Sexuality, and Power in Melanesia*, edited by L. Butt and R. Eves, 41–59. Honolulu, Hawai'i: University of Hawai'i Press.

Nanda, S. 1998. *Neither Man nor Woman: The Hijras of India*. Belmont, CA: Wadsworth Publishing Company.
Nguyen, Vinh-Kim. 2010. *The Republic of Therapy: Triage and Sovereignity in West Africa's Time of AIDS*. Durham, NC: Duke University Press.
Nichter, M. 2008. *Global Health: Why Cultural Perceptions, Social Representations, and Biopolitics Matter*. Tucson, AZ: The University of Arizona Press.
Nunes, João. 2014. 'Questioning Health Security: Insecurity and Domination in World Politics'. *Review of International Studies* 40, no. 5: 939–960.
Nuño, N. 2016. 'The Use of "Life-Enabling" Practices among Waria: Vulnerability, Subsistence and Paradoxes in Contemporary Jogjakarta'. In *Intimate Economies: Bodies, Emotions and Sexualities on the Global Market*, edited by S. Hofmann and A. Moreno. Basingstoke, UK: Palgrave Press.
Nuño, N. 2017a. 'El acceso y la atención sanitaria como reivindicaciones socio-políticas. Reconstruyendo la salud global desde los márgenes'. *Revista de Antropologia Social* 26, no. 1: 73–91.
Nuño, N. 2017b. 'Las dimensiones olvidadas de los programas de VIH dirigidos a las waria de Jogjakarta, Indonesia'. *Desacatos. Revista de Antropologia Social* 54: 122–137.
Nuño, N. 2017c. 'Redefiniendo las identidades waria en la Indonesia contemporánea'. *Revista de Dialectología y Tradiciones Populares* 72, no. 1: 103–123.
Obrist, Brigit, Iddy Mayumana and Flora Kessy. 2010. 'Livelihood, Malaria and Resilience: A Case Study in the Kilombero Valley, Tanzania'. *Progress in Development Studies* 10, no. 4: 325–343.
Oetomo, Dedé. 2000. 'Masculinity in Indonesia: Genders, Sexualities and Identities in a Changing Society'. In *Framing the Sexual Subject: The Politics of Gender, Sexuality, and Power*, edited by Richard Parker, Regina Maria Barbosa and Peter Aggleton, 46–59. London: University of California Press.
Oetomo, Dedé. 2002. 'Now You See It, Now You Don't: Homosexual Culture in Indonesia'. *International Institute for Asian Studies Newsletter*. Accessed 9 August 2019. https:// https://www.iias.asia/the-newsletter/newsletter-29-autumn-2002.
Oinas, Elina. 2019. 'HIV Politics and Structural Violence: Access to Treatment and Knowledge'. In *Gender, Global Health and Violence: Feminist Perspectives on Peace and Disease*, edited by Tiina Vaittinen and Catia Confortini. London and New York: Rowman & Littlefield.
O'Manique. 2004. *Neoliberalism and AIDS Crisis in Sub-Saharan Africa: Globalization's Pandemic*. Basingstoke, UK: Palgrave MacMillan.
Ong, A. 1995. 'Making the Biopolitical Subject: Cambodian Immigrants, Refugee Medicine and Cultural Citizenship in California'. *Social Science & Medicine* 40, no. 9: 1243–1257.
Ong, Aihwa. 2007. 'Neoliberalism as a Mobile Technology'. *Transactions of the Institute of British Geographers* 32, no. 1: 3–8.
Ong, Aihwa and Stephen Collier. 2008. *Global Assemblages: Technology, Politics, and Ethics as Anthropological Problems*. New York: Wiley-Blackwell.
Oriol, Joan P. 2006. 'Teoría y práctica del desarrollo. Cambios en las variables de la 'ecuación del desarrollo' en los últimos 50 años'. *Revista del CLAD Reforma y Democracia*, no. 36: 1–17.

Parker, R. G., D. Easton and C. H. Klein. 2000. 'Structural Barriers and Facilitators in HIV Prevention: A Review of International Research'. *AIDS* 14 Suppl 1: S22–S32.

Peletz, Michael G. 2011. 'Gender Pluralism: Muslim Southeast Asia since Early Modern Times'. *Social Research: An International Quarterly* 78, no. 2: 659–686.

Petryna, Adriana. 2002. *Life Exposed. Biological Citizens after Chernobyl*. Princeton: Princeton University Press.

Petryna, Adriana and Joao Biehl, eds. 2013. *When People Come First: Critical Studies in Global Health*. Princeton: Princeton University Press.

Pfeiffer, James and Mark Nichter. 2008. 'What Can Critical Medical Anthropology Contribute to Global Health?' *Medical Anthropology Quarterly* 22, no. 4: 410–415.

Philpott, A., W. Knerr and V. Boydell. 2006. 'Pleasure and Prevention: When Good Sex Is Safer Sex'. *Reproductice Health Matters* 14, no. 28: 23–31.

Prabawanti, C., L. Bollen, R. Palupy, G. Morineau, P. Girault, D. E. Mustikawati, N. Majid, Nurhayati, E. R. Aditya, A. S. Anartati and R. Magnani. 2011. 'HIV, Sexually Transmitted Infections, and Sexual Risk Behavior among Transgenders in Indonesia'. *AIDS and Behavior* 15, no. 3: 663–673.

Prozorov, Sergei. 2007. 'The Unrequited Love of Power: Biopolitical Investment and the Refusal of Care'. *Foucault Studies* 4: 53–77.

Rabeharisoa, V. 2006. 'From Representation to Mediation: The Shaping of Collective Mobilization on Muscular Dystrophy in France'. *Social Science & Medicine* 62: 564–576.

Ramin, B. 2007. 'Anthropology Speaks to Medicine: The Case HIV/AIDS in Africa'. *Mcgill Journal of Medicine* 10, no. 2: 12–32.

Reisner, Sari L., Tonia Poteat, JoAnne Keatley, Mauro Cabral, Tampose Mothopeng, Emilia Dunham, Claire E. Holland, Ryan Max and Stefan D. Baral. 2016. 'Global Health Burden and Needs of Transgender Populations: A Review'. *The Lancet* 388, no. 10042: 412–436.

Rose, Nikolas. 1999. *Powers of Freedom: Reframing Political Thought*. Cambridge: Cambridge University Press.

Safitri, D. M. 2013. 'The Politics of Piety in the Pondok Pesantren Khusus Waria Al-Fattah Senin Kamis Yogyakarta. Negotiating the Islamic Religious Embodiment'. In *Islam in Indonesia: Contrasting Images and Interpretations*, edited by J. Burhanudin and K. Van Dijk. Amsterdam: Amsterdam University Press.

Sahu, D. Arvind Pandey, Ram Manohar Mishra, Niranjan. Saggurti, Shekhar. Setu and Indra Raj Singh. 2014. 'An Appraisal of Sexual Behaviors, STI/HIV Prevalence, and HIV Prevention Programs among Truckers in India: A Critical Literature Review'. *World Journal of AIDS* 4: 206–218.

Sanahuja, J. A. 2007. '¿Más y mejor ayuda? La Declaración de París y las tendencias en la cooperación al desarrollo'. In *Guerra y conflictos en el Siglo XXI: Tendencias globales. Anuario 2007–2008 del Centro de Educación e Investigación para la Paz (CEIPAZ)*, edited by Manuela Mesa. Madrid: CEIPAZ.

Singer, M. 1996. 'A Dose of Drugs, a Touch of Violence, a Case of AIDS: Conceptualizing the SAVA Syndemic'. *Free Inquiry in Creative Sociology* 24, no. 2: 99–110.

Singer, M. C., P. I. Erickson, L. Badiane, R. Diaz, D. Ortiz, T. Abraham and A. M. Nicolaysen. 2006. 'Syndemics, Sex and the City: Understanding Sexually

Transmitted Diseases in Social and Cultural Context'. *Social Science & Medicine* 63, no. 8: 2010–2021.

Sumartojo, E. 2000. 'Structural Factors in HIV Prevention: Concepts, Examples, and Implications for Research'. *AISA* 14 Suppl 1: S3–S10.

Taha, Nur'Ain. 2012. 'Let Me Be a Servant of God: A Study of Pondok Pesantren Khusus Waria Senin-Kamis in Yogyakarta'. Southeast Asian Studies, National University of Singapore.

Thabrany, H. 2008. 'Politics of National Health Insurance of Indonesia: A New Era of Universal Coverage'. European Conference on Health Economics, Rome, 23–26/7/2008.

Thomsen, S., M. Stalker and C. Toroitich-Ruto. 2004. 'Fifty Ways to Leave Your Rubber: How Men in Mombasa Rationalise Unsafe Sex'. *Sex Transm Infect* 80, no. 6: 430–434.

United Nations. 2000. 'United Nations Millennium Declaration'. General Assembly, 08/09/2000.

United Nations. 2014. *The Millenium Development Goals Report*. New York: United Nations Press.

United Nations Programme on HIV/AIDS. 2004. *Report on the Global AIDS epidemic. 4th global report*. Geneva: UNAIDS.

United Nations Programme on HIV/AIDS. 2012. *Republic of Indonesia: Country report on the Follow up to the Declaration of Commitment on HIV/AIDS (UNGASS)*. Reporting period 2011–2012. Indonesian National AIDS Commission. Geneva: UNAIDS.

Valentine, David. 2007. *Imagining Transgender: An Ethnography of a Category*. Duke: Duke University Press.

van de Pas, Remco. 2016. 'Global Health in the Anthropocene: Moving beyond Resilience and Capitalism Comment on "Health Promotion in an Age of Normative Equity and Rampant Inequality"'. *International Journal of Health Policy and Management* 6, no. 8: 481–486.

Warner, J. and J. Gabe. 2004. 'Risk and Liminality in Mental Health Social Work'. *Health, Risk & Society* 6, no. 4: 387–399.

Winter, Sam, Milton Diamond, Jamison Green, Dan Karasic, Terry Reed, Stephen Whittle and Kevan Wylie. 2016. 'Transgender People: Health at the Margins of Society'. *The Lancet* 388, no. 10042: 390–400.

Wuijts, S., H. H. van den Berg, J. Miller, L. Abebe, M. Sobsey, A. Andremont, K. O. Medlicott, M. W. van Passel and A. M. de Roda Husman. 2017. 'Towards a Research Agenda for Water, Sanitation and Antimicrobial Resistance'. *Journal of Water and Health* 15, no. 2: 175–184.

Chapter 4

'I Cannot Know That Now I Have Cancer!': A Structural Violence Perspective on Breast Cancer Detection in Uganda

Deborah Ikhile, Linda Gibson and Azrini Wahidin

> Before my aunt died, I looked at her breast then she told me, 'I have breast cancer'. She told me this after going to the hospital before being admitted. She told me, 'I have breast cancer, but I don't know what I am going to do'. That time I was young, that time has been long. I was young I didn't know anything about it because when she told me, she told me 'I'm not going to die of any other disease but only breast cancer'. I told her 'don't worry we will go to Mulago'. We went to Mulago and there they checked her; they examined her and told her the cancer was all over her body. She told me 'look at my breast'. Her breasts were like yellow, she was dark skinned, but her breasts were yellow inside them because they were infected. They all had swollen things, they were very big that she could not even wear these bras. Whenever she looked at them, she was like 'aha aha these are not my breasts'. (Alice, focus group discussion, 16 April 2015)

Alice[1] is a peer educator in Kajjansi town council who lost her aunt to breast cancer. Alice's narrative provides an insight into the lived experiences of breast cancer and how they are socially constructed in Uganda. Alice's description of her aunt's advanced breast cancer is not uncommon as breast cancer among women in Uganda is mostly diagnosed at advanced stages – usually stages III or IV, when the cancer has spread from the breasts to other organs of the body (Grady 2013),[2] consequently reducing their chances of survival.

    The above narrative draws on a primary case study conducted by Deborah Ikhile[3] in 2015, investigating the barriers to early detection of breast cancer in Ssisa sub-county, now Kajjansi town council, Uganda (Ilaboya 2015). Kajjansi town council is a semi-rural area in Wakiso district located within the central part of Uganda. Although the district is engulfed within what is known as greater Kampala, there is a huge discrepancy between rural settings like Kajjansi town council and the capital city Kampala. The focus in the original case study was to investigate why breast cancer is detected late. Like other sub-Saharan African (SSA) countries, in Uganda, most women present at health facilities when the cancer has reached an advanced stage (Ilaboya, Gibson and Musoke 2018, 1–10). The aim of the study was to understand the perceptions of women in Kajjansi town council and other key informants as to the reasons for late detection, presentation and, consequently, late diagnosis.

This chapter explores the findings from that research, using a structural violence perspective. By applying a structural violence lens, we seek to provide a deeper understanding and analysis of global health and development landscapes within the context of breast cancer detection for women in Uganda. We argue that late detection of breast cancer is embedded within structural drivers of health at local, national and global levels. These structural drivers disadvantage women and, in turn, hinder their ability to detect breast cancer early. We also suggest that the social construction of breast cancer as an individual and subjective experience can also be a form of structural violence. This is because the social construction of breast cancer perpetuates a victim-blaming narrative, which relies on women's individual compliance to breast cancer detection measures, rather than emphasizing the need for supportive social and political structures that would enable women to detect breast cancer early.

The chapter begins by providing a general context of global and national trends in breast cancer and breast cancer detection. It then offers an explanation as to the application and conceptualisation of structural violence from a global health and development perspective. We follow with the study's methodology and an analysis of the barriers that women face when seeking early detection of breast cancer. We present these barriers by first describing the landscape of breast cancer detection and then exploring the underlying drivers of the existing landscape, using structural violence as an analytical lens. The chapter concludes by recommending approaches to address structural violence in relation to breast cancer detection in women. Our recommendations include taking a health promotion approach and arguing for gender responsive policies.

BACKGROUND

The global epidemiological transition from infectious (communicable) diseases, which dominated the nineteenth century, to non-communicable diseases (NCDs) (Cockerham 2007) such as cancer, cardiovascular diseases and diabetes is well recognised in the global health community (Allen and Feigl

2017, e129–e130). The implication of this transition is that countries like Uganda now grapple with what is increasingly known as the double burden of communicable (e.g. HIV/AIDs) and NCDs (e.g. breast cancer) (Agyei-Mensah and Aikins 2010, 879–897). Although breast cancer is a global public health issue which poses individual, societal and economic burdens (Boyle and Howell 2010, S7), its impact is not equally felt because of higher mortality associated with breast cancer in SSA women. Unequal mortality rates, in turn, indicate that socioeconomic and racial/ethnic disparities exist in relation to breast cancer mortality.

The most recent global estimates for cancer reveal that, in 2018, breast cancer incidence[4] among women in Africa was approximately 168,690 with associated 74,072 deaths (Global Cancer Observatory n.d.). These numbers are likely to be an underestimation, as the region lacks adequate systems for reporting breast cancer cases (Brinton et al. 2014, 467–478). That said, these figures indicate a high rate of mortality (approximately 50%) from breast cancer compared to regions like Europe and North America, where breast cancer mortality rates are approximately 26 per cent and 18 per cent, respectively[5] (Global Cancer Observatory n.d.). This high rate of mortality is attributed to a number of factors, including, but not limited to late detection, poor infrastructure, insufficient funding and low knowledge of breast cancer detection measures particularly among women and health providers in rural settings (Brinton et al. 2014, 467–478; Ilaboya 2015).

Early detection and diagnosis of breast cancer followed by prompt treatment increases the chances of survival, as it ensures that the disease is identified and treated early before it becomes advanced and incurable (World Health Organization 2007). Common measures for detecting breast cancer include breast self-examination (BSE), clinical breast examination (CBE) and ultrasound and mammography screening (Yip et al. 2008, 2244–2256). The effectiveness and significance of some of these measures for early detection for breast cancer are, however, fraught with myriad contentions.[6] For instance, in 1991, UK Chief Medical Officer Sir Donald Acheson announced that BSE was ineffective and could give a false sense of security to women (Austoker 2003, 1–2). It is now discredited as an effective early detection measure in countries of the global north, and the American Cancer Society no longer recommends BSE or CBE as adequate means for early detection (American Cancer Society 2015). Instead, breast awareness, that is, familiarity with one's breasts as well as alertness to the signs and symptoms of breast cancer, is being encouraged among women (ibid.). Conversely, while mammography screening is regarded as the 'gold standard' for breast cancer detection, Corbex, Burton and Sancho-Garnier (2012, 428–434) consider it ineffective for low resource settings. It is at best contentious elsewhere as well (see Gøetzsche 2012).

Despite these debates, early detection remains the cornerstone of breast cancer control (Anderson et al. 2008, 2221–2243) especially in low resource countries like Uganda. The breast cancer detection services that we referred to during the research include breast awareness, BSE and CBE. A discussion of the reasons why these methods continue to form the basis for breast cancer control in low resource settings is outside of the scope of this chapter. Nevertheless, it is important to note that these are the low-cost measures recommended by the WHO (World Health Organization 2017) and the Breast Health Global Initiative (Yip et al. 2008, 2244–2256) for early detection in primary health care in such settings.

STUDY METHODOLOGY

The methodology for this study was qualitative in nature and underpinned by a social constructionist philosophy, that is, the study was conducted with an assumption that realities are socially constructed. Therefore, the accounts provided in this chapter do not claim to paint the complete picture of breast cancer detection in Kajjansi community. Instead, they represent the context-specific and compelling voices of women, which are often neglected in research as well as global health policies (see Harman, this volume).

Ilaboya (2015) conducted five semi-structured interviews with women; two focus groups with women's groups; and seven semi-structured interviews with selected key informants from the Ministry of Health, Uganda Cancer Institute, Makerere University and Uganda Women's Cancer Support Organisation. The use of multiple qualitative methods enabled triangulation of the data and enhanced credibility (Baum 2008) of the study. While the numbers of interviews were small, this was the first piece of research undertaken in Uganda to explore the issue of barriers to breast cancer detection. Participants were purposively sampled based on the following criteria: being a woman; no known history of breast cancer (as the focus of the study was on perceptions of the general population around breast cancer detection); known professional or researcher in cancer-related fields.

For the analysis of data from the original research, Ilaboya (2015) carried out thematic analysis of the data through manual coding. The process of thematic analysis used followed three steps as adapted from Bazeley (2013), including transcription, familiarisation with the data and coding/identification of themes. Ilaboya then synthesised the identified themes and underscored them by verbatim extracts from participants' responses. The key findings from the study were that barriers to early detection of breast cancer operate at individual, community, organisational and policy levels (Ilaboya 2015; Ilaboya, Gibson and Musoke 2018).

Individual level barriers that emerged from the study were mostly associated with knowledge, attitudes, practices and beliefs. Lack of awareness and limited knowledge were prominent and closely linked to fear and fatalism. At the community level, poverty and transportation obstacles were identified as the main barriers. The organisational level mostly centred on health system constraints and competing healthcare burdens in the country. In terms of cancer facilities, the cancer unit at Mulago was the only national referral facility for cancer care. Primary health centres around Kajjansi town council were reported to be ill-equipped as they do not provide breast cancer services. At the policy level, absence of guiding national cancer policy was identified as the major barrier.

In this chapter, we discuss the findings from Ilaboya's study from a structural violence perspective. The focus of our analysis takes a double-layered approach: the first layer centres around the landscape and individual barriers to breast cancer detection. Using structural violence as analytical lens, the second layer of analysis provides an understanding of the underlying structural drivers that hinder early breast cancer detection among women in Uganda. Underpinning the argument throughout the chapter is a critical analysis of how structural violence manifests itself, barring women's access to breast cancer detection services in Uganda.

STRUCTURAL VIOLENCE, GLOBAL HEALTH AND DEVELOPMENT

As all the chapters in this volume show, gendered violence in global health can take varying forms including physical, sexual, emotional, verbal, symbolic, epistemic, cognitive, visual, representational and structural forms. Our focus is on the structural form of violence (see also Nuño; Tanyag; Reuterswärd; Finley; Vaittinen; Harman, in this volume). We recognise that the health systems in most low resource settings do not allow women any choice or opportunity to detect breast cancer earlier (Ilaboya, Gibson and Musoke 2018), despite the acknowledgement that early detection is an integral component of breast cancer control in these settings. Drawing on Galtung's (1969, 167–191) work on structural violence (see Confortini and Vaittinen, this volume; also Reuterswärd, this volume), Paul Farmer introduced the concept of structural violence in global health and development in 2005. In Farmer's (2005) conceptualisation, the structural violence of denied opportunities, economic deprivation, colonialism, violent despots (and the powers supporting them) and international financial organisations harm the health of billions of people who are so distant that they are glibly and uncomprehendingly referred to as living in a 'third world'. In a later publication, Farmer et al. (2006, e449) define structural violence as:

> social arrangements that put individuals and populations in harm's way. The arrangements are structural because they are embedded in the political and economic organization of our social world; they are violent because they cause injury to people (typically, not those responsible for perpetuating such inequalities).

Farmer's anthropological work has been influential in documenting the narratives and stories of people living in poverty and suffering ill health and the structural determinants that keep them poor. Farmer's use of the concept has been critiqued for being largely descriptive (Stephens 2005), as well as – more recently – for being out of date and poorly theorised (Hirschfeld 2017, 156–162). Nevertheless, Farmer's work has contributed to an emerging social model to analyse global health and development issues (see also Harman, this volume). Moreover, several public health scholars have subsequently used the concept to analyse structural violence in mental health nursing (Choiniere et al. 2014, 39–50); patients with sickle cell disease (Bahr and Song 2015, 648–661); HIV in South Africa (Mills 2016, 85–95); and ebola in Sierra Leone (Wilkinson and Leach 2015, 136–148), for example.

With the exception of Mills (2016) – who provides an ethnographic account of HIV in women's bodies and lives, highlighting the intersection between structural and interpersonal violence – what is lacking in these previous publications are the gendered and feminist aspects of structural violence. Other work (e.g. Wilkinson and Leach 2015) lacks a critical exploration of the structural dimensions of health. Our chapter aims to critically investigate these dimensions of global health discourse, particularly around a gendered NCD – breast cancer. In the following section, we analyse the barriers to breast cancer detection as follows: first, we describe the landscape of breast cancer detection as perceived by the women who participated in the study; we then use the concept of structural violence as an analytical tool, to better understand the underlying factors that shape this landscape.

BARRIERS TO BREAST CANCER DETECTION IN KAJJANSI TOWN COUNCIL

In her previous research, Ilaboya (2015) has established that the existing landscape of breast cancer among women in Kajjansi town council is characterised by limited knowledge, anxiety and fear. While some of the women in this study had heard of breast cancer, none of them knew how to detect it. In addition, awareness of the risk factors,[7] signs and symptoms of breast cancer was generally low among the women who participated in the study. The perceptions of the women in relation to knowledge are summarised in figure 4.1.

These quotes (figure 4.1) represent the questions asked and narratives of the women in Kajjansi town council who participated in the study. The quotes show how some of the women perceive breast cancer as a disease that springs up on them with no control over it. The women expressed helplessness towards their inability to detect breast cancer.

Another key individual finding was that women were extremely fearful. Their fear was manifested in five different ways – fear of death, fear of losing the breast, fear of stigma, fear of big hospitals (e.g. the Uganda Cancer Institute) and fear of the unknown. During the focus group discussions, when asked what might prevent a woman from detecting breast cancer, one of the women stated that: 'Some women, they fear the disease [so much that] they can't even check their breast . . . they fear to know those things about cancer . . . they fear to die' (Beatrice, focus group discussion, 16 April 2015). The other women in the focus group discussion nodded in agreement that fear was indeed a key challenge.

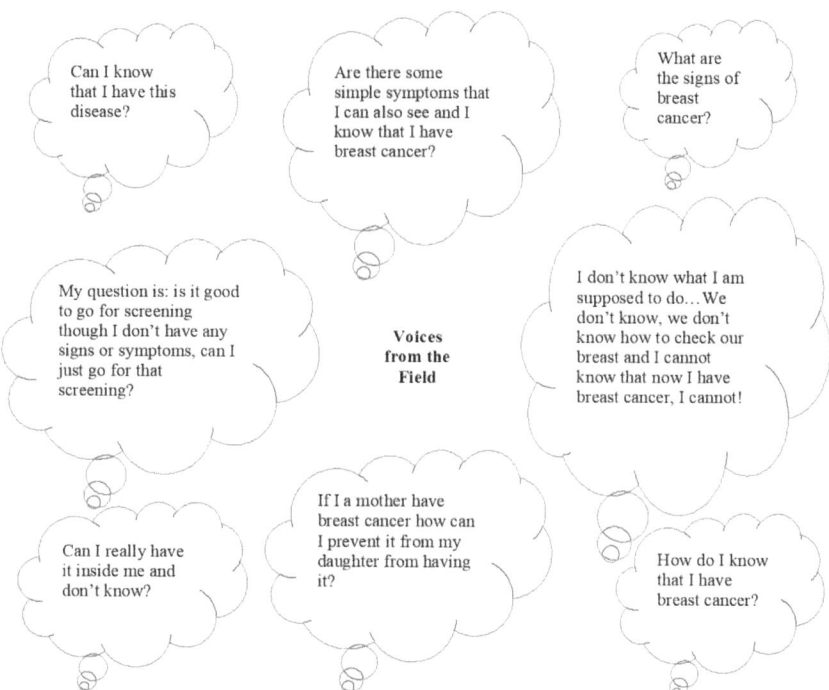

Figure 4.1. Voices of women from the field around low knowledge of breast cancer

However, it is somewhat myopic to simply state that women are not knowledgeable about breast cancer, or that they fear the disease. Doing so only draws attention to what happens on the surface, without paying adequate attention to the structural drivers around the challenges that women face around breast cancer detection. In the following section, we turn to analyse these through the lens of structural violence.

Structural Violence and Breast Cancer Detection

Using a structural violence lens, our second layer of analysis provides understanding on how structures and institutions engender inequity around access to breast cancer detection services. The existing reality of women in relation to access to breast cancer detection services in Kajjansi town council is perpetuated by structural violence. Structural violence can, in this context, be regarded as an indirect form of violence exhibited at global, national and local levels. As elaborated further, our analysis of the interviews and focus group discussions conducted further indicate that structural violence is manifested at three levels:

1. Local level – primary healthcare system infrastructure;
2. National level – lack of prioritisation and political will for breast cancer and
3. Global level – global health governance and influence of international donors.

Poor Primary Healthcare Infrastructure

At the local level, the most prominent health system barrier is poor primary healthcare infrastructure. The study participants indicated that health centres in Kajjansi town council were ill-equipped to detect breast cancer, consequently resulting in late detection and late diagnosis. This is because the three government-funded health centres in Kajjansi focus mostly on communicable diseases, and as such lack capacity for providing breast cancer services.[8] The consequence of the health centres' focus on communicable diseases is that women within the community who may have signs and symptoms of breast cancer do not get diagnosed early. Such women have to travel far distances to the national referral facility – Uganda Cancer Institute in Kampala (the capital city) – to be screened for breast cancer, and progress to breast cancer treatment in cases where the diagnosis for breast cancer is positive.

Travelling to Kampala for breast cancer screening has its own challenges. Not only are the roads in poor condition but travelling from Kajjansi to the Uganda Cancer Institute costs about 20,000 Uganda shillings (approximately

USD 5). Generally, individuals living is Kajjansi have to walk to a main road or board a *boda boda*[9] to where they can board public transportation to Kampala. This health system challenge was not only reported by the women but also acknowledged by key informants, who stated that

> the biggest problem [around early detection of breast cancer] is lack of awareness but also beyond lack of awareness the current [primary] health facilities in this country are not very prepared to provide the services needed at least for detection. (Ben, Key Informant, Semi-structured interview, 15 April 2015)

> If a girl or woman has breast cancer it will not be detected early enough because of the health system challenge. Personally, I've always felt bad when I'm telling the patient that they presented late because what did I do to help them present early? What have we done? What has the [health] system done to help them present early? (Juliet, Key Informant, Semi-structured interview, 15 April 2015)

Although private hospitals were identified by the research participants as being able to provide general breast cancer detection services, women have to pay to access these services. This in itself is problematic as a majority of these women and their households rely on subsistence farming as their major source of income (Uganda Bureau of Statistics 2016). Although exact costs were not provided, a recent publication by Novartis (n.d.) showed that the cost for a clinical breast examination in a private hospital in northern Uganda cost 25,000 Uganda Shillings (approximately USD 7). This cost is high for a woman living in Uganda, where the median monthly income for households involved in agriculture is 150,000 Uganda Shillings (approximately USD 40) (Uganda Bureau of Statistics 2018).

Low Prioritisation for Breast Cancer Intervention

At the national level, structural violence around early detection of breast cancer is manifested through low prioritisation of breast cancer on the national health agenda. This was highlighted during the study by a key informant, who stated:

> I don't think there's been a breast cancer screening or awareness campaign done in rural parts of Uganda because there are more pressing issues like WASH [Water, Sanitation and Hygiene] ... in those rural areas .... I think that's one of the major problems as to why there are not very many campaigns done in the country generally.... We are focusing more on the common diseases – malaria, cholera, typhoid. We don't focus on breast cancer. So, people don't know about breast cancer, there are more important diseases we are fighting with ... it is just of recent that we are seeing noncommunicable disease cases increasing but it has been majority communicable diseases. The focus has been there that's

why you see that very many people in the villages now even have mosquito nets freely and we just have only one mammography machine, yet the cases of breast cancer are on the rise. (Caroline, Key Informant, Semi-structured interview, 21 April 2015)

The prioritisation of breast cancer could be contested, as it is often argued that SSA countries such as Uganda still suffer from a wide range of communicable diseases such as HIV/AIDS, malaria and diarrheal diseases, for example, and so do not have the resources to deal with the rising burden of breast cancer and other NCDs. In the case of breast cancer in Uganda, access to early detection services for breast cancer is not a priority in a health system that is overwhelmed by and structured to respond to the burden of communicable diseases.

Although Uganda has an NCD unit, at the time of the research in 2015, there was no guiding national policy for cancer. The 2010 Uganda Health Policy and the Health Sector Strategic Plan III 2010/11–2014/15 – the national health policy documents developed to guide the strategic focus for the health sector – identify cancer as a health issue. However, they make no reference to breast cancer and do not articulate set guidelines for cancer management. The lack of a national cancer policy to provide national guidance across the continuum of cancer care reflects a lack of political commitment. It also fails to follow the WHO's requirement for its member countries to put in place a national cancer control plan (see World Health Organization 2002, 2005), in order to provide strategic guidance on how each country would tackle the growing burden of cancer.

On the other hand, the country cannot be solely held responsible for not prioritising cancer, as health priorities are steered by international agencies. One of the biggest challenges of political action and prioritisation in the health sector is funding (Glassman et al. 2012, 13–34). As shown in the next section, health in Uganda is still largely donor-driven. This creates a state of affairs whereby funding commitments are not necessarily matched to health system strengthening, but instead respond to a set of health agendas set by international funding organisations (cf. Nuño, this volume). Consequently, this hampers early and long-term investment to build strong, comprehensive and resilient health systems at primary care levels.

Global Health Governance and Influence of International Donors

Structural violence at the global governance level is manifested through international donors and funding bodies, which directly or indirectly drive health priorities in most SSA countries and other developing regions of the world. This is not specific to breast cancer but seen in other diseases as well. For example, Whyte et al. (2013, 140–166), while focusing on HIV/AIDS care in Uganda, demonstrate the reliance of the Ugandan health system on international aid projects, 'the projectified landscape of care' (Whyte et al. 2013, 140). In countries such as Uganda, NGOs compete for funding for health projects in order to gain access to resources, materials and identity to provide care as partners of the state. Priorities in terms of the provision of resources are then shaped by political interests and contestations over which NGO projects should be supported, and this, in turn, shapes the landscape of care. Consequently, the healthcare system is based around funding priorities and not necessarily driven by community needs. The influence of international donors was also highlighted by one of Ilaboya's study's key informants who stated that 'in most of these low-income countries, healthcare tends to be driven by the donor community so much' (John, Key Informant, Semi-structured interview, 13 April 2015).

Another area through which structural violence is manifested at global governance level is through a focus on treatment research and facilities. This was indicated by one of the study participants who stated that 'these funding bodies focus on funding individuals maybe who have been identified as suffering from breast cancer, so they don't exactly focus on creating awareness that much. . . . That's why we are seeing these women may not know about breast cancer' (Caroline, Key Informant, Semi-structured interview, 21 April 2015).

While it is well known that early detection followed by prompt treatment increases chances of survival, focus on treatment only without investing in early detection strategies indicates a reactive stance. Traditionally, global responses to health challenges have been more often reactive efforts, whereby international organisations coordinate themselves and draw up action plans after an outbreak has occurred – as in the case of ebola, for instance (Wilkinson and Leach 2015, 136–148). The implication of this reactive stance is that national health systems are not supported to be comprehensive, as international funders focus on specific health programmes (ibid.) rather than comprehensive disease programmes. Although focus on treatment is important for breast cancer, treatment alone will not reduce the number of breast cancer cases diagnosed at advanced stages.

As shown in figure 4.2, the existing reality and perceptions of women around breast cancer in Kajjansi are driven by external factors, including poor primary healthcare infrastructure, national policies and global governance. These different levels construct the realities of women in Kajjansi town council around breast cancer detection. Our analysis of the case of breast cancer detection in Uganda demonstrates how configurations of structural violence can filter through the wider determinants of health. Women, in this case, are deterred or hindered from accessing healthcare services early, largely

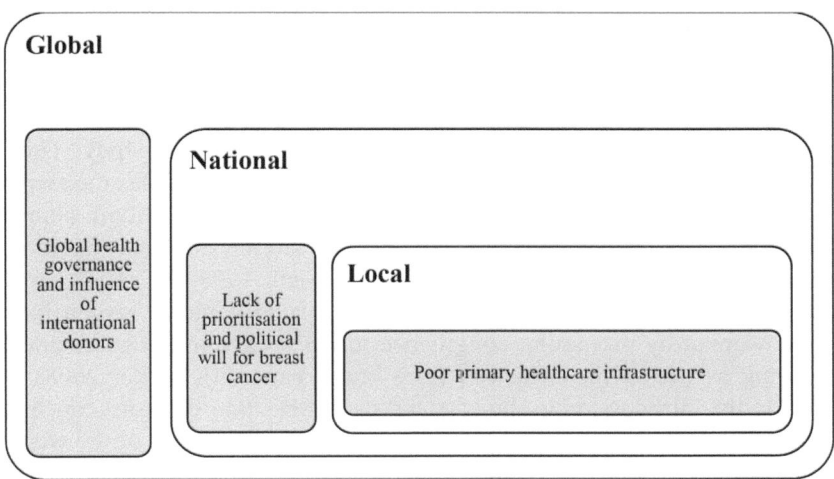

Figure 4.2. Illustration of structural violence analysis of barriers to breast cancer detection

because they fear breast cancer and are unaware about how it can be detected or treated. Women are unaware and fear breast cancer because breast cancer detection services are not available at primary healthcare level, making the services beyond women's reach financially and geographically. Breast cancer services are unavailable at primary healthcare level due to low prioritisation of the disease at the national level. Finally, national health priorities are largely driven by global health governance and international funding architecture, which do not adequately support the creation and strengthening of comprehensive cancer programmes.

In sum, the configuration and framing of the existing health infrastructure, low political will and the global health governance system exert a form of violence that serves to prohibit/deter women from detecting breast cancer early. Past studies on the barriers of breast cancer detection have generally focused on individuals (e.g. Mittra 2011, 121–122; Robb et al. 2014, 1–6), that is, the manifestation of fear and low knowledge among women. Our analysis in this chapter takes a step further and recognises the influence of more powerful structural drivers, which are commonly referred to as the structural determinants of health in contemporary global health discourse.

The need to recognise the wider determinants of health has been consistently made over the past twenty years (World Health Organization 2008), with an emerging call for social scientists to contribute critical theoretical insights (Kickbusch 2012, 5–7). The recognition of these structural determinants was clearly articulated in the influential WHO Commission on the

Social Determinants of Health Report in 2008. This report has been lauded for its recognition that health is socially constructed (Navarro 2009, 5–16).

However, the social construction of health can still be a form of structural violence, when the focus is solely on the experiential level – as was the common perception/narrative among the participants of our study. This is because presenting breast cancer as an individual problem places the responsibility for breast cancer care on individuals, perpetuating a victim blaming culture that holds the woman as the culprit for late breast cancer detection, or even breast cancer incidence (Lantz and Booth 1998, 907–918). In the case of breast cancer detection, this culture places a moral responsibility on the woman by promoting compliance to BSE, CBE and mammography screening as life-saving measures from breast cancer (Klawiter 2008). As stated in the introduction to this chapter, early detection of breast cancer on its own is ineffective and does not automatically save the life of the woman unless prompt diagnostic, treatment and support services are in place. Therefore, there is a need for a concerted effort, which does not only focus on the woman but seeks to address the different levels through which structural violence manifests itself.

ADDRESSING STRUCTURAL VIOLENCE IN BREAST CANCER DETECTION

To address structural violence in breast cancer detection, we recommend a combination of global social action, health promotion and gender responsive policies. Community social action has been a key approach for grass-root, bottom-up approach to health, especially as seen in the case of HIV/AIDS global social action. Historically, the AIDS activism model, which drew on patient representation and empowerment (Wachter 1992, 128–133; see also Oinas, this volume), was instrumental in creating a platform for women's voices and securing funding for breast cancer in the United States (Lantz and Booth 1998, 907–918). Similarly, breast cancer control in the global north has been predominantly driven by feminist activists and breast cancer advocacy campaigns. These actions were at the forefront of grounding scientific research, community awareness and progress into breast cancer treatments, and have been successful in driving breast health agenda in the United States (Klawiter 2008). A well-known example is, for instance, RavenLight's bold display of her one-breastedness, while marching in the 1993 San Francisco Lesbian-Gay-Bisexual-Transgender Pride Parade (Klawiter 2008). While breast cancer can now be publicly and openly discussed in this part of the world, it remains a subject of taboo still fraught with fear in places like Kajjansi.

Nevertheless, Uganda has also recognised success in using health promotion strategies to deal with infectious disease outbreaks through the use of community engagement strategies (Nyamwaya 2003, 85–87), what Beattie has called the collective negotiated approach (Beattie 1991, 162–172). In the case of Uganda, this approach garnered international attention from donors to increase resources to facilitate prevention, treatment and care for people living with HIV/AIDS (Smith and Whiteside 2010, 1–8). However, what is missing from Uganda's health promotion response to HIV/AIDS is a gender perspective (see Harman 2011). Although, there is a recognition of gender in the Uganda National Strategic HIV/AIDS Plan, this recognition does not necessarily translate to better outcomes especially as the strategic plan was identified to be inadequate in articulating how the gender perspective can be achieved (Harman 2011, 213–228).

Therefore, there is a need for gender responsive policies in order to address the vulnerabilities found in women, and also challenge the structures that maintain those vulnerabilities (World Health Organization 2010). The value of implementing gender responsive policies in breast cancer care is that not only would services be made available for breast cancer control but women would also be encouraged to access and use the services, which, in turn, would prevent women from dying if early detection and early diagnosis occurs.

NEW DIRECTIONS FOR GLOBAL HEALTH AND CANCER?

To conclude, this chapter has provided critical insights of how structural violence is rooted at various institutional levels and operates as a diverse set of policies and practices that shapes and influences the experiences of women, in relation to access to breast cancer detection services in Kajjansi town council. The chapter has shown that the challenges around breast cancer detection are manifested at the individual level as indicated by low knowledge of the women around breast cancer detection and fear of breast cancer. However, these individual factors are driven by underlying macro- level drivers of structural violence which are created at global, national and local levels.

Therefore, we argue for an approach by the global community that recognises the value of community action and a health promotion approach that ensures public policies around breast cancer control are gender responsive and fit for context and purpose. We would also suggest the concept of structural violence needs to be fully theorised in the global health field, particularly in order to understand gendered power relations at the local, national and global level. This is not just a question of theoretical analysis, but the reduction and elimination of gendered structural violence requires a more robust public policy response. In order to understand women's experiences of the lack of access to breast cancer care in Uganda, one needs to understand why there is a lack of political will and governance frameworks to invest in breast cancer care and how services can be made more accessible.

NOTES

1. Pseudonyms used for anonymity and confidentiality.
2. At stage III, breast cancer has spread beyond the breast and into lymph nodes and muscles. Metastasis (stage IV) happens when the cancer has spread to distant parts of the body (e.g., the brain, bones, lung and liver).
3. The study was independently conducted by Deborah Ikhile (in 2015, Deborah Ilaboya). However, access to the study site in Uganda was provided through the institutional Partnership between Nottingham Trent University School of Social Sciences, UK, and Makerere University School of Public Health, Uganda. The findings from the study have been previously presented entirely as part of Deborah Ikhile's master's dissertation (Ilaboya 2015) and recently published in *Globalization and Health* (Ilaboya, Gibson and Musoke 2018).
4. Breast cancer incidence refers to the number of new breast cancer cases occurring within a population in a specified period. It is presented either as an absolute number of cases per annum or as a rate per 100,000 persons per annum (Bray et al. 2018). The figure presented for breast cancer incidence in this chapter is an absolute number of estimated breast cancer cases in 2018.
5. Breast cancer incidences for these regions are higher than in SSA. From the 2018 global cancer statistics, the European and North American regions had breast cancer incidence of approximately 522,513 and 262,347, respectively.
6. It has to be noted that early detection is itself an ambiguous concept (Panieri 2012, 283–290). Often referred to as secondary prevention (Kolak et al. 2017, 549–553), it is not prevention at all, but rather the identification of the disease before it spreads beyond the breasts.
7. Breast cancer does not have definitive causes, so its occurrence is associated with risk factors. However, there is a critical literature around the concept of risk in relation to breast cancer. See Klawiter (2008) chapter 3 which discusses the biopolitics of breast cancer and the repositioning of seemingly healthy women within the population as risky subjects.
8. Data from ongoing doctoral study by Ikhile.
9. *Boda boda* refers to a motorcycle.

REFERENCES

Agyei-Mensah, Samuel and Ama de-Graft Aikins. 2010. 'Epidemiological Transition and the Double Burden of Disease in Accra, Ghana'. *Journal of Urban Health* 87, no. 5: 879–897.

Allen, Luke N. and A. B. Feigl. 2017. 'What's in a Name? A Call to Reframe Non-Communicable Diseases'. *The Lancet Global Health* 5, no. 2: e129–e130.

American Cancer Society. 2015. 'American Cancer Society Releases New Breast Cancer Guidelines'. https://www.cancer.org/latest-news/american-cancer-society-releases-new-breast-cancer-guidelines.html. Accessed 7 September 2019.

Anderson, Benjamin O., Cheng-Har Yip, Robert A. Smith, Roman Shyyan, Stephen F. Sener, Alexandru Eniu, Robert W. Carlson, Edward Azavedo and Joe Harford. 2008. 'Guideline Implementation for Breast Healthcare in Low-Income and Middle-Income Countries: Overview of the Breast Health Global Initiative Global Summit 2007'. *Cancer* 113, no. 8: 2221–2243.

Austoker, Joan. 2003. 'Breast Self Examination: Does Not Prevent Deaths Due to Breast Cancer, But Breast Awareness Is Still Important'. *BMJ: British Medical Journal* 326, no. 7379: 1–2.

Bahr, Nathan C. and John Song. 2015. 'The Effect of Structural Violence on Patients with Sickle Cell Disease'. *Journal of Health Care for the Poor and Underserved* 26, no. 3: 648–661.

Baum, Frances. 2008. *The New Public Health*. 3rd ed. Oxford: Oxford University Press.

Bazeley, Patricia. 2013. *Qualitative Data Analysis: Practical Strategies*. London: SAGE.

Beattie, A. 1991. 'Knowledge and Control in Health Promotion: A Test Case for Social Policy and Social Theory'. In *The Sociology of Health Service*, edited by J. Gabe, 162–172. London: Routledge.

Boyle, Peter and Antony Howell. 2010. 'The Globalisation of Breast Cancer'. *Breast Cancer Research* 12, no. 4: S7.

Bray, Freddie, Ferlay Jacques, Soerjomataram Isabelle, Siegel Rebecca, Torre Lindsey and Jemal Ahmedin. 2018. 'Global Cancer Statistics 2018: GLOBOCAN Estimates of Incidence and Mortality Worldwide for 36 Cancers in 185 Countries'. *CA Cancer Journal for Clinicians* 68, no. 6: 394–424.

Brinton, Louise A., Jonine D. Figueroa, Baffour Awuah, Joel Yarney, Seth Wiafe, Shannon N. Wood, Daniel Ansong, Kofi Nyarko, Beatrice Wiafe-Addai and Joe Nat Clegg-Lamptey. 2014. 'Breast Cancer in Sub-Saharan Africa: Opportunities for Prevention'. *Breast Cancer Research and Treatment* 144, no. 3: 467–478.

Choiniere, Jacqueline A., Judith A. MacDonnell, Andrea L. Campbell and Sandra Smele. 2014. 'Conceptualizing Structural Violence in the Context of Mental Health Nursing'. *Nursing Inquiry* 21, no. 1: 39–50.

Cockerham, William C. 2007. *Social Causes of Health and Disease*. Cambridge, UK: Polity.

Confortini, Catia C. and Tiina Vaittinen. 2019. 'Introduction: Analysing Violences in Gendered Global Health'. In *Gender, Global Health and Violence: Feminist Perspectives on Peace and Disease*, edited by Tiina Vaittinen and Catia Confortini. London and New York: Rowman & Littlefield.

Corbex, Marilys, Robert Burton and Hélène Sancho-Garnier. 2012. 'Breast Cancer Early Detection Methods for Low and Middle Income Countries, a Review of the Evidence'. *The Breast* 21, no. 4: 428–434.

Farmer, Paul. 2005. *Pathologies of Power: Health, Human Rights, and the New War on the Poor*. Berkeley: University of California Press.

Farmer, Paul E., Bruce Nizeye, Sara Stulac and Salmaan Keshavjee. 2006. 'Structural Violence and Clinical Medicine'. *PLoS Medicine* 3, no. 10: e449.

Finley, Laura. 2019. 'Domestic Violence and Public Health: Beginning Steps for Creating More Just and Effective Community Responses'. In *Gender, Global Health and Violence: Feminist Perspectives on Peace and Disease*, edited by Tiina Vaittinen and Catia Confortini. London and New York: Rowman & Littlefield.

Galtung, Johan. 1969. 'Violence, Peace, and Peace Research'. *Journal of Peace Research* 6, no. 3: 167–191.

Glassman, Amanda, Kalipso Chalkidou, Ursula Giedion, Yot Teerawattananon, Sean Tunis, Jesse B. Bump and Andres Pichon-Riviere. 2012. 'Priority-Setting Institutions in Health: Recommendations from a Center for Global Development Working Group'. *Global Heart* 7, no. 1: 13–34.

Global Cancer Observatory. n.d. 'Cancer Today'. Accessed 12 December 2018. http://gco.iarc.fr/today/home. Accessed 7 September 2019.

Gøetzsche, Peter C. 2012. *Mammography Screening: Truth, Lies and Controversy*. London and New York: Radcliffe.

Grady, Denise. 2013. 'Uganda Fights Stigma and Poverty to Take on Breast Cancer'. *The New York Times*, 15 October 2013. https://www.nytimes.com/2013/10/16/health/uganda-fights-stigma-and-poverty-to-take-on-breast-cancer.html. Accessed 7 September 2019.

Harman, Sophie. 2011. 'The Dual Feminisation of HIV/AIDS'. *Globalizations* 8, no. 2: 213–228.

Harman, Sophie. 2019. 'Violence and the Paradox of Global Health'. In *Gender, Global Health and Violence: Feminist Perspectives on Peace and Disease*, edited by Tiina Vaittinen and Catia Confortini. London and New York: Rowman & Littlefield.

Hirschfeld, Katherine. 2017. 'Rethinking "Structural Violence"'. *Society* 54, no. 2: 156–162.

Ilaboya, Deborah Evho. 2015. *Investigating the Perceived Barriers to Early Detection of Breast Cancer in Central Uganda, Using a Multilevel Approach*. M.A. thesis. Nottingham Trent University.

Ilaboya, Deborah, Linda Gibson and David Musoke. 2018. 'Perceived Barriers to Early Detection of Breast Cancer in Wakiso District, Uganda Using a Socioecological Approach'. *Globalization and Health* 14, no. 9: 1–10.

Kickbusch, Ilona. 2012. '21st Century Determinants of Health and Wellbeing: A New Challenge for Health Promotion'. *Global Health Promotion* 19, no. 3: 5–7.

Klawiter, Maren. 2008. *The Biopolitics of Breast Cancer: Changing Cultures of Disease and Activism*. Minneapolis: University of Minnesota Press.

Kolak, Agnieszka, Marzena Kamińska, Katarzyna Sygit, Agnieszka Budny, Dariusz Surdyka, Bożena Kukiełka-Budny and Franciszek Burdan. 2017. 'Primary and Secondary Prevention of Breast Cancer'. *Annals of Agricultural and Environmental Medicine* 24, no. 4: 549–553.

Lantz, Paula M. and Karen M. Booth. 1998. 'The Social Construction of the Breast Cancer Epidemic'. *Social Science & Medicine* 46, no. 7: 907–918.

Mills, Elizabeth. 2016. '"When the Skies Fight": HIV, Violence and Pathways of Precarity in South Africa'. *Reproductive Health Matters* 24, no.47: 85–95.

Mittra, Indraneel. 2011. 'Breast Cancer Screening in Developing Countries'. *Preventive Medicine* 53, no. 3: 121–122.

Navarro, Vicente. 2009. 'What We Mean by Social Determinants of Health'. *Global Health Promotion* 16, no. 1: 05–16.

Novartis. n.d. 'Living with Breast Cancer in Uganda'. Accessed 7 June 2019. https://www.novartis.com/stories/access-healthcare/living-breast-cancer-uganda.

Nyamwaya, David. 2003. 'Health Promotion in Africa: Strategies, Players, Challenges and Prospects'. *Health Promotion International* 18, no. 2: 85–87.

Oinas, Elina. 2019. 'HIV Politics and Structural Violence: Access to Treatment and Knowledge'. In *Gender, Global Health and Violence: Feminist Perspectives on Peace and Disease*, edited by Tiina Vaittinen and Catia Confortini. London and New York: Rowman & Littlefield.

Panieri, Eugenio. 2012. 'Breast Cancer Screening in Developing Countries'. *Best Practice & Research Clinical Obstetrics & Gynaecology* 26, no. 2: 283–290.

Reuterswärd, Camilla. 2019. '¡Malas Madres, Malas Mujeres, Malas Todas! The Incarceration of Women for Abortion-Related Crimes in Mexico'. In *Gender, Global Health and Violence: Feminist Perspectives on Peace and Disease*, edited by Tiina Vaittinen and Catia Confortini. London and New York: Rowman & Littlefield.

Robb, Kathryn A., Simon Alice E., Miles A and Wardle Jane. 2014. 'Public Perceptions of Cancer: A Qualitative Study of the Balance of Positive and Negative Beliefs. *BMJ Open* 4, no. 7: 1–6.

Smith, Julia H. and Whiteside, A. 2010. 'The History of AIDS Exceptionalism'. *Journal of the International AIDS Society* 13, no. 47: 1–8.

Stephens, Carolyn. 2005. '*Pathologies of Power: Health, Human Rights and the New War on the Poor* Review of *Pathology of Power*, by Paul Farmer'. *International Journal of Epidemiology* 34, no. 3: 718.

Tanyag, Maria. 2019. 'Replenishing Bodies and the Political Economy of SRHR in Crisis and Emergencies'. In *Gender, Global Health and Violence: Feminist Perspectives on Peace and Disease*, edited by Tiina Vaittinen and Catia Confortini. London and New York: Rowman & Littlefield.

Uganda Bureau of Statistics. 2016. The National Population and Housing Census 2014 – Main Report. Kampala, Uganda. https://unstats.un.org/unsd/demographic/sources/census/wphc/Uganda/UGA-2016-05-23.pdf. Accessed 7 September 2019.

Uganda Bureau of Statistics. 2018. Uganda National Household Survey 2016/2017. Kampala, Uganda; Uganda Bureau of Statistics. https://www.ubos.org/onlinefiles/uploads/ubos/pdf%20documents/UNHS_VI_2017_Version_I_%2027th_September_2017.pdf. Accessed 7 September 2019.

Vaittinen, Tiina. 2019. 'Exposed to Violence While Caring: From Caring Self-Protection to Global Health as Conflict Transformation'. In *Gender, Global Health and Violence: Feminist Perspectives on Peace and Disease*, edited by Tiina Vaittinen and Catia Confortini. London and New York: Rowman & Littlefield.

Wachter Robert. 1992. 'AIDS, Activism, and the Politics of Health'. *New England Journal* 326, no. 2: 128–133.

Whyte, S. R., M. I. A. Whyte, L. Meinert, L. and J. Twebaze. 2013. 'Therapeutic Clientship: Belonging in Uganda's Projectified Landscape of AIDS Care'. In *When

People Come First: Critical Studies in Global Health, edited by J. Biehl and A. and Petryna, 140–166. Princeton, NJ: Princeton University Press.

Wilkinson, Annie and Melissa Leach. 2015. 'Briefing: Ebola – Myths, Realities, and Structural Violence'. *African Affairs* 114, no. 454: 136–148.

World Health Organization. 2002. *National Cancer Control Programmes: Policies and Managerial Guidelines*. Geneva: World Health Organization.

World Health Organization. 2005. *Resolution WHA58.22. Cancer Prevention and Control*. Fifty-Eighth World Health Assembly, Geneva, 16–25 May 2005. http://apps.who.int/medicinedocs/en/d/Js21323en/. Accessed 7 September 2019.

World Health Organization. 2007. *Cancer Control: Knowledge into Action. WHO Guide for Effective Programmes: Early Detection*. Geneva: World Health Organization.

World Health Organization. 2008. *Closing the Gap in a Generation: Health Equity through Action on the Social Determinants of Health: Commission on Social Determinants of Health Final Report*. Geneva: World Health Organization.

World Health Organization. 2010. *Gender, Women and Primary Health Care Renewal: A Discussion Paper*. Geneva: World Health Organization.

World Health Organization. 2017. *Guide to Cancer Early Diagnosis*. Geneva: World Health Organization.

Yip, Cheng-Har, Robert A. Smith, Benjamin O. Anderson, Anthony B. Miller, David B. Thomas, Eng-Suan Ang, Rosemary S. Caffarella, Marilys Corbex, Gary L. Kreps and Anne McTiernan. 2008. 'Guideline Implementation for Breast Healthcare in Low-and Middle-Income Countries'. *Cancer* 113, no. S8: 2244–2256.

Chapter 5

HIV Politics and Structural Violence: Access to Treatment and Knowledge[1]

Elina Oinas

'*Amandla*!', echoed the activist women's forceful outcry in one of the massive rallies against President Thabo Mbeki's HIV politics in South Africa on the streets of Cape Town in 2003, evoking the spirit of the anti-apartheid struggle. By shouting the well-known '*Amandla-awethu*' slogan, with their fists raised high in the air, the women connected their fight for medication to a long line of struggles about power: 'power', *amandla* in the Xhosa language, to *awethu*, 'the people', 'us'. The women marching on the streets made a case for HIV being political. Their message, underlining the connection between health, death, and politics, was radical at the time, when AIDS was seen as a result of personal sin or stupidity – reckless sex without condoms. A month later, the image of one of the women, Kebareng Moeketsi, was on one of the flyers used by the activists. Moeketsi died at the age of thirty-three, only a year before the medicines were made available through the public sector healthcare system in South Africa.

In the rallies and meetings of the early 2000s, the energy of the Treatment Action Campaign (TAC) movement was palpable and inspiring, yet the people were also seriously sick and dying, sometimes only weeks after attending a rally. Remarkably, despite the hundreds of deaths, there was a sense of victory around the movement. 'Mobilise and mourn!' was another important slogan derived from the anti-apartheid 'Don't Mourn! Mobilise!'. This reformulation was a way of paying tribute to the historical political struggle, not only showing continuity in the fight against political violence but also pointing to the personal and emotional side of the illness: in the face of this epidemic, there must be room for mourning (Jungar and Oinas 2010, 183).

While it might be fair to state that the field of peace and violence research is seldom concerned with health, in the field of global HIV policies, the themes of violence and even genocide have been central (Oinas and Jungar 2008). This is largely due to the tight links between activism and HIV science, as shown by the South African TAC and also evident in the earlier phases of HIV research (Epstein 1996). In the 1990s US, gay men's health movements and medical science joined forces in unique ways, blurring the boundaries between scientist insiders and lay outsiders in a way that had never been seen before in medical history, claims Epstein (1996). Thus, from the moment AIDS became a matter of public attention, questions of state violence through negligence and inattention were raised.

Regarding the axis of geopolitical structural violence of the North-South divide, HIV was an exception there too. In 2001, HIV became the first health issue brought before the UN Security Council. Currently, in the *UNAIDS 2016–2021 Strategy* (UNAIDS 2015), peace is one of the items mentioned in its eight key result areas. In general, research on the origins, historical and social contexts, as well as the concrete forms of genocide and related acts of mass violence in the global South has often focused on the economy, poverty, colonisation, and colonial rule, not health as a matter of violence. Yet, already a decade ago, Henning Melber (2008, 10) underscored the 'need to include forms of gender-based violence, consequences of ecologically changing environments as a result of human interventions and the effects of climate change for the survival of people (and the threat to it), as well as other effects of structurally induced violence – such as HIV/AIDS and its non-treatment' – in the issues crucial for genocide research.

That existing life-saving medications were not made available for the poor in Africa was defined by activists as genocide in the early 2000s. This was before academics turned their attention to the link between access to medicine and social justice and the so-called new materialist turn (Oinas and Jungar 2008). The TAC, against all odds, was victorious, leading to a re-negotiation of international patent laws and the introduction of antiretroviral treatment (ART) through public health care in South Africa in 2004 (Fassin 2007). The global shift in the HIV policy landscape during the 2000s was the result of an assemblage of a wide array of concurring phenomena, yet one of the important ones was the global struggle of activist women living with HIV in South Africa (Jungar 2011).

This chapter discusses the landscape of HIV activism and politics since the 2000s (see also Biehl 2007; Campbell 2003; Comaroff 2007; Fassin 2007; Nattrass 2004; Robins 2004, 2006). It argues that global health politics is a field of tremendous political contestation and tension, one that, in the case of HIV, uses the discourse of violence and political power. HIV challenges the vast literature on medicalisation that views medicine and public health interventions as technical and depoliticising (Conrad 2007). Reflecting upon the themes of the book, this case demonstrates why it is important to articulate global injustices as forms of violence, and how such articulations may result in positive changes for global health politics.

Recent threats to the goal of universal access to ART underline the key difficulty in global health care: it is a process with no end or permanent victory. It demands a constant discussion on the value and nature of life, on whose life matters, and a constant negotiation regarding political accountability for the costs. In this process, people living with HIV play a crucial role not only in any successful policy or treatment intervention but also in formulating what constitutes global justice and peace in the context of health care.

The case of HIV in South Africa shows that within structural violence of inequality, there are (at least) three different aspects of violence: the *material*, the *symbolic*, and the *epistemic*, and that all of them have embodied consequences. The theoretical stance I present in this chapter employs a poststructuralist conceptualisation of power and violence, drawing loosely on Gayatri Chakravorty Spivak's (1988) broad notion of epistemic violence, where she critically deconstructs the Foucauldian framework to consider the discursive construction of the subaltern 'other'. This chapter does not dwell on existing debates on theories of violence; instead, I will use Spivak's notion as a tool to read the different types of violence I detected during the empirical analysis.

For the sake of analytical clarity, I choose to make some grave simplifications, apparent for everyone with knowledge of Spivak's complex framework. While Spivak's epistemic violence is a broad term, it is here compartmentalised into three different aspects of structural violence. Structural *material* violence, drawing rather bluntly from the Marxist tradition, refers to the systematic denial of material resources to certain groups of people, with consequences to their embodiment. With *symbolic* violence, I refer to the way structural material violence is rendered natural, often by a systematic denial of rights, subjectivity, and citizenship for certain groups of people while others continue enjoying them (cf. Reuterswärd's discussion of cultural violence, this volume). While Pierre Bourdieu (1984) is regarded as the master of the analysis of how class distinction draws on symbolic violence (cf. Lukić and Lotherington this volume), the one who explicitly underlines the discursively denied subjectivity as epistemic violence is Spivak (1988), the main source of inspiration here (but see also, for example, Cornell and Panfilio 2010).

For the sake of analytical precision, the violence of being denied full humanity is here named symbolic, and the last component, the *epistemic*, refers explicitly to knowledge systems that exclude people from legitimate, hegemonic knowing and understanding, and denies them the possibility to engage in authoritative knowledge production. Science is one such system which is analogous to Spivak's example, the colonial legal system. The distinction between the material, the symbolic, and the epistemic is an attempt to be clear in my analytical work, yet I acknowledge that any one of these elements always already comprises the others too, so the difference lies in the foregrounding by the analyst. Dissecting these endless entanglements, however, may well be at the very core of feminist research on gendered violence in global health. As this entire volume suggests, feminist scholarship and activism in both peace and global health have the capacity to seek such dis-entanglements. It is only by disentangling the different forms of violence that we make them fully visible and, as a consequence, make lessening or eliminating violence possible (see Confortini and Vaittinen, this volume).

Empirically, this chapter has its beginning on the streets of Cape Town where TAC marched against government negligence in 2002, and it ends in a gentrified downtown office complex in Johannesburg in late 2017, where an hour-long, catch-up interview with high-level leaders of the movement took place. The first round of fieldwork with the TAC activists in 2002–2003 included eight months of ethnographic observation of the public appearances of the movement in South Africa with Katarina Jungar, whose PhD study expands our shared project (Jungar 2011). The second set of data, interviews with volunteer treatment counsellors and HIV patients, I collected in a township in the Western Cape near Cape Town in 2009 and 2012. Here I enquired about the influence of activists' discourse and movement politics on the daily work and lives of the people living with HIV and attempting to support an ART programme in their community.[2]

In their rallies, TAC highlighted that, when the actual *material goods, the pills*, are denied to poor people, that is, when they cannot access existing life-saving medicines, such abandonment also signals *denied subjectivity* (Biehl 2007; Comaroff 2007). In my reading, this constitutes the interlinkage between material and symbolic violence. Their marches for the constitutional right to health care demanded a symbolic recognition of the poor and the marginalised as viable subjects, citizens with rights. Feminist scholarship further adds the elements of the everyday and epistemic violence to the study of structural violence. First, it demands attention to the more mundane acts against violence that are overshadowed by the vocal protests and marches. While political movements are crucial, everyday resistances should be highlighted too, based on the motto 'the private is political', argued the early women's health movement (Boston 1972). In my analysis, the grassroot work of voluntary HIV counsellors consists of subtle, everyday acts against structural violence and as explicit articulations against both material and symbolic violence, in contexts where the material violence of poverty takes the shape of everyday danger and aggression within communities. Anti-violence work on a daily basis also involves the refusal to accept the label of what Spivak (1988) calls *the subaltern*, and hence it can be read as action against symbolic violence. Second, while the voluntary HIV counsellors' work involves both of the aforementioned levels of work with violence, additionally, it highlights the third aspect of violence in the context of health: the potential epistemic violence of biomedicine if it is not translated to be attuned to the circumstances and the prevailing structural violence of the everyday in the community.

STRUCTURAL VIOLENCE OF A VIRUS?
THE GLOBAL AIDS EPIDEMIC AS CONTEXT

Since the early 1980s, the HIV epidemic has been a remarkable case with an unusually mediatised global health policy interest. Yet, it is also an epidemic where global inattention and structural abandonment of the ill in the global south can be witnessed in the statistics of millions of (unnecessary) deaths (UNAIDS 2015). To date, there still is no vaccine or cure for HIV, but since the late 1990s, ART, a complex medication that needs to be taken daily for the rest of one's life, enables living with HIV in a manner that resembles life with many other chronic illnesses, such as diabetes (Cameron 2005). Shortly after the introduction of the first lines of ART, access to medication became a highly political issue, gaining momentum in the global south in the early 2000s.

Media and science alike operated within a risk-group framework, thus launching a series of symbolic exclusions from early on. In the early 1980s, media attention focused on depicting a shocking, unknown, gay men's disease. HIV quickly became a universal concern with overly liberal sexual behaviours, and then an epidemic that changed sex education for young people globally, often engaging different religious authorities to take a firm stand alongside health and medical experts. Towards the mid-1990s, pharmaceutical innovations and the availability of treatment weakened northern alarmism. Media attention disappeared and shifted to Africa only, while discursively HIV was depicted as less of a threat in the global north (Patton 1997). By isolating the actual and potential HIV risk to clusters and risk groups, new boundaries of risk were constantly drawn (for the violent impacts of this on marginalised groups, see Nuño, this volume). While the virus can be transmitted to anyone, risk-group-thinking focused on gay men, sex workers, drug users, and Africans. Africa as a continent (or a country, one could ironically add) became one massive risk group (Patton 1997).

South Africa has a special place in the history of the epidemic because of its uniquely rapid growth rate, from a minimal HIV+ population at the end of the apartheid era in the early 1990s to the largest HIV+ population in the world by the early 2000s. In the hardest-hit region, KwaZulu Natal, the statistics in the early 2000s estimated every third pregnant woman to be HIV+ and life expectancy to fall by twenty years within a few decades (Fassin and

Schneider 2003). That this catastrophic turn took place right after the end of apartheid that had inspired so much hope across the globe, during the first years of democracy, was stunning and led to a passive, inadequate political response to the epidemic (Fassin 2007). The political delay in implementing effective HIV policy was a deliberate choice by President Thabo Mbeki, despite massive protests. It led to a catastrophic death toll – according to one study (Chigwedere et al. 2008), more than 330,000 unnecessary deaths occurred in 2000–2005, putting a precise number to the mass suffering due to inaction. While public health policy is seldom a topic attractive to the media, Mbeki, who came to power after Nelson Mandela, was soon in the global limelight as the president who failed the poor because of his explicit 'AIDS denialism'.

President Mbeki was notoriously suspicious of 'western medicine' and allied himself with dissident scientists who doubted both the existence of the virus and ART as a safe intervention (Nattrass 2011). During the 1990s and early 2000s, ART programmes were introduced only with private funding or by international actors, leaving most poor people with no medication. While activists and researchers were outraged by the government's lack of initiative, the history of racist violations in the name of public health may help to understand Mbeki's reluctance to resort to expensive drugs (Fassin 2007). In one of his widely quoted speeches, the frustrated Mbeki stated: 'Convinced that we are but natural-born, promiscuous carriers of germs, unique in the world, they proclaim that our continent is doomed to an inevitable mortal end because of our unconquerable devotion to the sin of lust' (Mbeki 2001).

In many ways, the arguments President Mbeki used highlight juxtapositions which are familiar to the medicalisation literature in sociology: either AIDS has to do with poverty, being a social illness, or with sexuality; being a behavioural problem or a racist stereotype; or it is a biomedical condition and is then relegated only to experts. Mbeki operated on the level of suspicion: perhaps the epidemic is just a racist social construct and the political leadership can continue remedying the true ills of the nation, such as inequality, poverty, and an economy that needed restructuring (Hoad 2005). The activists, in contrast, attempted to introduce a line of thinking that was radical and challenging, and resembled a more complex feminist politicising epistemology of embodiment (Thompson 2005): medicine is far from a technical practice; it is a socio-political intervention and can both enhance and undermine democracy (Jungar and Oinas 2010). If poor people are not seen as worthy of medication, they are denied their citizenship, argued activists, referring to the new constitution (Achmat 2004). Both the Mbeki administration and the activists shared the view that HIV was not a single apolitical biological entity but a construct that carried with it the history of racism.

The first clinics around Cape Town offering treatment for poor people were initiated as political responses to government reluctance, using alternative funding sources. For example, Doctors without Borders (MSF) introduced the famous Khayelitsha ART programme to show the government and the entire world, including doubtful scientists and funders, that ART could work in resource-poor settings (Interview with MSF in 2009; cf. Coetzee 2004). Some clinics were founded based on scholarly – biomedical or public health – interests, often with developmental aspirations (cf. Sariola and Simpson 2019). The focus on ART was radical, as most HIV interventions in the global south at the time focused on prevention and sexual behaviour. Shifting the focus to care and treatment demanded a shift in discourse, and there were no guarantees that it would work.

After four years of protests, the South African government introduced ART in its national HIV/AIDS policy in late 2003. Since 2004, the rapid change has been remarkable, even if activists have continued to campaign for better implementation of the new policy. From less than 50,000 people on ART in 2004, South Africa quickly became the largest ART provider in the world, with 1.79 million people on ART in 2012 (Johnson 2012, 22–23). A major shift in the epidemic took place, both in the country and globally, although HIV by no means was defeated. The number of people living with HIV in South Africa was hoped to have stopped growing around 2006 and remained first rather stable, at less than five million (Johnson 2012, 25). In 2018, however, the total number of people living with HIV in South Africa is estimated at approximately 7.52 million. For adults aged fifteen to forty-nine years, an estimated 19 per cent of the population is HIV positive (Statistics SA 2018). This recent increase in cases is all the more worrisome considering that globally the number of new infections has dropped. Especially the number of children becoming infected has dramatically declined by 30 per cent worldwide, a shift that has mostly to do with healthcare improvements, the availability of treatment for mothers and pregnant women, and increased awareness among pregnant women, according to UNAIDS (UNAIDS 2010). UNAIDS, however, warns about the lack of adequate funding and decreasing interest on the global scale, putting the successful trajectory at risk (UNAIDS 2015).

Overall, it is fair to say that the 2000s were a remarkable era in the history of epidemiology: although catastrophic outcries of unmanageable emergency and hopelessness characterised the mid-1990s (Epstein 2006, 15), today there is clear evidence that many of the 2000s massive interventions have worked. The HIV epidemic deemed too difficult to deal with – due to issues of sexuality, stigma, and weak infrastructure in places where the problem was most urgent – was by the end of the 2000s no longer viewed as a looming global disaster. It still created personal tragedies and national challenges, but it was shown to be manageable too, as long as there was political will and funding. Politics, science, and individual health go hand in hand, the statistics of the 2000s show. Rather straightforward public health measures such as treatment and care were enabled by the sense of urgency created among local, national, and international activism but also among the media, international actors, national politicians, and funders – and the statistics did change. Behind public health programmes lies an enormous effort by activists, patient movements, experts, politicians, and funders – and individuals affected by HIV. The framing of the HIV epidemic as explicit violence was crucial in the shift.

CIVIL DISOBEDIENCE, GENOCIDE, AND A POLITICISED JAR OF PILLS

To get an understanding of how a single health issue became successfully framed as a key question for democracy, peace, and justice, it is worthwhile to pause in February 2003. TAC made a daring decision to charge individual politicians with homicide – 600 homicides a day, to be precise. Two ministers, Manto Tshabalala-Msimang, the minister of health, and Alec Erwin, the minister of finance, were personally sued. Their alleged crime was the failure to respond to the HIV/AIDS epidemic in South Africa, leading to preventable deaths. In addition, TAC started a 'civil disobedience campaign', a political campaign that has a very strong symbolical meaning in South Africa. The decision to use civil disobedience, a tool that was used in the anti-apartheid struggle, was a bold step in the new democracy, with the still-very-popular ANC in government (cf. Friedman and Mottiar 2006).

The activists' message was that these two individuals were personally responsible for the lives lost every day. The campaign also pointed at the political machinery, addressing the government as a whole, as an institution, accountable for deaths in the country. In 2003, the focus was on the South African leadership, but activists addressed the international community too. Linking health, suffering, and death to larger social structures was novel. The TAC speeches depict the 'embodiment of violence' that I analyse as a multi-level approach to violence: connections were drawn between cells and viruses, community violence, and national and global politics. Multiple intersecting layers of violence (cf. Tanyag, this volume) were highlighted at all TAC events: global intellectual property rights and a neoliberal, bio-economic order were discussed in the same meetings where community stigma was addressed; viral cells and capitalism were seen as interlinked; treatment literacy and biomedical basics were woven with political jingles. Women dancing with a jar of pills and singing anti-apartheid melodies brought the history of racism to the question of medication.

Accusations of criminal acts aimed at politicians who did not show commitment to leadership in the face of the AIDS epidemic – that is, a political standpoint being interpreted as a crime – had previously not been taken to court. D'Adesky (2004, 7) documents a case where the Malawian activist Chatinka Nwoma, during a rally at the Durban AIDS conference in 2000,

> grabbed the microphone, pointed to a building behind her where World Bank officials and drug company experts were discussing the cost-effectiveness of global AIDS treatment, and shouted to a sea of African faces like hers: 'There is a crime being committed here! You cannot have 42 million people dying and have the issue be about money!'

Similarly, the Wola Nani activist Gary Lamont used the following language in a speech on the South African government's lack of policy regarding ART provision to pregnant women: 'Every month that the government withholds these drugs is a cumulative act of genocide for thousands' (Fassin 2007, 52), also indicating a crime committed by a government. Eventually, TAC dropped the threat to pursue the legal case when the political campaign was successful.

The civil disobedience campaign highlighted the two components of the activists' view on state violence: structural violence consists of the material elements of denied health care, poverty, and other material social injustices, as well as the symbolic element of exclusion from the realm of worthy citizens. In a lecture given by Zackie Achmat (2004, 10), a founding member of TAC and its spokesperson at the time, a long list of interlinked issues was present, including discourses on sexuality and gender inequality:

> We die because of excessive drug company profiteering. We die because our governments are in denial of the seriousness of the HIV epidemic by governments and bureaucratic procrastination and equivocation. We also die because men have greater access to resources and power than women; because rich countries invest substantially more in war than in public goods, and because many global corporations live outside the law of global human rights. We die because religious dogma and reactionary traditionalism suppress sexual freedom and because some African leaders label homosexuality unAfrican. And we die because we cannot buy life-saving medicines. Unlike some of our neighbours in the north, we cannot afford to buy life.

The quote is an illustration on how structural violence has a multitude of interlinked actors and acts that enforce it and enable it to continue. Achmat asserted that embodiment is shaped by global biopolitics, that power/knowledge networks enable certain subjectivities, and that the implications are local and personal (cf. Nuño, this volume). In the following, material, symbolic, and epistemic elements of violence come together in individual bodies, death, and suffering:

> Our bodies are the evidence of global inequality and injustice. They are not mere metaphors for the relationship between inequality and disease. But our bodies are also the sites of resistance. We do not die quietly. We challenge global inequality. Our resistance gives us dignity. In the Treatment Action Campaign (TAC), the voices of our comrades, friends and children echo around the world to resist injustice. Our voices demand life even as our bodies resist death. (Achmat 2004, 13)

The TAC language often brought up oppositions between the rich and poor, politicians and patients, pharmaceuticals and poor people, and government ministers and citizens. But TAC both utilised and challenged dichotomous models of thinking typical for political struggles. A polarising set-up between the power of the government versus lay civil society thus appeared in some statements but was also constantly revoked. Sometimes a juxtaposition of 'us' and 'them' was there, sometimes everyone was part of the 'nation' or 'us'. A similar contradiction (or, rather, a double strategy) was applied regarding who was 'affected' by AIDS: sometimes there was a clear 'us' who were dying, sometimes 'everyone' was included. For example, the famous T-shirts stating 'HIV POSITIVE' that participants in TAC rallies wore indicated an erasure of difference between HIV-positive people and the others. The message was that everyone was affected by the epidemic. The T-shirt did not mark the identity of an HIV-positive person but a commitment to resistance. 'We all need treatment to be made available' (Cameron 2005, 130).

With the message that AIDS affected everyone, victims ceased to be a clearly defined group of subaltern 'others'. Rather, the epidemic compelled everyone to take responsibility – including government ministers. The government was implicated in a different way because of different access to resources and the possibility to make policy and budget decisions, but often the campaign pointed to the possibility for everyone to act and be part of a change.

The civil disobedience campaign's message against the symbolic violence of subalternity – that is, the outrage in the face of the denial of materialised citizenship rights in the form of existing medication – had an interesting outcome in terms of health promotion. There clearly was a link between effective HIV prevention and the move to challenge state violence against the poor when the state neglected health services. The fight against structural violence included de-stigmatising elements that contributed to HIV prevention because activism went beyond the individual-responsibility discourse that was typical of many HIV prevention discourses (Jungar and Oinas 2010). HIV prevention with an individualising agenda – 'you must stop *your* risky behaviour' – blames individuals for their infection. When the message is only that 'risky behaviour' causes the infection, it must have been the individual's own fault, leading to shame, silence, and secrets. In contrast, the politicising of structural violence by activists focused on structural issues that contributed to the risk factors underlying the potential for the epidemic to spread, including violent, gendered structures (cf. Ratele 2006; also Ikhile, Gibson and Wahidin, this volume in regard to breast cancer). In the individualising discourse, being open about one's status becomes very difficult, whereas in the politicised movement, being openly HIV positive was possible and brave. While in the former case, HIV-positive people were regarded as a risk towards innocent victims, in the latter case, the HIV positive themselves were framed as victims of structural violence. The victimhood itself was turned into political fuel: these were active, vocal, and rebelling victims, not silent, silenced subalterns (Jungar and Oinas 2011).

The success of TAC in challenging the Mbeki HIV policy in 2003 lay in its ability to define ART anew, moving away from medicine as a costly, technical, Western intervention to focus on the denial of the pill as material violence and the simultaneous symbolic violence of the denial of worthy citizenship. It may also be that in the activist campaign for ART, the progressive white middle class found a way to legitimately criticise the ANC and President Mbeki, something that otherwise was difficult during the first decade of democracy. The leadership of TAC tapped into the sentiments of the white healthcare professionals and rights activists. I argue that this may be connected to the subjective sense of loss and disorientation among the liberal white middle class that was hard to articulate. This segment of society supported the shift to democracy but found little means to be politically active in a complex, new political landscape. They agreed with the discourse that demanded space for the marginalised yet were feeling strangely alienated and voiceless themselves. This is a speculative argument, but if it has any value, it suggests that TAC was insightful in envisioning that the symbolic and material forms of violence experienced by the poor could be connected to the experience of symbolic violence of a formerly dominant but newly silenced voice in society – the educated middle class – when forming a mass movement. The different experiences of Mbeki's South Africa treating its citizens violently could be united behind a single legitimate cause, HIV. The deliberate choice of the first campaign, to focus on new-born babies, created a sense of unnecessary mass violence and a shared political goal in a divided nation.

GRASSROOTS INTERVENTIONS WITHIN MEDICAL PRACTICE

Having focused on HIV activism as a strong public voice against structural violence in South Africa in the first half of the 2000s, it became increasingly important for me to learn how people living with HIV but not actively involved in movements perceived the politicised HIV field. Thus, in my 2009–2012 study, I enquired how the political situation and 'treatment fury' affected the lives of people living with HIV who were also active in health care. To get some data on women dealing with HIV outside the movements, I conducted interviews with a group of patients who were acting as volunteer counsellors for other patients. I did not conduct the study ethnographically inside a clinic; rather, I interviewed the individuals about their views and daily life. These data, too, dealt with resistance to the material and symbolic aspects of structural violence but in more every day, practical ways, as feminist scholars have often claimed to be the case in women's mundane resistance (Honkasalo 2009). Furthermore, the data brought the element of epistemic violence to the fore. In contrast to the activist agendas, these interviewees had a more subtle and pragmatic approach to structural violence, yet the embodied consequences of violence were equally dramatic and palpable in the ways the volunteers spoke.

In a smaller scale compared to the activists, these women too formed a vocal support and advocacy group within the clinic where they volunteered as well as in the larger community. They described their lives, care, and survival as an entangled net of different relations that sustained them, and this entanglement included both human and non-human actors, for example, food, laboratory results, transport to the clinic and, last but not least, the pills. These entanglements of relations that produced healthier embodiments required a lot of work but not in an individualistic, heroic manner. The entanglements these women 'held together', as they put it, required a lot of knowledge, but such knowledge was not bookish or abstract. It was a matter of solidarity, of feeling, living, and doing together (Honkasalo 2009). Linda, one of the counsellors, described her motivation as follows: 'I was helped, so I wanted to help. I wanted to show to people that there is life after HIV, it is not so that once you get HIV you are going to die. As long as you are taking your medicines properly'. When I asked if it was easy for the patients to talk to her, she replied: 'Yes, because I disclose to them too. That's when I give them hope. If you are HIV positive, it is not so that you are going to die. So they take me as a sister' (Linda, interviewed 2009).

The way the interviewees described their engagement with HIV medicine, I suggest, is resistance against an understanding of them as passive subaltern victims with little resources and knowledge. This, I argue, is a strong stand against symbolic violence that 'others' poor women in the global south (Ahmed 2000; Spivak 1988). The interviewees spoke about their work in an apolitical manner, and the violence they mentioned was the material one on the streets and in the homes, but I argue that this precisely challenged two assumptions that every now and then emerge in social science discussions on health care: the dichotomy of medicine versus lay agency in medicalisation (Riska 2010) and the dichotomy of north versus south as the two poles in the axis of modernity (Ahmed 2000). Both assumptions are symbolically violent in their negation of viable subjects with capabilities and rights. Feminist literature and activism often criticise such dichotomies, but that repetitive act ends up reproducing the dichotomies. The voluntary counsellors' pride in their work with the doctors deconstructs dichotomising boundaries. The interviewees countered the symbolically violent representations of subaltern victims with disinterest; rather than debating this, they stubbornly insisted simply going on with their work. Their bypassing of the insulting, othering symbolic violence is in stark contrast with the vocal campaigns of the activists. The counsellors said, however, that they valued the movements and learned from them, sometimes attending workshops, so these stances were not oppositional to each other, just different in mode of operation.

The dichotomy of medical experts versus lay patients was simply set aside in the volunteers' way of speaking confidently of the importance of their work and their way of collaborating with the professional medical staff. Instead of maintaining dichotomies, lay counsellors created and maintained links between medical care, treatment knowledge, patients, and the wider community with a great effort, but, in their way of talking about their activities, with surprising ease. Fiona, one of the lay counsellors, asserted in an interview that 'doctors and counsellors here work together, as a team, as equal partners. They need us, we need them. Not like in the other clinics, where they [doctors] know. Here, it is sharing' (Fiona, interviewed 2009). They viewed their role in the HIV treatment as essential in successful care relations, thereby strongly resisting the kind of epistemic violence that devalorises or marginalises lay knowledge of medicine.

Thus, these uneducated women who could be defined as subaltern can also be seen as key nodes in the networks that, against all odds, curbed the spread of the pandemic during the 2000s (UNAIDS 2010, 7–8). Their voluntary work illustrates an implicit practice against symbolic and epistemic violence through the simultaneous presence of different levels of human and non-human relationality that enables sustainable care, knowledge, and survival. In the early years of the AIDS epidemic, patient activism, gay movements, and medicine collaborated in path-breaking ways (Epstein 1996); similarly, in the context of the South African slum, where uneducated patients and high-tech medicine interacted, important aspects of lay medicine collaborations were present. The non-human elements are important to underscore here, as seen in the previous chapter: without the actual pills and laboratories, people with HIV die.

TRAJECTORIES OF COUNSELLING PRACTICE: THE CLIENT, THE CLINIC, AND THE COMMUNITY

While all the interviews, not very surprisingly, emphasised the importance of volunteer counselling in a successful treatment programme, they recounted remarkably many elements as aspects of their work. All these I read as ways of countering structural violence. The activities addressed three different recipients of care: the client, the clinic, and the community. First, the most obvious and easily anticipated was support to the client. Second, the interviewees portrayed the counsellor as someone who engaged in knowledge generation about living with HIV and ART, thus informing doctors and cooperating with the medical staff in successful ART. The third direction of the activities was the contact with the community at large. This mainly involved the local community where the counsellors and clients lived and practiced. Only some of the interviewees touched upon global politics and their work against an unjust world order. The politicised context of the South African HIV epidemic (Fassin 2007; Nattrass 2004, 2007) was both present and absent in the interviews. The South African and global context of HIV and ART politics was often implicitly mentioned in the interviews, assuming I as a researcher in the field would know what inevitably framed the entire setting.

'I am a sister, priest, and a doctor', said Fiona about her work in her first interview with me in 2009. Peer support, meaning the interviewee's work with an individual client, was portrayed as the main focus of counselling, but this too intertwined with the other layers and involved several elements. I analysed peer support to deal with three separate areas of work: understanding and support for the *social realities* of living with HIV, that is, dealing with a rather demanding drug regimen in a certain community; dealing with the *psycho-social* issues related to diagnosis, survival, and treatment in everyday lives; and, lastly, *disclosure*, an issue that was discussed at length in each interview and seemed to be the key aspect in ART. Anyone on ART was expected to eventually 'disclose', that is, tell about his/her HIV+ status and the drugs to at least one person, but only when one was ready, as was said over and over again in the interviews. Discussions around disclosure involved a lot of practical advice about stigma, secrecy, integrity, and rights, knowledge that was highly contextual. The three elements guiding the counsellors' work were all connected to violence, also to the often-individualised psycho-social aspect due to the violence of stigma and the structural, material violence of poverty. Only when the material violence was mentioned as a central theme and not as something to downplay could the language of hope be brought up and effectively challenge the symbolic violence.

Both the counsellors and the medical professionals I talked to stressed the importance of peer support, grasping the everyday realities of the clients in their communities. Fiona also began with mentioning hope: 'It is so much about hope. Counsellors are examples. They are patients too, and they are open about it. They have lived through all that, they know'. For Fiona, knowing about the social realities on the ground was the crucial difference between the doctors and the peer counsellors: 'They know the circumstances where people live; they understand what they talk about. You don't even need to say yourself, a counsellor can anticipate things. You are not scary. You share the language, community' (Fiona, interviewed 2009).

The counsellors said that their knowledge of the larger issues, like how poverty works in the shacks, allowed them to give accurate advice and support and even to anticipate the questions that the clients would ask or might not dare to ask. For example, the way South African welfare grants – which may be the only income for an extended family – are conditional may mean that, when the ART starts working and one recovers, one may lose the grant. This dilemma, if not addressed well in counselling, may risk the entire programme, cost lives, and create resistant strands of the virus due to juggling with the pills when facing desperate circumstances. The counsellors acknowledged the material, structural violence in the everyday life of a township with their own situated knowledge and the epistemic translation of ART. This is also an example of how the human and non-human entanglements resist the coming together of multiple forms of violence: material violence needs to be taken seriously for the symbolic violence not to happen – and for the treatment to work in the body.

The interviews indicated that the questions clients asked were of medical nature, but the volunteer counsellors felt fully equipped to answer. A lot of the questions dealt with side effects, infections, and worries about the possibility of getting pregnant again (Richey 2011). They were universal yet also highly contextual, situated questions. The counsellors' point of view on the side effects of medication seemed different and complementary to the answers the doctors gave, as most doctors did not live through those physical sensations and did not know the context of the concern, or lacked the language. 'We can even help the doctors', said Fundiswa. She also reminded me of the importance of knowing the many rumours to be able to counter them: there were 'too many stories that antiretrovirals are dangerous, change their bodies' (Fundiswa, interviewed 2009). As some people did not respond well, and some died despite ART, or some simply had too-high expectations regarding the medicine, there tended to be rumours that this or that was caused by the medicine. A local peer voice was able to tell 'that the doctor is not Jesus' (Fundiswa, interviewed 2009) and strengthen the motivation to stay on ART.

When asked about the major difficulties in achieving good ART, the answers mainly touched upon socioeconomic issues, varying from poverty, unemployment, alcoholism, and crime to lack of transport between homes and the clinics and airtime for mobile phones – a rich variety of levels of structural, material violence manifesting in the everyday. Here, it would be easy to overemphasise the enormous difficulty of the allegedly 'white' medicine, as it sometimes was named, to even start to grasp the realities of the black township dwellers, a gap that still, and increasingly, is the reality in post-apartheid South Africa. Eve, the research assistant, repeated daily to me: 'You know, there is still apartheid in South Africa' (Field Notes 2009). In these violent circumstances, the medical staff alone was not best-equipped to do the work around coping with and understanding the illness, diagnosis, and care in everyday context, but in collaboration with activists and peer counsellors, epistemic violence was held at bay. Indeed, it was emphasised often that biomedical knowledge did not feel alien or difficult for the counsellors. Thus, I argue that biomedicine should not be considered 'western', or foreign, in itself, even if it needs to be attuned to the realities on the ground – anywhere. A feminist critique of biomedical knowledge and its potential for epistemic violence should always account for the intersections of violence that go beyond monolithic identifications of the 'west'.

THE POTENTIAL EPISTEMIC VIOLENCE OF BIOMEDICINE

For Fiona, the counsellor had a double role: on the one hand, the counsellors represented the clinic in the homes of people; on the other, they represented the people at the clinic. When I interviewed the leading ART programme director in a university hospital, Dr. O., she also mentioned that, the real key to their success as an HIV clinic was the counselling programme. However, she also noted that this aspect had not been studied in the otherwise well-researched and documented ART practice. 'What is this ingredient that makes this difference that makes it work? We have decided that it is friendship' (Dr O., interviewed 2009). It is revealing that the richness of the counsellors' work and the complexity of social relations they deal with were reduced to vague 'friendship'. There clearly was appreciation in Dr O.'s way of viewing the counsellors' capacities; Dr. O. told me she was personally involved in initiating the programme and called it crucial.

That such a key element was never properly studied and documented, let alone published in a medical journal by her research group, however, testifies to the limits of the scope of biomedical science. This leading medical researcher did not comprehend the social aspect of the treatment to be a medical issue; the social matters were mentioned with appreciation but relegated to the non-medical domain, to the socio-technical administration side separate from the actual research. This separation of domains that some researchers analyse as gendered-masculine hard science versus gendered-feminine care of the patient, regardless of the gender of the scientist (Riska 2010), in my view, caters to epistemic violence, as it, in the long run of ART research, renders the knowledge and context of the patients irrelevant.

In the South African case, the usage of the notion 'friendship' can be read as a possibly well-meaning acknowledgement of not really comprehending social lives across the racialised divide, a polite recognition of difference typical for post-apartheid South Africa. While this may be a sign of respect and distance that indicates non-intrusion and appreciative non-sameness (cf. Ahmed 2000), it is also a gesture that confirms academic biomedicine's inability to engage with the social context. The interviews show that the intricate web of community relations taking place in ART management had a pattern and meaning that should not be reduced to 'friendship', however much 'friendship' was a positive attribution. The cosy term belittles and feminises the highly needed expertise of the volunteers. Yet, while the leadership delegated 'the social' to volunteer counsellors' domain only, the medical staff on the ground were said to be fully cooperative. The interviews indicate that the medical staff embraced the counsellors' knowledge of the community, patients' needs, and language. Thus, while the research-side of the programme dismissed and denied the medical importance of the context by not studying it, therefore signalling the epistemic violence of half-hearted half-engagement, in the concrete daily life of ART, such epistemic violence was countered and renegotiated.

The statement by this director was ambivalent but descriptive of the realities in HIV medicine. The counsellors were in the first place granted a central role in the programme due to the recognition that township conditions have medical relevance, but the programme was not documented, and only a while later the counsellor programmes were cancelled in the majority of sites. By being a volunteer programme, it exploited the cheap labour of the patients, not offering them proper employment. Yet, such voluntary workers' presence might have been the only way of communicating between communities and clinics due to lack of diversity and numbers among educated healthcare staff – indicating the deeper roots of structural violence in the entire education system, when so few of the educated healthcare workers in general at the time came from the communities most impacted by HIV. Something crucial in the social embeddedness of the programme was lost when everyone involved in the clinic was required to be on an employment contract only, and professional skills and qualifications became the primary recruitment criteria. The loss of counselling programmes, I argue, is an unfortunate resignation in the face of structural, material, and epistemic violence that underpins social life and medical practice in South Africa.

Peer counselling and support groups are necessary in order to counteract the epistemic violence of academic biomedicine, when there is an enormous gulf in living conditions between clients and doctors. It is not a question of a one-way translation but of a thorough engagement with local knowledge systems that also inform medicine. Biomedical science's lack of engagement with the everyday life on the ground and the health consequences of the political conditions people live in can be seen in recent statistics: in Africa, the number of people on ART has grown in exemplary ways, but the statistics on a major biomedical indicator of success, the suppressed viral load, are still lower than expected. The pills are there, but they work less well than they scientifically should (UNAIDS 2015). This indicates that, in spite of access to ART, something is still missing. Research on material, symbolic, and epistemic violence in ART can explain the missing link.

I argue that the potential epistemic violence inherent in biomedicalisation can be challenged by practices of engagement, like in the voluntary counselling programme, where a socially embedded negotiation of ART took place. Instead of imposing medical authority on people living with HIV, something that mainstream sociology of health and illness criticises (Conrad 2007), the peer counsellors were an access point that generated new modes of situated knowledge about living with ART and HIV. They contextualised the medical knowledge and transformed it into local realities (e.g. Das and Das 2007) in collaboration with the trained clinic staff.

In the classic view of medicalisation research, the ART programme and the counsellors visiting homes could be seen as biomedicalising and pharmacologising intrusions in the community (Conrad 2007; Martin and Gabe 2011; Riska 2010; Williams). Yet the activists and counsellors alike argued that with the HIV epidemic, biomedicine is already unavoidably present (cf. Whyte et al. 2002). Despite a wide range of modes of structural violence, the township dwellers are already 'cyborgs', socio-technological hybrids (Haraway 1985), and any claim that Western biomedicine is alien to them was treated as foolish by the peer counsellors. While their bodies 'bear witness to global injustices' (Achmat 2004), they are also evidence of the uselessness of the developed world versus third-world distinction in terms of patients' 'will to life' (Biehl 2007).

The counsellors' peaceful responses to epistemic and symbolic aspects of structural violence come together in the claim that HIV treatment can be managed also by uneducated poor people in a township in the global south (Jungar and Oinas 2010). For the participants living with HIV, ART was an enabling force, an extremely sought-after asset, not a threatening colonisation of the life-world (Zola 1972). They did not want to resort to African traditional medicine only; the pills represented hope, dignity, and justice. Having said this, it is important to bring the issue of epistemic violence to the fore. Without local activists and counsellors, the treatment programme would have probably been much more alien and inaccessible for the community.

The contextualising and politicising component of counselling and activism translated ART to local needs and practices, and reduced stigma. Following Charis Thompson (2005), it is clear that the issue here is not *if* a social process is biomedicalising or not, but what the political *effects* of biomedical practices are – for example, ART as social justice, as in staying alive just like the richer neighbours.

Simi, one of the women I interviewed in 2009, talked more about the girls' football team she coached than about the ART I actually asked her to tell me about. Her life did not revolve around her HIV status. However, the framework of our conversation was all the time clear for both of us. Without the treatment she would die. Had she needed the drugs five years earlier, when the health minister still recommended garlic and beetroot instead of costly Western medicines, she would not have been there telling me how she collects shoes for her team, or avoiding the topic of ART she was already used to and found nothing remarkable about. The simple view that medicine is an enterprise that enables life, as advocated by activists who remind us that they would die if deprived of medicines (Fassin 2007; Jungar and Oinas 2010; Nattrass 2007; Robins 2004, 2006), is, I claim, in fact a radical claim about structural violence. It is sometimes made through an insistence to speak about football rather than grief.

The TAC activists and the counsellors did not themselves use the concept of potential epistemic violence of biomedicine. The activist discourse needed to defend its agenda against accusations of ART being too difficult, complicated, or 'scientific' for Africans. Due to racist stereotypes, they had to downplay the need to translate and contextualise medicine. TAC presented a rather straightforward, respectful 'pure science' account (Oinas and Jungar 2008) to also counter the political agenda of dissident science. For example, the following quote, discussed by Jungar (2011, 82), was typical for the time: 'It is not simple to use these medications because you have to take them for the rest of your life. But if a person like me who does not have two degrees in science or any other subject can take them, anyone who wants to live can learn about them and take them well' (Ncapayi, TAC activist).

STRATEGICALLY SUBALTERN CYBORG EMBODIMENT AND THE STRUCTURAL MATERIAL VIOLENCE IN DENIED HIV TREATMENT

In this chapter, I suggested a three-dimensional view on structural violence: first, that the absence of pills signifies *material* violence; second, that the absence of pills for some citizens but not for others signifies *symbolic* violence of denied rights and humanity; and third, that the absence of engagement with local realities and knowledge practices, that is, a denied translation of biomedical knowledge, signifies *epistemic* violence. The 2000s showed a remarkable shift towards the better in all these aspects. Now, approaching a new decade, with a shift towards colder winds in global solidarity, a focus on violence is more important than ever.

A situation where only a part of the global population has access to life-saving medication indicates material violence against the less-fortunate ones, argued the vocal cries of HIV activists in South Africa in the early 2000s. Such an optimist approach to medicine as a right may seem naïve to the most critical, but I argue that it does not require abandoning the critical approach to medicine as biopower (Agamben 1998; Comaroff 2007; Foucault 1980; Rabinow 2011), nor the critique of neoliberal capitalism in new development practices that render political problems technical or consumerist (Richey and Ponte 2010). The HIV activists who advocated a more explicit attention to questions of *access* to biomedical treatment suggest that these are questions of not only material but symbolic violence because, when denied the material reality of the antiretroviral medication, one's rights, citizenship, entire subjectivity, and humanity are also put in question. My research suggests, furthermore, that alongside material and symbolic violence, healthcare systems should also be concerned about the potential *epistemic* violence inherent in biomedicine, if it does not seriously engage with the everyday lives and politics on the ground.

The politics and practices of ART of HIV are a network of relations that involves a variety of actors and layers. Activists and volunteers are key figures in global politics of health and social justice through both symbolic and epistemic – and practical – work against structural violence. The volunteer HIV counsellors I interviewed for my research explained their care work and their own treatment management in terms that constantly drew links between the knowledge and ability to utilise a high-tech biomedical, anti-retroviral HIV treatment regimen with more traditionally sociological components, such as social support for negotiating poverty and crime. In their accounts, different elements of care and survival smoothly intertwined in this setting, with little need to create hierarchies in expertise or authority, in western or southern patients. For them – the hybrid subaltern cyborgs of a township – biomedicine is not alien, foreign, or 'western' in itself as it was claimed by President Mbeki to be. It is a set of knowledges, tools, and practices that can be learned, understood, translated, and elaborated on by people living with HIV. In their activism, the focus of action was not an individual subject in a neoliberal, modernist sense (Butler 1990, 1993; Martin 2006; Richey 2011); nor authority over medical expertise. Rather, their anti-violence work was geared towards solidarity, life, and hope, a hope that required a multitude of relational, collective agencies to be sustained (Campbell 2003; Das and Das

2007; Honkasalo 2009; Whyte et al. 2002), a hope that effectively rejected subalternity. While the activists were more vocal and strategic about subalternity, and the counsellors more pragmatic than explicitly political, in both cases, the different elements of violence were central.

ART and peer counselling are not magic bullets that erase the epidemic of HIV. Yet, currently, while still waiting for better means of intervention, they are crucial politico-epidemiological tools in the fight against a massive catastrophe both on personal and global levels. ART captures the crux of health care: there is no cure nor quick fix for the vulnerability of the physical body; survival and dignified life are thoroughly political questions that are never resolved once and for all. Currently, the success of the 2000s global HIV management is possibly heading towards a downward spiral again (UNAIDS 2015), making the urgency to connect it to violence even more crucial.

Social science scholarship on medicine is traditionally more likely to approach medicine critically than to address issues of material and epistemic access to biomedicine. If academic approaches remain limited to a mere critique, academics are also complicit in culpable homicide, the activists might argue. If social science does not address the vital dimensions of health care – and the lack thereof as violence – the way activist agendas do, social and political sciences will continue the problematic tradition of not taking the materiality of life seriously.

NOTES

1. Acknowledgements: This research was possible thanks to the Academy of Finland funding (79687, 258235, 320863) as well as the Nordic Africa Institute, for the 2006–2009 part. Tiina and Catia, editors of this book: thank you for the long journey, your tremendous input and labour, wise comments, insights, and advice. This is the end of an era: I have had this theme for one-third of my lifetime, and this will be the final text, now moving on to other topics. From all of my heart and intellect I wish to thank the activists in the movements and clinics for their work and for sharing a tiny part of it with me. Elizabeth Seabe has been an invaluable colleague in so many ways. Without Katarina Jungar urging me to join her on our first HIV project, and without the following years of collaboration, my life would be quite different now – tack! My chapter in this book is dedicated to my brave kids travelling with me all this way, but this one goes especially to Theo, the funny, clever boy of six, afraid of roaring lions in Cape Town; and, of course, to Penni, my main academic companion.

2. While the first data, with the movement, were observational, the second data set with the volunteers was composed of interviews. I visited the clinics for a few weeks at a time, conducting semi-structured interviews of thirty to sixty minutes with twenty volunteers.

REFERENCES

Achmat, Zackie. 2004. 'HIV and Human Rights: A New South African Struggle'. John Foster Lecture 2004. Accessed 24 April 2019. http://www.rothschildfostertrust.com/materials/lecture_achmat.pdf.

Agamben, Giorgio. 1998. *Homo Sacer: Sovereign Power and Bare Life*. Stanford: Stanford University Press.

Ahmed, Sara. 2000. *Strange Encounters: Embodied Others in Post-coloniality*. London: Routledge.

Biehl, João. 2007. *Will to Live: AIDS Therapies and the Politics of Survival*. Princeton: Princeton University Press.

Biehl, João, Byron J. Good and Arthur Kleinman. 2007. 'Introduction: Rethinking Subjectivity'. In *Subjectivity: Ethnographic Investigations*, edited by João Biehl, Byron J. Good and Arthur Kleinman, 1–23. Berkeley: University of California Press.

Bourdieu, Pierre. 1984. *Distinction: A Social Critique of the Judgement of Taste*. London: Routledge & Kegan Paul.

Butler, Judith. 1990. *Gender Trouble: Feminism and the Subversion of Identity*. New York: Routledge.

Butler, Judith. 1993. *Bodies That Matter: On the Discursive Limits of 'Sex'*. New York: Routledge.

Cameron, Edwin. 2005. *Witness to AIDS*. London: IB Tauris.

Campbell, Catherine. 2003. *'Letting Them Die': How HIV/AIDS Prevention Programmes Often Fail*. Bloomington, IN: Indiana University Press.

Chigwedere, Pride, George R. III Seage, Sofia Gruskin and Tun-Hou Lee. 2008. 'Estimating the Lost Benefits of Antiretroviral Drug Use in South Africa'. *JAIDS Journal of Acquired Immune Deficiency Syndromes* 49, no. 4: 410–415.

Coetzee, David, Andrew Boulle, Katherine Hildebrand, Valerie Asselman, Gilles Van Cutsem and Eric Goemaere. 2004. 'Promoting Adherence to Antiretroviral Therapy: The Experience from a Primary Care Setting in Khayelitsha, South Africa'. *AIDS* 18, Suppl 3: 27–31.

Comaroff, Jean. 2007. 'Beyond Bare Life: AIDS, (Bio)Politics, and the Neoliberal Order'. *Public Culture* 19, no. 1: 197–219.

Confortini, Catia C. and Tiina Vaittinen. 2019. 'Introduction: Analysing Violences in Gendered Global Health'. In *Gender, Global Health and Violence: Feminist Perspectives on Peace and Disease*, edited by Tiina Vaittinen and Catia Confortini. London and New York: Rowman & Littlefield.

Conrad, Peter. 2007. *The Medicalization of Society: On the Transformation of Human Conditions into Treatable Disorders*. Baltimore: The John Hopkins University Press.

Cornell, Drucilla and Kenneth Michael Panfilio. 2010. *Symbolic Forms for a New Humanity: Cultural and Racial Reconfigurations of Critical Theory*. New York: Fordham University Press.

d'Adesky, Anne-Christine. 2004. *Moving Mountains: The Race to Treat Global AIDS*. London: Verso.

Das, Veena and Ranendra K. Das. 2007. 'How the Body Speaks: Illness and the Lifeworld among the Urban Poor'. In *Subjectivity: Ethnographic Investigations*, edited by João Biehl, Byron Good and Arthur Kleinman, 66–97. Berkeley: University of California Press.

Epstein, Helen. 2006. *The Invisible Cure: Africa, the West, and the Fight against AIDS*. London: Penguin Books.

Epstein, Steven. 1996. *Impure Science: AIDS, Activism, and the Politics of Knowledge*. Berkeley: University of California Press.

Fassin, Didier and Helen Schneider. 2003. 'The South African Politics of AIDS: Beyond the Controversies'. *British Medical Journal* 326: 495–497.

Fassin, Didier. 2007. *When Bodies Remember: Experience and Politics of AIDS in South Africa*. Berkeley: University of California Press.

Foucault, Michel. 1980. *Power/Knowledge: Selected Interviews and Other Writings 1972–1977*. New York: Pantheon Books.

Friedman, Stephen and Shauna Mottiar. 2006. 'Seeking the High Ground. The Treatment Action Campaign and the Politics of Morality'. In *Voices of Protest*, edited by Richard Ballard, Adam Habib and Imraan Valoodia, 23–44. Scottsville: University of KwaZulu-Natal Press.

Gilbert, Leah and Liz Walker. 2002. 'Treading the Path of Least Resistance: HIV/Aids and Social Inequalities – A South African Case Study'. *Social Science & Medicine* 54, no. 7: 1093–1110.

Gramsci, Antonio. 1992. *Prison Notebooks*. New York: Columbia University Press.

Haraway, Donna. 1991. *Simians, Cyborgs and Women: The Reinvention of Nature*. New York: Routledge.

Hoad, Neville. 2005. 'Thabo Mbeki's AIDS Blues: The Intellectual, the Archive, and the Pandemic'. *Public Culture* 17: 101–127.

Honkasalo, Marja-Liisa. 2009. 'Grips and Ties: Agency, Uncertainty and the Problem of Suffering in North Karelia'. *Medical Anthropology Quarterly* 23, no. 1: 51–69.

Ikhile, Deborah, Linda Gibson, and Azrini Wahidin. 2019. '"I Cannot Know That Now I Have Cancer!" A Structural Violence Perspective on Breast Cancer Detection in Uganda'. In *Gender, Global Health and Violence: Feminist Perspectives on Peace and Disease*, edited by Tiina Vaittinen and Catia Confortini. London and New York: Rowman & Littlefield.

Johnson, Leigh. 2012. 'Access to Antiretroviral Treatment in South Africa, 2004–2011'. *The Southern African Journal of HIV Medicine* 13, no. 1: 22–27.

Jungar, Katarina. 2011. *Long Live! South African HIV-Activism, Knowledge and Power*. Turku: Åbo Akademi University Press.

Jungar, Katarina and Elina Oinas. 2010. 'A Feminist Struggle? South African HIV Activism as Feminist Politics'. *Journal of International Women's Studies* 12, no. 1: (No page numbers). https://vc.bridgew.edu/jiws/vol11/iss4/13/. Accessed 7 September 2019.

Jungar, Katarina and Elina Oinas. 2011. 'Beyond Agency and Victimization: Re-Reading HIV and AIDS in African contexts'. *Social Dynamics* 16, no. 3: 248–262.

Lukić, Dragana and Ann Therese Lotherington. 2019. 'Fighting Symbolic Violence through Artistic Encounters: Searching for Feminist Answers to the Question of

Life and Death with Dementia'. In *Gender, Global Health and Violence: Feminist Perspectives on Peace and Disease*, edited by Tiina Vaittinen and Catia Confortini. London and New York: Rowman & Littlefield.

Martin, Emily. 2006. 'The Pharmaceutical Person'. *Biosocieties* 1, no. 3: 273–287.

Mbeki, Thabo. 2001. Address by President Mbeki at the Inaugural ZK Matthews Memorial Lecture, University of Fort Hare, 12 October 2001. Accessed 10 April 2019. https://omalley.nelsonmandela.org/omalley/index.php/site/q/03lv03445/04lv04206/05lv04302/06lv04303/07lv04304.htm.

Melber, Henning. 2008. 'Introduction: Revisiting the Heart of Darkness – Explorations into Genocide and Other Forms of Mass Violence'. *Development Dialogue* no. 50: 7–11. Accessed 24 April 2019. http://www.daghammarskjold.se/wp-content/uploads/2008/12/Development_dialogue_50_web.pdf.

Nattrass, Nicoli. 2004. *The Moral Economy of AIDS in South Africa*. Cambridge: Cambridge University Press.

Nattrass, Nicoli. 2007. *Mortal Combat: AIDS Denialism and the Struggle for Antiretrovirals in South Africa*. Scottsville: University of KwaZulu-Natal Press.

Nattrass, Nicoli. 2011. 'Defending the Boundaries of Science: AIDS Denialism, Peer Review and the Medical Hypotheses Saga'. *Sociology of Health and Illness* 33, no. 4: 507–521.

Nuño, Néstor M. 2019. 'Rethinking Global Health Priorities from the Margins: Health Access and Medical Care Claims among Indonesia's *Waria*'. In *Gender, Global Health and Violence: Feminist Perspectives on Peace and Disease*, edited by Tiina Vaittinen and Catia Confortini. London and New York: Rowman & Littlefield.

Oinas, Elina and Katarina Jungar. 2008. 'A luta continua! South African HIV Activism, Embodiment and State Politics'. *Development Dialogue* no. 50: 239–258. Accessed 24 April 2019 http://www.daghammarskjold.se/wp-content/uploads/2008/12/Development_dialogue_50_web.pdf.

Patton, Cindy. 1997. 'Inventing "African AIDS"'. In *The Gender/Sexuality Reader: Culture, History, Political Economy*, edited by Roger N. Lancaster and Micaela di Leonardo, 387–405. New York: Routledge.

Rabinow, Paul. 2011. *The Accompaniment: Assembling the Contemporary*. Chicago: University of Chicago Press.

Ratele, Kopano. 2006. 'Ruling Masculinity and Sexuality'. *Feminist Africa* 6: 48–64.

Reuterswärd, Camilla. 2019. '¡Malas Madres, Malas Mujeres, Malas Todas! The Incarceration of Women for Abortion-Related Crimes in Mexico'. In *Gender, Global Health and Violence: Feminist Perspectives on Peace and Disease*, edited by Tiina Vaittinen and Catia Confortini. London and New York: Rowman & Littlefield.

Richey, Lisa Ann. 2011. 'Antiviral but Pronatal? ARVs and Reproductive Health: The View from a South African Township'. In *Reproduction, Globalization, and the State*, edited by Carole H. Browner and Carolyn F. Sargent, 68–82. Durham: Duke University Press.

Richey, Lisa Ann and Stefano Ponte. 2011. *Brand Aid: Shopping Well to Save the World*. Minneapolis: University of Minnesota Press.

Riska, Elianne. 2010. 'Gender, Medicalization and Biomedicalization Theories'. In *Biomedicalization: Technoscience, Health, and Illness in the U.S.*, edited by Clarke

Adele E., Laura Mamo, Jennifer Ruth Fosket, Jennifer R. Fishman and Janet K. Shim, 147–170. Durham, NC: Duke University Press.

Robins, Stephen. 2004. '"Long Live Zackie, Long Live": AIDS Activism Science and Citizenship after Apartheid'. *Journal of Southern African Studies* 30, no. 3: 651–672.

Robins, Stephen. 2006. 'From "Rights" to "Ritual": AIDS Activism in South Africa'. *American Anthropologist* 108, no. 2: 312–323.

Sariola, Salla and Bob Simpson. 2019. *Research as Development: Clinical Trials, Collaboration and Bioethics in Sri Lanka*. London: Routledge.

Spivak, Gayatri Chakravorty. 1988. 'Can the Subaltern Speak?' In *Marxism and the Interpretation of Culture*, edited by Cary Nelson and Lawrence Grossberg, 271–313. Urbana: University of Illinois Press.

STATS SA. 2018. *Statistical Release P0302: Mid-Year Population Estimates 2018*. Accessed 24 April 2019. https://www.statssa.gov.za/publications/P0302/P0302 2018.pdf.

Tanyag, Maria. 2019. 'Replenishing Bodies and the Political Economy of SRHR in Crisis and Emergencies'. In *Gender, Global Health and Violence: Feminist Perspectives on Peace and Disease*, edited by Tiina Vaittinen and Catia Confortini. London and New York: Rowman & Littlefield.

Thompson, Charis. 2005. *Making Parents: The Ontological Choreography of Reproductive Technologies*. Cambridge, MA: MIT Press.

UNAIDS. 2010. 'UNAIDS Report on the Global AIDS Epidemic 2010'. Accessed 24 April 2019. http://www.unaids.org/globalreport/Global_report.htm.

UNAIDS. 2015. '2016–2021 Strategy'. Accessed 24 April 2019. http://www.unaids.org/sites/default/files/media_asset/20151027_UNAIDS_PCB37_15_18_EN_rev1.pdf.

Whyte, Susan R., Sjaak van der Geest and Anita Hardon, eds. 2002. *Social Lives of Medicines*. Cambridge: Cambridge University Press.

Williams, Simon, Paul Martin and Jonathan Gabe. 2011. 'The Pharmaceuticalisation of Society? A Framework for Analysis'. *Sociology of Health and Illness* 33, no. 5: 710–725.

Zola, Irving Kenneth. 1972. 'Medicine as an Institution of Social Control'. *Sociological Review* 20, no. 4: 487–504.

Part II

VIOLENCES ENTANGLED

Chapter 6

Fighting Symbolic Violence through Artistic Encounters: Searching for Feminist Answers to the Question of Life and Death with Dementia

Dragana Lukić and Ann Therese Lotherington

> *I was at the F ward in the nursing home. One of the residents was Tiffany Doggett, who played the part of an angel in the American series 'Orange Is the New Black'. Tiffany saw how Gilbert [another resident] wanted to open a window, but no matter the effort, he couldn't! He became afraid and stepped back. So Tiffany immediately went towards the window and opened it, stepping out on the balcony and gazing at Siri [a nurse in nursing clothes] who was standing across. Siri, calm and confident that the 'patient' would listen, said: 'Come on, Tiffany! Come on, do not go there!' But Tiffany did not obey. She looked at Siri in the eyes and thought: 'No, I do not want to! Because you should learn how it is to be accused of something you feel no guilt for'. Suddenly she jumped over the banister to her death. Her intention was to prove that she was present, that she knew what she was doing, and to demonstrate for Siri how it feels like to become a dementia patient. Siri would have to understand and take the consequences for what had happened; because now, it would be Siri's fault that one 'patient' jumped and that she lost control over her. It was her fault but also an institutional mistake. It was the system to blame for Tiffany's jump, and for the ward's lack of fresh air that had triggered the situation. The tension between the glass of window and Tiffany's hands made creaking sounds, which then, suddenly, disappeared.*

This dramatic situation took place in a dream the first author had during her fieldwork in a nursing home for people with dementia in May 2017. A claustrophobic atmosphere during some days at the nursing home overwhelmed her and affected her dreams. She felt a clear cut between 'them' and 'us' in dementia care – from 'their' point of view. This problematic us-them binary within dementia care and research is the pivot of this chapter. *They* – people living with dementia – are those who do not pass as *one of us*. *They* do not comply with the neoliberal ideal of ageing well – the demand for a disembodied, self-contained autonomous individual – and hence cannot pass as fully 'response-able' humans (Latimer 1999, 2018). In Dragana's dream, Tiffany did not follow the scripted 'them' but stepped back and jumped, and paradoxically produced herself as response-able.

Suicide is a fatal act of agency, while at the same time an effect of the us-and-them binary that powerfully stigmatises 'them'. In this chapter, we problematise how this binary in imaginations of dementia produces and reproduces suicide and euthanasia as the last response-able act for people who fail to be 'fully human'. People with Alzheimer's disease (AD) or other dementias (ADD) fall into this category. Worldwide, ADD is emerging as a health 'epidemic' that affects more than 46 million people and will affect 123 million by 2050 (World Alzheimer Report 2015). There is no cure on the horizon. Even so, the bulk of research funds worldwide is devoted to biomedical and pharmaceutical research situating the disease within individuals' brains as if the brains were isolated from the body and the environment. This biomedical understanding of ADD obscures the relational, material-semiotic, multisensorial human-non-human practices that challenge the dominance of such an understanding (Åsberg and Lum 2010; Haraway 1997; Lukić 2019). In concord with neoliberal ideals of the autonomous, response-able individual and a market-based logic of care as choice (Mol 2008 [2006]), the biomedical understanding of dementia is dominant both within health care and among the general public, producing the disease as deficiency and decay, potentially contributing to stigmatisation (Bond 1992). Suicide or suicidal thoughts are not uncommon effects of stigmatisation among people with ADD and next of kin alike (O'Dwyer et al. 2015; Purandare et al. 2009), and this is a feminist concern.

In 2015, a special issue of the journal *Feminism and Psychology* (Vol. 25:1), entitled *Suicide and Assisted Dying: Reflections on Sandra Bem's Death*, addressed feminist contributions to the 'right to die' debate in the case of the death of feminist scholar Sandra Bem. In this issue, Sue Wilkinson (2015) suggests that the right to suicide or assisted suicide is a feminist issue for people with ADD. Wilkinson argues that people who wish to end their lives before they lose their decision-making capacities and awareness of themselves, their loved ones, and the environment should be allowed to do so. Elderly women, in particular, have been socialised to comply with paternalistic, masculinist traditions; therefore, they should not be compelled to subordinate their desire to die to desire of their doctors (or daughters) to keep them alive as long as possible (Wilkinson 2015). Davis (2015) supports the claim that health professionals should not monopolise the decision to die. In the editorial for this issue, Kitzinger (2015) suggests, in agreement with Parks (2000, 32), that women's request to die may be dismissed as irrational due to their supposed self-denial and virtue of caring for others, not to be cared for. In contrast, in the same issue, other feminists argue for improved dementia care as a better solution than institutionalising the right to die (Andrews 2015). From the standpoint of feminist ethics, Tulloch (2015), in turn, criticises the implicitly male Cartesian model of a rational, disembodied, independent self as a norm that advances masculine attributes and behaviours over feminine attributes and behaviours. Furthermore, Callahan (2015, 112) addresses how a naturalised symbolic power of male domination utilises violence that opens a space for suicidal decisions for people living with ADD 'under the banner of increasing individual choice'.

We take this debate as our starting point, but argue that, with no way to cure the on-going and devastating brain damages, neither helping people to end their lives nor alleviating the burden of the disease through better care fully problematises the biomedical understanding of ADD. We do not see in these solutions much room for appreciating a life together in difference: for 'dwelling alongside and cherishing ... difference' (Latimer 2018,16). Hence, despite good intentions, the positions in the special issue have the potential to contribute to the production and reproduction of stigma through picturing life with a dementia diagnosis as a life not worth living. Our worry is that the positions could inadvertently produce fear among those afflicted and strengthen the image of the person with the diagnosis as 'the diagnosis only'.

By transcending the common biomedical foundation of the disease, and questioning the neoliberal logic of individualised autonomy, our aim is to offer new understandings of ADD. We approach this endeavour *first* via two previously told stories about women with Alzheimer's disease. The first story is about professor of psychology and feminist pioneer Sandy Bem, who died by suicide in May 2014 (Henig 2015). The second story is about a fictitious Professor of Linguistics, Alice Howland, whom we get to know in the popular novel and film adaptation *Still Alice* (Genova 2015 [2007]; *Still Alice* 2014). Alice considers suicide, but does not succeed.

Second, we comparatively analyse the stories using a feminist understanding of Bourdieu's (2001) theory of symbolic violence linked to Latimer's (2018) concept of stigma. We draw on feminist materialist theories and feminist visual studies of technoscience (Åsberg and Lum 2010) that defy hierarchical binaries between mind and body, self and other, subject and object, human and non-human, and are attuned to study differences enacted in practices. We demonstrate how the biomedical understanding of dementia, underpinned by a neoliberal masculinist order of the autonomous responseable individual and a neoliberal logic of care as choice (Mol 2008), reinforces symbolic gendered violence, rendering suicide a rational choice.

Third, through a merging of the theoretical concepts and the stories, we actualise 'being alongside' AD (Latimer 2013) by proposing different enactments of ADD. We suggest that artistic entanglements in everyday life are helpful for the development of different understandings of what cognition and connectivity might be, not only for people with ADD, but for everyone.

We retell the stories about the two women, Sandra Bem and Alice Howland, for three reasons: first, dementia figures globally as a feminised disease. Across the globe, women are disproportionally affected by ADD, both as people with the diagnosis and as next of kin (GADAA 2017). Since age is the strongest risk factor for developing ADD, and women live longer than men, more women than men will develop and live with ADD; they also more often bear the consequences of the disease alone (Bartlett et al. 2016). Worldwide, women account for more than two-thirds of the family carers and a majority of formal carers, performing feminised, devalued, overloaded, racialised, healthcare, and lowest-paid, social care jobs (GADAA 2017). In general, females next of kin experience a higher burden of care than males next of kin – also due to the aggressive behaviours of their male partners living with dementia (Lotherington et al. 2018) – while at the same time receiving less support than males next of kin (Gibbons et al. 2014). In addition, women with dementia receive less formal or informal support than men with dementia, and because women's spouses in heterosexual relationships are often not willing to care for them, they are institutionalised sooner (Bartlett et al. 2016). Consequently, women are more prone to stigmatisation (GADAA 2017). In spite of this, gender perspectives on stigma within dementia research are missing, and so are relational gender perspectives in policy guidelines and strategies worldwide (Bartlett et al. 2016; GADAA 2017).

Second, in the stories we relate, both Sandy and Alice strived to fulfil the neoliberal masculine ideal of being an independent, strong, active, free individual. Then they got AD. To continue to live this ideal, they chose suicide as a means of maintaining control over their lives, their loved ones, and the environment. Third, both stories provide knowledge about dementia, but in different ways. While Sandy Bem's story complies with the common understanding of dementia as deficit, Alice's story offers new possibilities of dwelling alongside dementia in artistic encounters, cherishing differences and breaking hierarchical dualisms between the biomedical and the artistic knowledge of dementia (Lukić 2019).

SANDY BEM: SUICIDE AS AN OPTION AND ASSISTED SUICIDE AS A POSSIBILITY

'The Last Day' is a story about Sandy Bem, as told by Robin M. Henig in the *New York Times Magazine* of 17 May 2015. Sandy Bem was a feminist pioneer, psychology professor and director of the Cornell University Feminist,

Gender, and Sexuality Studies Programme, who published a number of books on gender identities. Sandy was married to professor of psychology, Daryl, with whom she had a daughter, Emily, and a son, Jeremy. The Bems were known as an unusual couple, travelling worldwide to give public talks on gender stereotypes. They raised their children in a gender-neutral way, and shared household duties equally. However, when Emily and Jeremy grew older, Sandy felt that Daryl did not take enough responsibility at home. Therefore, the Bems went through a friendly separation after twenty-nine years of marriage, while Daryl continued visiting the family. When Sandy was diagnosed with mild amnestic cognitive impairment – a condition that in most cases progresses to AD within 10 years – she decided to end her life:

> She felt terror at the prospect of becoming a hollowed-out person with no memory, mind or sense of identity, as well as fury that she was powerless to do anything but to endure it. With Alzheimer's disease, she would write, it is 'extraordinarily difficult for one's body to die in tandem with the death of one's self'. . . . The prospect of mental decay was particularly painful for Sandy, whose idea of herself was intimately entwined with her ability to think deeply and originally. (Henig 2015, 38)

Sandy first told Daryl about her decision, then the other family members. No one opposed her. The question was when. She wanted as much joy as possible without waiting too long. She discussed this problem with Daryl who, after the diagnosis, became closer to her than ever before. He accompanied her to doctors' appointments, and Sandy was surprised at how attentive, gentle and emotive he had become. In spite of this 'gift' of tenderness and attention, she would never have accepted living with dementia (Henig 2015, 39). On the other hand, Daryl was surprised that Sandy's cognitive decline did not affect his feelings for her, and that their relationship rather heightened as the disease progressed. Daryl became, again, a central person in Sandy's life.

When Emily gave birth to Felix – Sandy's and Daryl's grandson – Sandy was thrilled: 'She told Emily that her "new brain" might actually make her better suited to being a grandmother than her focused, hyper-analytical "old brain"' (Henig 2015, 41). Sandy babbled songs and stories to Felix, without bothering about her memory loss. Emily liked her 'newer' mother. It had been hard to grow up with a hyper-critical one. She hoped this 'newer Sandy' would quit the suicide idea: 'Who should make the decision to die, the old Sandy or the new one?' (Henig 2015, 41). In this case, the 'old one' did.

Sandy appreciated sentient pleasures, but prioritised her ability to think critically and believed that this ability was a reflection of her true autonomy. After having read two books on 'dying with dignity' that Daryl brought her, she decided on a liquid substance controlled in the USA, called pentobarbital – a barbiturate that veterinarians use to euthanise animals and physicians for assisted suicides – to do the deed for her. She followed the instructions from one of the books and ordered the drug from a foreign supplier. Her younger sister Bev – who had been diagnosed with ovarian cancer a year before Sandy was diagnosed – offered the alternative that Sandy could have the drugs she might get from her doctor in Oregon, as Bev would not need them. For a long time, Sandy envied Bev's option to have her request to die accepted.[1]

Even though she had enough savings to prolong her treatment for AD, and be with Felix for one more year, her condition deteriorated, and she felt that she was losing control. Prolonging the treatment with expensive medications 'for Felix's sake' was not worth her savings (Henig 2015, 54). Therefore, she realised that time had come, and asked Daryl which date it should be. He chose 20 May. Nobody except Emily dared to challenge her decision. Emily was angry at everybody, particularly her father, because he was thinking 'so pragmatically about her mother's death' (Henig 2015, 54). However, the day before Sandy died, Emily admired her mother for choosing the right moment. On her last day, five years after receiving the diagnosis, Sandy printed an email called 'Ending' that she had written to Daryl nine months earlier, telling him why she wanted to die and stating that nobody was responsible for her death but herself. On the printout, she marked the date 20 May 2014, with the declaration: 'The time has come to end my life. I love you, Daryl' (Henig 2015, 56). After 5:30 pm, she wanted only Daryl to be in the room with her. She poured a glass of pentobarbital and a glass of wine, and asked Daryl twice which glass is the wine, which is the drug and if she could combine the wine and the drug. ' "That's not a good idea", Daryl answered. "You don't want to fall asleep before you've drunk it all"' (Henig 2015, 56). She died peacefully in her home on 20 May 2014 at the age of sixty-nine.

ALICE AND LYDIA: ARTISTIC ENTANGLEMENTS

We learn about Alice Howland in Lisa Genova's bestselling novel *Still Alice* (2015) and Glatzer's and Westmoreland's popular film adaptation, *Still Alice* (2014). Alice is a fifty-year-old honoured expert in linguistics and professor at Columbia University (*Still Alice* 2014). She is happily married to John, a professor in biomedicine, also at Columbia. They have three grown-up children: Anna, Tom, and Lydia. After some memory glitches and incidents of disorientation, Alice goes to the doctor and is diagnosed with early onset AD – a rare, but familial, disease probably also affecting her children. In a genetic test, it turns out that Anna carries the same gene mutation, while Tom's test is negative and Lydia refuses to be tested.

For a long time, Alice and John have disagreed about Lydia's path as a stage actress in Los Angeles (*Still Alice* 2014). Alice admires Anna and Tom for choosing 'real careers' in law and medicine and feels that Lydia is losing valuable time performing on the stage in LA (*Still Alice* 2014, 00:07:22). The tension between Alice and Lydia culminates when Alice finds out that John has been financially supporting Lydia's theatre company without informing her (*Still Alice* 2014). However, with the progression of Alice's disease, and Lydia's inclusion of her mother into her drama practices, the relationship between Alice and Lydia flourishes. In particular, reviewing plays with Lydia buttresses Alice's memory as she can talk over the scenes without having to compete, as she always does with John (Genova 2015). As they analyse the plays together, Alice comes to appreciate the strength of Lydia's intellect and emotions, feel Lydia and love her in a different way than before. At the same time, Lydia practises her roles while anticipating Alice's affection. As Alice's ability to speak declines, her ability to track 'body language and unspoken feelings' heightens (Genova 2015, 191). Lydia recognises Alice's inability to speak as an 'enviable skill' for an actor, who has to express actions and feelings without speaking (Genova 2015, 191). When Alice visits Lydia's theatre for the first time while she is playing the piece Alice had helped her to practise (Genova 2015), she finds it easy to empathise with the character Catharine, whom Lydia plays (Genova 2015; *Still Alice* 2014). Moved by the play, Alice acknowledges Lydia's acting skills off the stage, without realising that she is speaking to her own daughter (*Still Alice* 2014). No matter how defeating are the signs of her mother's decline, Lydia appreciates that Alice sincerely recognises her talent.

Inspired by Lydia's play, and following her encouragement, Alice writes a manuscript, hoping to deliver the most influential speech of her life at an Alzheimer's Association conference (Genova 2015). In comparison to her previous and famous speeches about linguistics worldwide, this time Alice is the subject of her own speech. She stands at the centre of the stage, advocating for people living with AD, emphasising their agency, and that they always are more than the disease, more than others' perceptions of them. She stresses that she is not a victim of AD, but that she is struggling to stay connected with the world and with her 'old ambitious self', who was 'fascinated with communication' (*Still Alice* 2014, 01:07:59).

As AD progresses, Alice's relationship with John declines. In her neurologist's office and without John as her closest advocate, Alice feels guilty for becoming an unreliable AD patient (Genova 2015). However, Alice begins to wonder if John, and not AD, triggers her decline (Genova 2015), while John cannot accept the situation of Alice being seriously ill and in need of him. He hates that AD is happening to them (*Still Alice* 2014). Alice hates it too. She would rather have cancer because then she would not feel like a social outcast. Beside social support, with cancer she would also deserve John's attention, as in his job he is dedicated to find a cure for cancer (Genova 2015; *Still Alice* 2014). Instead of taking the opportunity to be with her on a sabbatical for one year, John chooses to follow his career and moves to another city, leaving Alice with caretaker Elena, and Lydia, who decides to move back home. With tears in his eyes, John admits to Lydia: 'You are a better man than I am' (*Still Alice* 2014, 01:26:12).

Because of John's behaviour and Alice's own fear of burdening her family (Genova 2015), Alice decides to visit a nursing home for people living with dementia to see if this would be a place for her to live. She sees apathetic, elderly female residents in wheelchairs with no group activities and no loved ones around (*Still Alice* 2014). She realises that, for a young and physically fit person like her, a nursing home is not the answer. She imagines the fatal end with dementia: her body curled up in the foetal position, not able to swallow and, therefore, developing pneumonia (Genova 2015, 109). This is not the life she wants, so she secretly sets up her criteria for the timeliness of her suicide (*Still Alice* 2014): when she is no longer able to do the things she enjoyed in life, like eating ice-cream – 'when the burden of her disease exceeded the pleasure of that ice cream' (Genova 2015, 132) – she would want to die. She creates a memory test similar to the one her doctor and the neuropsychologist use (Genova 2015). When she is no longer able to pass that test, the time will have come. To be sure of fulfilling her plan, Alice records and stores a video of herself on her computer, addressing her future self:

> Hi Alice, I am you and I have something very important to say to you. So, I guess that you've reached that point, the point that you can no longer answer any of the questions. So, this is the next logical step. I am sure of it. In your bedroom, there is the dresser with a blue lamp, open the top drawer, in the back of the drawer there is a bottle with pills in it. It says take all pills with water. Now there are a lot of pills in the bottle but it is very important that you swallow them all. OK? And then, lay down and go to sleep. And do not tell anyone what you are doing. [After finishing the video, she types] 'When you can no longer answer these questions, go to a folder on your computer labelled Butterfly'. (*Still Alice* 2014, 01:19:51)

Alice calls the video 'Butterfly' because she once told Lydia that like the life of a butterfly, life with AD is short, but may be beautiful and worth living (S*till Alice* 2014). One day, Alice accidentally opens the video 'Butterfly', but after several attempts to proceed with the instructions, she drops the box of sleeping pills and they spill all over the floor (*Still Alice* 2014). Her suicidal plan fails. However, this does not seem to worry her too much as life goes on and she appreciates the pleasures of life in the moment. The film shows Alice confidently holding Anna's new-born twins, eating ice-cream with John, and discussing plays with Lydia. Even after her language is gone, she continues helping Lydia practise her theatre monologues. Both the book and the film conclude with a scene in which Lydia is reciting a part of the play to Alice, and Alice sees her as 'the actress', because she cannot remember Lydia's name (Genova 2015, 326). Lydia's interest is to figure out what Alice thinks about the play, focusing on her feelings and emotions, rather than narrative, coherence, and words:

> Alice watched and listened and focused beyond the words the actress spoke. She saw her eyes become desperate, searching, pleading for truth. She saw them land softly and gratefully on it. Her voice felt at first tentative and scared. Slowly, and without getting louder, it grew more confident and then joyful, playing sometimes like a song. Her eyebrows and shoulders and hands softened and opened, asking for acceptance and offering forgiveness. Her voice and body created an energy that filled Alice and moved her to tears. (Genova 2015, 326)

In an immediate closeness to Lydia's face and lips' movements asking from Alice to express what the play was about, Alice articulates, searching for words that are mostly already lost for her, the word 'Love' (*Still Alice* 2014, 01:30:29; Genova 2015). Lydia repeats, confirms to her mother: 'Yes . . . it was about love', acknowledging a physically mutual feeling as well as their comprehension of the meaning of the play (*Still Alice* 2014, 01:30:37; Genova 2015).

SANDY AND ALICE: SUICIDAL AGENTIAL CUTS

Our analysis of the two stories problematises hierarchical binaries in which we see locations of symbolic violence in 'agential cuts'. Drawing on quantum physics, feminist philosopher Karen Barad (2007, 140) defines 'agential cuts' as enactments of particular space-time-matters within phenomena that emerge as effects of material-discursive intra-actions. Barad (2007, 33, emphasis in the original) defines intra-action as '*mutual constitution of entangled agencies*'. To be entangled is to lack individual self-contained existence (Barad 2007, ix). Hence, 'intra-actions' presuppose inseparable agencies that emerge through mutual and dynamic processes of becoming, in contrast to 'interactions' that presuppose pre-existence of individual self-sustained agencies. Cartesian cuts enact inherent hierarchical and static distinctions between an individualised subject and object and other hierarchical distinctions, in contrast to agential cuts that enact 'inherent ontological (and semantic) indeterminacy' not pre-existing as individual entities but resolving as '*exteriority-within-phenomena*' (both quotes from Barad 2007, 140, emphasis in the original). Barad (2007, 140, 72) defines phenomena as 'diffraction patterns'

(Haraway 1997, 16), that is, iterative, material-discursive 'patterns of difference that make a difference' in particular space-time-matters cuts.

In what follows, we analyse particular agential cuts in Sandy's and Alice's stories of living/dying with dementia. Doing so, we demonstrate how the symbolic gendered violence that is co-constituted within these cuts is also structurally maintained (Bourdieu 2001), with physical, harmful effects, one extreme of which is suicide. Finally, we propose a different understanding of ADD as not necessarily harmful but potentially vitalising, producing joy and connectivity within creative art encounters.

Both Sandy and Alice are white, middle-aged, married women (one previously married), with higher education, higher-class status, and an American background, tying the stories to Western Euro-American biomedical visions of ADD (Åsberg and Lum 2009) that make the contemplation of suicide possible. Public debates on euthanasia are in general a white-educated-privilege, where the opinions of subordinated groups by race, class, and gender are invisible and deviant. Jennings and Talley (2003), for instance, have demonstrated that people with racialised backgrounds are more likely to oppose euthanasia, because of both their collective history of abuse, and their lack of trust in the medical profession. Less-educated people and elderly women also tend to oppose euthanasia. Future research on euthanasia should, therefore, pay attention to intersections between race, class, and gender, as well as other cultural differences (Jennings and Talley 2003). In different socio-cultural environments, ADD and suicide might not be issues at all (Hulko 2009).

Sandy and Alice also share a common background as worldly, honoured intellectuals cherishing their cognitive mastery as their main defining feature. They dread losing the ability to think and use their brains intellectually – a feature that Rooney (2017) describes as associated with the mind, in opposition to the body, in Western philosophical tradition. The mind figures as the centre of our thinking that 'owns the body' and controls its movements through the environment (Vaittinen 2017, 138). In the history of Western philosophy and modern political thinking, mind is commonly associated with masculinity and the body with femininity (Grosz 1994; Vaittinen 2015). Likewise, the biomedical understanding of ADD situates the disease within the brain as an isolated, self-referential organ set apart from the body and the environment (Åsberg and Lum 2009). In contrast, indigenous worldviews, some religious worldviews, and feminist materialist theories subsequent to those views suggest an understanding of thinking as an entanglement of mind, body, and the environment (Mortimer-Sandilands 2008). As the most dominant in the environment of the contemporary West, the biomedical understanding of ADD thus shapes our thinking, potentially making us understand ADD as a deficit, overshadowing other realities of life with the disease (Moser 2008).

Here we see symbolic gendered violence as elaborated in Bourdieu's *Masculine Domination* (2001). Masculine domination, Bourdieu argues, is a paradigmatic form of symbolic violence that acts as an insidious, omnipresent, and subtle domination by masculine virtues, durably maintained via institutions as logical universal calculations. Masculine domination – the androcentric world order – revolves around the hierarchical primary opposition of male/female, followed by the secondary oppositions of top/bottom, public/private, outside/inside, big/small, strong/weak, and mind/body. Such a world order prioritises masculinist virtues at the top of all hierarchies, while exposing vulnerable gendered human beings, women in particular, to symbolic violence. This means, effectively, erasure, silencing, and de-valorisation of all that is coded as feminine – violence reminiscent to cultural violence (Reuterswärd, this volume) and epistemic violence (Confortini and Vaittinen; Féron, this volume). Within this order, the dominant is masculinised with symbols of virility, honour, and duty, while the dominated is feminised. This naturalises the sexes and their relations, and potentially humiliates men who do not conform to the symbolic power and authority of the dominant masculine ideal (Bourdieu 2001, 22; cf. Nuño; Féron, this volume). On the other hand, masculinised women may achieve intellectual independence but still be placed as objects into a 'double bind' (Bourdieu 2001, 67). Acting according to a dominant masculine ideal necessarily *defeminises* these women, leaving them with the only options to participate in the masculine order or leave (Bourdieu 2001, 68) – perhaps by suicide.

Hence, symbolic violence is already material – it is, to apply Barad's terminology, *material-discursive* violence. It acts 'at the deepest level of the body' through 'familiarisation' with established dispositions, in which the dominated may feel systematic self-denigration, taking the 'form of bodily emotions – shame, humiliation, timidity, anxiety, guilt – or *passions* and *sentiments* – love, admiration, respect' (Bourdieu 2001, 38). Therefore, being in relationships of domination is not a matter of choice or constraint (Bourdieu 1992, 168). Rather, it is a mode of living (or dying) that is made possible upon the acceptance of structures of domination that are not imposed by force but taken as self-evident. Both Sandy and Alice accept the biomedical understanding of AD as an abject failure of personhood (cf. Latimer 1999). While for Alice a quickly deteriorating memory is the criterion for suicide, for Sandy it is a sense of losing control over her life. Both criteria adhere to the elusive neoliberal (white masculine) autonomous capitalist ideal (more on this later) of response-ability and able-bodiedness, which require constant body work and brain elasticity to age successfully (Latimer 2018). This biomedical understanding produces self-sustaining, autonomous subjects with an isolated brain as the centre for the formation of subjectivity (Åsberg and Lum 2010; Lukić 2019). In such a rationalistic hegemonic order, suicide becomes an option, and neglect of care a naturalised possibility. This is shown, for instance, by Purandare et al. (2009), who underscore that the risk of suicide is elevated in younger persons with dementia, as they are more aware of the disease and are still able to take care of, and make decisions for themselves.

The stigma associated with a dementia diagnosis is so strong that suicidal ideation often emerges shortly after a diagnosis has been disclosed (Erlangsen et al. 2008). Latimer (2018) explains stigma as an effect of complex entanglements of biomedical, political, and cultural practices evolving from dementia's relationship with ageing – perceived as the individual's abject failure in the context of neoliberal world making. This ageing-dementia relation – the process of ageing entangled with the processes of becoming 'the demented other' – figures as a 'double jeopardy', particularly in Euro-American biomedicalised culture (Greengross 2014, 6 in Latimer 2018). This relation leads to a cultural and social magnification of becoming the hollowed-out person in a zombie state (Behuniak 2010), finally suffocating from pneumonia (which both Alice and Sandy fear).

The ageing-dementia relation is a failure in the masculine, neoliberal symbolic order, because it represents an unavoidable downward spiral, subverting the ideal of the highly cherished youthfulness of modernity. This stigma affects everybody who fails to enact the active, vigorous, and self-sustained ideal of 'successful aging', producing misfits with internalised feelings of guilt and weakness. According to Latimer (2018, 2), 'growing old badly', that is, failing to remain response-able, emerges as the biggest sin. The stigma that emerges with the ageing-dementia relation, then, operates as a series of *agential cuts*: they are enacted as effects of material-discursive intra-actions with ADD, sustained through media representations, public discourse, and healthcare institutions, while legitimising the use of medicalisation for reduced costs and enhanced profitability. Taken together, these political and cultural practices violently transform people with ADD into non-humans (Latimer 2018).

Early on, in the doctor's office, Sandy brings up her final decision about suicide, while Alice carries her decision secretly alone. Neither uses physical pain as a reason, but mainly each underscores the fear of losing her sense of identity (Sandy) and becoming a burden of care (Alice). Steinbock (2005) affirms that suffering and losing a sense of autonomy and control over one's own life are the main reasons for suicide requests among people in general, rather than pain. Clear Lewis (2010), a disabled activist, points out that the usual response to suicidal people is not to help them die but to help them live better lives. From a disability studies perspective, if debility is the reason why a person may be granted assistance in dying, then it means that persons with disabilities and their lives are less valuable. The clear-cut distinctions between a healthy and diseased 'self', as between able-bodied and disabled individuals, are grounded in the linear 'peak-and-decline ideology' (Gullette 2017, 4), in which gradual decline and ageing with a disease are inevitable. Gullette (2017) argues that the neoliberal rational order generates ageism, producing 'incitements to suicide' as the norm for the elderly, particularly women, insofar as they are the majority. The neoliberal order pushes people with disabilities to 'choose' death (Shildrick 2015). This, we argue, is symbolic violence at the heart of gendered symbolic orders of health and life.

Both Sandy and Alice make the clear-cut distinction between the 'older self' and 'self with AD', where the 'older self' – the more rational, liberal, independent self – is the one to make the suicide decision. However, the 'older self' cannot predict when the diseased self will stop enjoying life and when the right moment to die will be. Alice thinks that no longer enjoying an ice-cream would be one important sign. However, she continues enjoying ice-cream even after her suicide attempt. Feeling that she is losing control and capacity to end life with AD, Sandy asks Daryl to decide a right date. Hence, the coherent self in which both Sandy and Alice believe – isolated from the environment and from others – does not exist. The 'self' is never static, and agency is not an attribute of the body, or the rational mind. Rather, as Karen Barad (2007) emphasises, agency emerges in 'intra-actions' with*in* the environment, not in relation to an environment that is external to an individuated 'self'.

THE NEOLIBERAL STRUCTURES OF SYMBOLIC VIOLENCE

The violence of the biomedical understanding of dementia is not only embedded in circulating terminology regarding life with ADD (e.g. dignity or not) but also in the rationalist logic of choice (Mol 2008). Therefore, the symbolic gendered violence in question reshapes not only our language, culture, and bodies but also how we live and the decisions we make. Indeed, to return to Bourdieu (2001, 83), symbolic gendered violence is maintained via institutions (the state, nursing homes, family, etc.) that are de-historicising and permanently preserving masculine domination. Following neoliberal ideology, the state is presently dismantling welfare services for elderly citizens in Western, democratic ageing societies (Andersson and Kvist 2015; Burke 2015; Tronto 2017; Vaittinen 2017), thereby cutting off collectivity (Bourdieu 1998). Neoliberal ideology celebrates the abstract self-centric, self-realising, able-bodied, white male independent individual (Burke 2015), focusing on the accumulation of wealth and excluding all those who are seen as intruders disrupting (his) independence (Code 1991, 77).

Such individualist ideology values isolation, separation, and the formal sameness of individuals whose 'interdependence is at best *manageable* if carefully regulated; at worst it is straightforwardly menacing' (Code 1991, 80). Those who do not fit in these ideals are alienated as 'others'. In such a reality, people living with dementias are always in deficit, in need not only of constant care but also of third-party mediation between their needs and the market logic of choice. They emerge as a burden doomed always to fail to become accountable as 'human' and 'normal' autonomous individuals according to a medical norm (Moser 2011). In contrast, a logic of care is preoccupied with liveable, unpredictable bodies entangled with a more-than-human environment *interfering* with a disease, figuring out how to craft care to create a good balance and live better *with* a disease. The logic of care does not impose a limit, give up, or say no to 'unprofitable' patients (Mol 2008).

To come back to our analysis of Sandy's and Alice's stories, both calculate the financial and emotional prospects of the disease. Sandy will not, even if she could, financially cover the cost of further treatment of her AD. She does not want to be *that* Sandy. Alice, on the other hand, cannot imagine herself ageing in a nursing home after she visits a stereotypical home that does not allow for connectivity and joy. What Alice saw was probably a nursing home in which the effects of work pressure and lack of resources, which were likely a result of constant neoliberal cuts, only sustained the biological functions of life (Hoppania and Vaittinen 2015). Having internalised the symbolic order of (neo)liberal individualism, she does not want to end her life in a nursing home that is founded on hierarchical relations and procedures, in which bodies with AD would not pass as full humans but as dependent 'others'. Her rejection of the biomedical culture in the nursing home delivers, therefore, a critique of the neoliberal masculinist symbolic order, while paradoxically strengthening agential individualisation. Hence, she rather produces herself as agential, as Tiffany did. Yet, as we emphasise towards the end of this chapter, life with dementia – also in nursing homes – can be otherwise (see also Vaittinen, this volume).

AD is surrounded with such a stigma that Alice and Sandy would rather have had cancer. Therefore, both prefer death to a life with AD. They both act as response-able citizen-consumers, choosing a medical product (pentobarbital for Sandy, sleeping pills for Alice) to attempt ending their lives. While Sandy shares her suicidal decision with family members, Alice develops her suicide plan secretly because she fears the reactions of her family. Sandy's decision to die is 'both enabled through, and constrained by, the relational and legal contexts in which she live[s]' (Peel and Harding 2015, 38). Suicidal decisions are also effects of intimate relationships in which next of kin are deeply involved and need more time to learn to cope with ADD (Martin 2015), or to go through another exit, as John does. John continues to live a life that is in line with the dominant, masculine, independent, biomedical ideal of life, prioritising his own career in cancer research over life with Alice – and dementia. John's choices are in line with the biomedical quest for a cure (Falcus 2014) that surpasses the relational and emotional dimensions of life. Hence, as Falcus (2014) suggests, John's crying at the end enacts the failure of this quest and the failure of the biomedical understanding of AD.

We learn from Sandy's story that AD strengthens her relationship with Daryl, but even so, suicide triumphs. Drawing on Bourdieu's (2001, 109–112) understanding of love within the symbolic violent order – the supreme and most subtle and invisible form of masculine domination based on trust and disinterestedness – we suggest that their love relationship co-constitutes symbolic gendered violence. As AD progresses, Sandy takes on a position of the dominated female in her relationship with Daryl, as she leaves it to him to decide the last day of her life, and relies on his help to end her life. Alice's relationship with John also co-constitutes symbolic gendered violence as Alice inevitably falls into the dominated position of a dependent AD patient, with internalised feelings of guilt as imposed on both Alice and her intimate others by the surrounding biomedical culture. Feelings of guilt are an effect of stigma, the symbolic and material ageing-dementia relation that affects both Alice and Sandy. This stigma makes them 'choose' suicide, a 'choice' that is amplified within relationships of domination, and the symbolic gendered violence that circulates through them.

ENACTMENTS OF BEING ALONGSIDE DEMENTIA(S)

Bypassing suicide as a matter of concern, Sandy and Alice's stories demonstrate how AD is *enacted* differently in particular space-time-matter cuts of 'being alongside' the disease. Here, we find Mol's (2002, 32) term 'enactment' useful, as it connotes the disease 'being done' differently within different situated practices. 'Enactment' disrupts the binaries of subject/object, epistemology/ontology, culture/nature, and goes well with Barad's ontology of agential realism, particularly the intra-actions of space-time-matters in agential cuts.

We read Sandy and Alice's stories of living with dementia and seeking to control death as an enlightening series of differently situated agential cuts – that is, specific resolutions of *indeterminacy* between the subject and object, and other hierarchical distinctions (Barad 2007) – which delineate meanings of AD. Here, each space-time-matter cut emerges as an enactment of AD as a phenomenon intertwined with other enactments that go 'beyond choice' (Mol 2002, 178). Enactments of AD then intra-act and are never a coherent whole – AD is never a coherent whole, but in *constant ongoing processes of becoming*. With this understanding, we see the potential to disrupt the biomedical comprehension of AD as timeless, spaceless, fixed, and universal. To do this and propose different – and hence liveable – AD enactments in particular space-time-matter cuts, we utilise Latimer's understanding of 'being alongside' dementia which breaks the dualistic humanist visions of the autonomous individual, allowing entities to emerge differently through multisensorial artistic encounters situated in time and space (cf. Vaittinen, this volume).

Latimer (2013) formulates 'being alongside' as a human-non-human animal relational encounter, in which both parties are being partially connected and partially divided, each preserving a sense of difference and mutuality. The parties are not becoming 'better humans', but are becoming differently through the encounter (Barad 2007). Hence, the relation enacted cherishes differences and differential becomings. Although Latimer uses this concept for studying human-non-human animal relations – sensitive to multisensorial post-humanist ways of living together respectful of differences – we adapt this concept to demonstrate how AD is enacted differently in Alice's and Sandy's stories within particular agential cuts.

For instance, in Sandy's story, the relationship between Sandy and Emily is strengthened after the Alzheimer's diagnosis. Using babbling sounds and emotions with her grandson, Felix, enables Sandy to communicate differently and hence *become differently* alongside Felix, transforming her from the critical 'old' Sandy to the 'new' Sandy which ultimately enacts AD as a mutual delight in an agential cut. Thus, using Barad's terminology, the encounter between Sandy and Felix delineates inherent ontological and semantic indeterminacy between them as the subjects of the encounter, and AD as the object that enables the encounter. In contrast to a/the Cartesian cut that enacts absolute separability (and independency) between subject and object (i.e. individual independence of Sandy and Felix from AD situated in Sandy's brain), this situated agential cut enacts 'local', 'contingent separability' *within* the encounter which creates conditions for objectivity (Barad 2007, 348, 350).

However magical they are, these moments are not enough for Sandy to endure the disease. Such very present perceptual moments are undermined in the context of a neoliberal rationalist ideology that values reflection over perception and requires a coherent, autonomous self, capable of rational comprehension and expression (Mortimer-Sandilands 2008). Therefore, not even the 'gift' of a renewed relationship with Daryl persuades Sandy to endure the disease. Her life with AD ends in an agential cut while being alongside Daryl. This agential cut resolves indeterminacy between the subjects (Sandy and Daryl), the object (AD), and the instrument (pentobarbital). We interpret this last cut in Sandy's life as 'choice' within a neoliberal masculinist individualist order, which perpetuates symbolic gendered violence.

However, Alice's story is more complex. We learn that the relationship between mother and daughter (Lydia) strengthens. In her artistic drama encounters with Lydia, Alice becomes Lydia's most reliable audience, and AD is enacted as an 'enviable skill' that evolves into a most influential speech at the Alzheimer's conference (Lukić 2019). The artistic intra-active encounters create a world in themselves (Latimer 2012) and the environment, while becoming differently alongside each other. In her artistic drama entanglements with Lydia, thanks to AD, Alice becomes differently abled to communicate beyond language and the meanings of words. Simultaneously, Lydia becomes the professional actress, whom Alice helps her to acknowledge. In the final space-time-matters cut, Alice *feels* what Lydia expresses by using her body, gesticulation, and different voice tonalities, becoming emotionally touched. Beyond the words, she realises and articulates the meaning of the play physically, inviting Alice to articulate the word love at a point when she has mostly lost the ability of verbal communication. They are together in a joint intra-active artistic drama entanglement, partially connected with different accomplishments. In this intra-active entanglement of which Alice and Lydia are subjects, AD – an object intertwined with the subjects – is enacted as enviable skill-professional actress.

All these different enactments within the two stories intermesh, and, eventually, the emergent entanglements determine the choices to be made (Mol 2002). In Sandy's case, the biomedical enactment of ending one's life to survive dementia dominates, while in Alice's case, artistic entanglements of being alongside Lydia defeat the understanding of her life as the life of a misfit. Lydia and Alice's relationship demonstrates that life with AD can be valuable to live, as we argue – also in nursing homes (see Vaittinen, this volume) – if we are tuned into multisensorial aspects of life that do not stigmatise 'them' as distinct from 'us'. Having done field work in a nursing home for a long time, Dragana also experienced lovely and joyful moments through artistic as well as care encounters. Luckily, the prologue that began this chapter was just a dream. Yet, we have seen how Tiffany's fatal act of response-able agency repeats in Alice's fictional and Sandy's factual stories.

ARTISTIC ENCOUNTERS AND THE
ART OF LIFE

In this chapter, we have argued that the symbolic gendered violence of a biomedical understanding of AD, amplified by a stigmatised ageing-dementia relation, produces suicide and assistance in suicide as choices. This violence affects all gendered human beings, particularly women. We find that the feminist 'right to die' movement is grounded in this biomedical understanding of AD, prescribing life with dementias as un-liveable. We build on a feminist debate on assisted suicide in *Feminism and Psychology*, to examine the symbolic gendered violence in dominant understandings of AD, and analyse how this violence affects Sandy and Alice, two women living with AD and seeking to control death. We propose that different enactments of AD emerge in multisensorial encounters of 'being alongside' dementia. We offer the examples of a multisensorial entanglement between Sandy and Felix – and their 'irrational' babbling, as an agential space-time-matter cut – and of the last liveable emotional entanglement between Sandy and Daryl – which ultimately dies the last day of Sandy's life.

Although we draw our analysis of symbolic violence using the factual narrative on Sandy's and her family's life with AD, we do not take an individualistic approach that would lead us to moralise about suicide or make judgements about actual people. The intention of exploring Sandy's 'choice' to die due to AD – and consequently the agential choices of other people living with AD to end their lives – is not to dismiss or reject these possibilities, but to problematise the individualisation of these choices within a neoliberal masculinist symbolic order. The point is that *we do not own our choices* even though we *do them* and choices are individually enacted. Our analysis focuses, rather, on the symbolic gendered violence that we encounter within the neoliberal order that we are part of. Therefore, our hope is that the analysis rather enlightens a multiplicity of situated 'choices' that each space-time-matters cut enacts.

We discuss the more profoundly multisensorial, artistic entanglement between Alice and Lydia. Given the latter example, as a conclusion, we propose that in the artistic encounters that extend connectivity beyond the cognitive abilities and able-bodiedness of the people involved, different possibilities for lives with dementias emerge. The world that Alice and Lydia create while being alongside AD situates AD in-between the limits of life and death for a moment, where having AD is just one of the meaningful experiences in life that is unfolding in-between the dreams of tomorrow and longings for the past (Lukic 2019; *Still Alice* 2014). In contrast to Sandy, Alice fails to die by suicide but lives on and continues to appreciate life in moments, making us see the value of arts in life – and perhaps value the art of life. The entangled, if sometimes conflicting, enactments of AD that we have described suggest that a life with the disease might be prosperous and worth living, even towards the end, and that artistic modes of knowing and producing new knowledge about AD should have legitimacy and validity, in feminist debates on global health and beyond.

NOTE

1. Physician-assisted dying has been legal in Oregon since 1997, but for people living with AD different regulations apply (Kitzinger 2015) and therefore Sandy may not have had her request to die accepted even if she would have lived in Oregon (Henig 2015). In the state of New York, where Sandy lived, terminally ill people do not have the right to physician-assisted dying.

REFERENCES

Andersson, Katarina and Elin Kvist. 2015. 'The Neoliberal Turn and the Marketization of Care: The Transformation of Eldercare in Sweden'. *European Journal of Women's Studies* 22 no. 3: 274–287.

Andrews, June. 2015. 'II. Keeping Older Women Safe from Harm'. *Feminism and Psychology* 25, no. 1: 105–108.

Åsberg, Cecilia and Jennifer Lum. 2009. 'PharmAD-Ventures: A Feminist Analysis of the Pharmacological Imaginary of Alzheimer's Disease'. *Body and Society* 15, no. 4: 95–117.

Åsberg, Cecilia and Jennifer Lum. 2010. 'Picturizing the Scattered Ontologies of Alzheimer's Disease: Towards a Materialist Feminist Approach to Visual Technoscience Studies'. *European Journal of Women's Studies* 17, no. 4: 323–345.

Barad, Karen. 2007. *Meeting the Universe Halfway: Quantum Physics and the Entanglement of Matter and Meaning.* Durham, NC: Duke University Press.

Bartlett, Ruth, Trude Gjernes, Ann Therese Lotherington and Aud Obstefelder. 2016. 'Gender, Citizenship and Dementia Care: A Scoping Review of Studies to Inform Policy and Future Research'. *Health and Social Care in the Community*, 1–13. https://doi.org/10.1111/hsc.12340. Accessed 7 September 2019.

Behuniak, M. Susan. 2010. 'The Living Dead? The Construction of People with Alzheimer's Disease as Zombies'. *Ageing & Society* 31, no. 1: 70–92.

Bond, John. 1992. 'The Medicalization of Dementia'. *Journal of Aging Studies* 6, no. 4: 397–403.

Bourdieu, Pierre. 1998. *Acts of Resistance: Against the New Myths of Our Time.* Cambridge: Polity Press.

Bourdieu, Pierre. 2001. *Masculine Domination.* Cambridge: Polity Press.

Bourdieu, Pierre and Loïc J. D. Wacquant. 1992. *An Invitation to Reflexive Sociology.* Cambridge and Malden, NJ: Polity Press.

Burke, Lucy. 2015. 'The Locus of Our Dis-Ease: Narratives of Family Life in the Age of Alzheimer's'. In *Popularizing Dementia: Public Expressions and Representations of Forgetfulness*, edited by Swinnen, Aagje and Schweda, Mark, 23–41, Bielefeld: Transcript Verlag.

Callahan, Sidney. 2015. 'III. A Feminist Case against Self-Determined Dying in Assisted Suicide and Euthanasia'. *Feminism and Psychology* 25, no. 1: 109–112.

Code, Lorraine. 1991. *What Can She Know? Feminist Theory and the Construction of Knowledge*. Ithaca and London: Cornel University Press.

Confortini, Catia C. and Tiina Vaittinen. 2019. 'Introduction: Analysing Violences in Gendered Global Health'. In *Gender, Global Health and Violence: Feminist Perspectives on Peace and Disease*, edited by Tiina Vaittinen and Catia Confortini. London and New York: Rowman & Littlefield.

Davis, Kathy. 2015. 'IX. Dying, Self-Determination, and the (Im)Possibilities of a "Good Death"'. *Feminism and Psychology* 25, no. 1: 143–147.

Erlangsen, Annette, Stevan H. Zarit and Yeates Conwell. 2008. 'Hospital-Diagnosed Dementia and Suicide: A Longitudinal Study Using Prospective, Nationwide Register Data'. *American Journal of Geriatric Psychiatry* 16, no. 3: 220–228.

Falcus, Sara. 2014. 'Storying Alzheimer's Disease in Lisa Genova's *Still Alice*'. *EnterText* 12: 73–94.

Féron, Élise. 2019. 'Élise. 2019. 'When Is It Torture? When Is It Rape? Discourses on Wartime Sexual Violence'. In *Gender, Global Health and Violence: Feminist Perspectives on Peace and Disease*, edited by Tiina Vaittinen and Catia Confortini. London and New York: Rowman & Littlefield.

GADAA (Global Alzheimer's and Dementia Action Alliance). 2017. 'Women and Dementia: A Global Challenge'. Published February 2017. Accessed 6 January 2018. https://www.gadaalliance.org/wp-content/uploads/2017/02/Women-Dementia-A-Global-Challenge_GADAA.pdf.

Genova, Lisa. 2015 (2007). *Still Alice*. London: Simon and Schuster.

Gibbons, Carrie, Joy Creese, Mun Tran, Kevin Brazil, Lori Chambers, Bruce Weaver and Michel Bédard. 2014 'The Psychological and Health Consequences of Caring for a Spouse with Dementia: A Critical Comparison of Husbands and Wives'. *Journal of Women and Aging* 26, no. 1: 3–21.

Greengross, Baroness S. 2014. 'Foreward'. In *A Compendium of Essays: New Perspectives and Approaches to Understanding Dementia and Stigma*, edited by Sally-Marie Bamford, George Holley-Moore and Jessica Watson, 6–7. London: ILC-UK.

Grosz, A. Elizabeth. 1994. *Volatile Bodies: Toward a Corporeal Feminism*. Bloomington and Indianapolis: Indiana University Press.

Gullette, M. Margaret. 2017. 'How Does Incitement Work When the Target Is Not an Adolescent, But Old People?' *International Network for Critical Gerontology*, Published 4 August 2017. Accessed 30 December 2017. http://criticalgerontology.com/incitement-suicide/.

Haraway, J. Donna. 1997. *Modest_Witness@Second_Millennnium: FemaleMan_Meets_OncoMouse*. New York and London: Routledge.

Henig, R. Marantz. 2015. 'The Last Day'. *The New York Times*, 17 May 2015.

Hoppania, Hanna-Kaisa and Tiina Vaittinen. 2015. 'A Household Full of Bodies: Neoliberalism, Care and "the Political"'. *Global Society* 29, no. 1: 70–88.

Hulko, Wendy. 2009. 'From "Not a Big Deal" to "Hellish": Experiences of Older People with Dementia'. *Journal of Aging Studies* 23: 131–144.

Jennings, K. Patricia and Clarence R. Talley. 2003. 'A Good Death?: White Privilege and Public Opinion: Research on Euthanasia'. *Race, Gender and Class* 10, no. 3: 42–63.

Kitzinger, Celia. 2015. 'I. Feminism and the "Right to Die": Editorial Introduction to the Special Feature'. *Feminism and Psychology* 25, no. 1: 101–104.

Latimer, J. Elizabeth. 1999. 'The Dark at the Bottom of the Stairs: Performance and Participation of Hospitalized Older People'. *Medical Anthropology Quarterly* 13, no. 2: 186–213.

Latimer, J. Elizabeth. 2012. 'Home Care and Frail Older People: Relational Extension and the Art of Dwelling'. In *Perspectives on Care at Home for Older People*, edited by Christine Ceci, Kristín Björnsdóttir and Mary Ellen Purkis, 35–61. New York and London: Routledge.

Latimer, J. Elizabeth. 2013. 'Being Alongside: Rethinking Relations amongst Different Kinds'. *Theory, Culture and Society* 30, no. 7/8: 77–104.

Latimer, J. Elizabeth. 2018. 'Repelling Neoliberal World-Making? How the Ageing-Dementia Relation is Reassembling the Social'. *The Sociological Review*, 66, no. 4: 832–856. https://doi.org/10.1177/0038026118777422. Accessed 7 September 2019.

Lewis, Clair. 2010. 'Clair Lewis: Disabled People Need Assistance to Live, Not Die'. *Independent*, 28 February 2010. Accessed 28 December 2017. http://www.independent.co.uk/voices/commentators/clair-lewis-disabled-people-need-assistance-to-live-not-die-1911313.html.

Lotherington, Ann Therese, Aud Obstfelder and Gøril Ursin. 2018. 'The Personal Is Political Yet Again: Bringing Struggles between Gender Equality and Gendered Next of Kin onto the Feminist Agenda'. *NORA – Nordic Journal of Feminist and Gender Research*, 1–13. https://doi.org/10.1080/08038740.2018.1461131. Accessed 7 September 2019.

Lukić, Dragana. 2019. 'Multiple Ontologies of Alzheimer's Disease in *Still Alice* and *A Song for Martin*: A Feminist Visual Studies of Technoscience Perspective'. *European Journal of Women's Studies*. https://doi.org/10.1177/1350506819831718. Accessed 7 September 2019.

Martin, Norah. 2015. 'VI. From the Theoretical to the Personal: Weighing Further Feminist Concerns on Physician-Assisted Suicide and Euthanasia'. *Feminism and Psychology* 25, no. 1: 124–130.

Mol, Annemarie. 2002. *The Body Multiple: Ontology in Medical Practice*. Durham, NC: Duke University Press.

Mol, Annemarie. 2008 (2006). *The Logic of Care: Health and the Problem of Patient Choice*. London and New York: Routledge.

Mortimer-Sandilands, Catriona. 2008. 'Landscape, Memory, and Forgetting: Thinking through (My Mother's) Body and Place'. In *Material Feminisms*, edited by Stacy Alaimo and Susan Hekman, 265–287, Bloomington: Indiana University Press.

Moser, Ingunn. 2008. 'Making Alzheimer's Disease Matter: Enacting, Interfering and Doing Politics of Nature'. *Geoforum* 39: 98–110.

Moser, Ingunn. 2011. 'Normalitetens grenser, pris og alternativer – funksjonshemning som levd realitet'. ['Limits, Price and Alternatives of Normality – Disability as Experienced Reality'.], *Tidsskrift for Den norske legeforening* 9, no. 10: 962–964.

Nuño, Néstor M. 2019. 'Rethinking Global Health Priorities From the Margins: Health Access and Medical Care Claims among Indonesia's *Waria*'. In *Gender, Global Health and Violence: Feminist Perspectives on Peace and Disease*, edited by Tiina Vaittinen and Catia Confortini. London and New York: Rowman & Littlefield.

O'Dwyer, T. Siobhan, Wendy Moyle, Melanie Zimmer-Gembeck and Diego De Leo. 2015. 'Suicidal Ideation in Family Carers of People with Dementia'. *Aging and Mental Health* 20, no. 2: 222–230.

Parks, A. Jennifer. 2000. 'Why Gender Matters to the Euthanasia Debate: On Decisional Capacity and the Rejection of Women's Death Requests'. *The Hastings Center Report* 30, no. 1: 30–36.

Peel, Elizabeth and Rosie Harding. 2015. 'VII. A Right to "Dying Well" with Dementia? Capacity, "Choice" and Relationality'. *Feminism and Psychology* 25, no. 1: 137–142.

Purandare, Nitin, Richard C. Oude Voshaar, Cathryn Rodway, Harriet Bickley, Allstair Burns and Nav Kapur. 2009. 'Suicide in Dementia: 9-Year National Clinical Survey in England and Wales'. *The British Journal of Psychiatry* 194: 175–180.

Reuterswärd, Camilla. 2019. '¡Malas Madres, Malas Mujeres, Malas Todas! The Incarceration of Women for Abortion-Related Crimes in Mexico'. In *Gender, Global Health and Violence: Feminist Perspectives on Peace and Disease*, edited by Tiina Vaittinen and Catia Confortini. London and New York: Rowman & Littlefield.

Rooney, Phyllis. 2017. 'Rationality and Objectivity in Feminist Philosophy'. In *The Routledge Companion to Feminist Philosophy*, edited by Ann Garry, Serene J. Khader and Alison Stone, 243–255. New York and London: Routledge.

Shildrick. Margrit. 2015. 'Death, Debility and Disability'. *Feminism and Psychology* 25, no. 1: 155–160.

Steinbock, Bonnie. 2005. 'The Case for Physician Assisted Suicide: Not (Yet) Proven'. *Journal of Medical Ethics* 31, no. 4: 235–241.

Still Alice. 2014. Glatzer, Richard and Wash Westmoreland. Stockholm: BSM Studio.

Tronto, Joan. 2017. 'There Is an Alternative: Homines Curans and the Limits of Neoliberalism'. *International Journal of Care and Caring* 1, no. 1: 27–43.

Tulloch, Gail. 2015. 'IV. Sandra Bem, Feminism, Assisted Suicide and Euthanasia'. *Feminism and Psychology* 25, no. 1: 113–117.

Vaittinen, Tiina. 2015. 'The Power of the Vulnerable Body: A New Political Understanding of Care'. *International Feminist Journal of Politics* 17, no. 1: 100–118.

Vaittinen, Tiina. 2017. *The Global Biopolitical Economy of Needs: Transnational Entanglements between Ageing Finland and the Global Nurse Reserve of the Philippines*. PhD diss. (published). Tampere Peace Research Institute and Tampere University Press: http://urn.fi/URN:ISBN:978-952-03-0505-5. Accessed 7 September 2019.

Vaittinen, Tiina. 2019. 'Exposed to Violence While Caring: From Caring Self-Protection to Global Health as Conflict Transformation'. In *Gender, Global Health and Violence: Feminist Perspectives on Peace and Disease*, edited by Tiina Vaittinen and Catia Confortini. London and New York: Rowman & Littlefield.

World Alzheimer Report. 2015. 'The Global Impact of Dementia: An Analysis of Prevalence, Incidence, Cost and Trends'. Republished with corrections October 2015. London: Alzheimer's Disease International. Accessed 1 June 2018. https://www.alz.co.uk/research/WorldAlzheimerReport2015.pdf.

Chapter 7

¡Malas Madres, Malas Mujeres, Malas Todas!: The Incarceration of Women for Abortion-Related Crimes in Mexico

Camilla Reutersward

Since the turn of the century, Latin America's restrictive and persistent abortion policies underwent unprecedented change. After decades of policy stasis, watershed liberalisations in Chile, Colombia and Uruguay eased previously conservative laws. At the same time, however, El Salvador, Honduras and Nicaragua among others restricted their already limited policies and, in some cases, outlawed abortion under all circumstances. Accompanying this uneven pattern of policy change has been a growing rate of incarcerations of women for abortion-related crimes. From El Salvador and Mexico in Central America to Brazil, Bolivia and Argentina in the Southern Cone, women have been prosecuted for alleged illegal abortions and on separate charges for aggravated homicide – accused of murdering their newborns. Between 1990 and 2008, 417 women received sentences for illegal abortions in Argentina (Carbajal 2016; Kane, Galli and Skuster 2014). In El Salvador, 129 women were prosecuted for abortion-related crimes in the first decade of the 2000s and in federal Brazil, 334 police reports in the Rio de Janeiro state involved illegal abortions between 2007 and 2011 (CIMAC Noticias 2017; Strochlic 2016). During the same time period, 775 abortion-related criminal investigations opened in Bolivia (Kane, Galli and Skuster 2014). In Mexico, cases such as Dafne McPherson, who miscarried in a mall bathroom in Querétaro and received a prison sentence of sixteen years accused of homicide, increasingly made media headlines (Agren 2017).

Incarcerations for abortion-related crimes began to receive international attention in 2010 when news broke of the impoverished indigenous women sentenced to over thirty years in prison for aggravated homicide in the state of Guanajuato in central Mexico. Now released from prison and nicknamed *Las Libres* [The Free] after *Centro Las Libres* [Centre of The Free], the Non-Governmental Organization (NGO) that successfully litigated their cases, the women's stories made news around the world. In interviews, *Las Libres* explained to journalists how obstetric emergencies had landed them in prison for aggravated homicide, a crime that carries sentences for up to thirty years. Investigations in the aftermath of the scandal found that 679 women were reported and convicted for the crime of abortion in Mexico between 2009 and 2011. At least 124 of those cases involved women sentenced for aggravated homicide (GIRE 2015; Martínez 2014). However, no reliable official statistics exist, and it is likely that more women are currently imprisoned on abortion-related charges.[1]

In Mexico, incarcerations for illegal abortions or aggravated homicide appear to have increased in the aftermath of restrictive legal change. Following Mexico City's legalisation of abortion in 2007, a rapid wave of conservative counter-reforms swept the Mexican states and ushered in restrictive change in seventeen states (Lopreite 2014). As I return to next, however, these reforms did not change the penal codes that govern abortion policy. Rather, local constitutions were amended to 'protect the right to life from the moment of conception' seeking to pre-empt future policy liberalisations.[2] The passage of such reforms or other types of restrictive legislation does not however imply strict enforcement. In fact, incarcerations for abortion-related crimes are a relatively recent phenomenon (Kane, Galli and Skuster 2014). In most of Latin America, states for decades – if not centuries – largely ignored the fact that women seek abortions regardless of its legal status and rarely invoked penal codes. Restrictive policies combined with little enforcement of criminal codes generated an industry of clandestine abortions with grave implications for maternal mortality. Notably, the region suffers from the world's highest number of maternal deaths from illegal abortions (Centre for Reproductive Rights 2015). Available data, however, suggests that states in Latin America did not begin to systematically prosecute women for abortion-related crimes until the first decade of the 2000s. What explains this sudden change?

This chapter explores the intersection of gender, global health and violence through the lens of incarcerations for abortion-related crimes in Mexico. I examine the multiple causes behind abortion-related sentences focusing on the state as the perpetrator of gender violence. Building on insights from feminist scholarship and using Johan Galtung's typology of violence as an analytic tool, I examine how the state through its gendered practices engages in multiple forms of violence that intersect to specifically target marginalised women. Direct or personal violence takes the shape of incarcerations in this chapter and stands in sharp contrast to indirect or structural violence. Also referred to as social injustice, structural violence is a process, a 'slow killer' expressed through inequality, above all in the distribution of power. It can include repressive structures, exploitation or marginalisation and more concretely, poverty or lack of education and health care. Cultural violence, by contrast, refers to aspects that motivate and legitimise acts of direct and structural violence. Oftentimes symbolic and built into all areas of social life – including in laws – cultural violence operates to make 'direct and structural violence look, even feel, right, or at least not wrong' (Galtung 1990, 291).

Focusing on incarcerations for abortion-related crimes highlights the ways in which the state as a gendered and gendering structure maintains control over women and their bodies via laws, policies and practices and perpetrates multiple forms of violence simultaneously. Galtung's framework provides a useful starting point for analysing the origin and reproduction of different forms of violence. However, his conceptualisation does not account for *who or which actor* that perpetrates violence and the multiple ways in which these different forms may intersect. Importantly, although Galtung acknowledges that structural violence arises from and is upheld by man-made systems, he defines it as lacking a subject or agent. But if we accept that 'structural violence is inequality, above all in the distribution of power' (Galtung 1969, 175), we should direct our attention to actor(s) with distributive capacities. The state, with its power to allocate resources, create policies and enforce sanctions, is one of them. By specifying the state as an actor that perpetrates structural, in addition to cultural and direct forms of violence, I depart from Galtung's 'neutral' conceptualisation to make visible how these forms of violence are mutually constituted, produced and reproduced.

The state has the capacity to subject citizens (and non-citizens) to violence. As Weber once claimed, it has monopoly over the means of violence within its territory. Moreover, it has the ability to shape and alter gender relations (Waylen 1998). Previous scholarship primarily centres on the state as a perpetrator of sexual violence during times of peace or conflict (e.g. Cohen 2013; Sanford, Stefatos and Salvi 2016). A limited number of works also examine abortion-related legal proceedings (e.g. Eggers 2018; Viterna and Guardado Bautista 2014). Few studies, however, examine state-perpetrated gender violence in the context of reproductive health policy and its implications. I focus on the causes behind incarcerations for abortion-related crimes and use Galtung's typology as an analytic tool, placing the state with its various actors, institutions and governance levels at the centre of the framework.

In this chapter, I show how incarcerations for abortion-related crimes result from the state's capacity to perpetrate direct, indirect and cultural violence simultaneously, and how such violence is motivated and legitimised by a systematic gender bias. In Mexico, I find that reforms that protect life from the moment of conception have created a climate of confusion and fear regarding abortion's legal status. Although such amendments do not alter penal codes, they are commonly interpreted to outlaw abortion. For fears of being prosecuted themselves, medical personnel, as a result, report women for suspected illegal abortions to a greater extent. Once investigations open, grave due process violations, lack of evidence and outdated methods characterise these legal proceedings that ultimately operate to incriminate the individual women on trial. Expectations related to motherhood and female sexuality are deeply implicated in these processes. Women perceived to transgress boundaries set by traditional gender roles by allegedly committing abortion-related crimes are punished with severe prison sentences. These interrelated forms of structural and cultural violence thus motivate and legitimise direct violence in the shape of incarcerations. Above all, they operate to target women already marginalised due to their location at the intersection of gender, race/ethnicity and socioeconomic class.

I draw on data collected during field research in four Mexican states – Guanajuato, Hidalgo, Mexico City and Yucatán – between 2015 and 2016. In each state, I conducted semi-structured interviews with legislators, bureaucrats and civil society actors on the topic of abortion policy. I also draw on archival sources including newspaper articles and NGO reports. In what follows, I provide a brief overview of feminist analyses of the state. Building on previous insights, I propose a framework to examine the multiple ways in which the state perpetrates gender violence. In subsequent sections, I apply this framework to the case of incarcerations for abortion-related crimes in Mexico. Using empirical evidence, I show how the state commits direct, indirect and cultural violence and how these different forms intersect to target marginalised women. I conclude with suggestions for future research.

THEORISING THE STATE AS A PERPETRATOR OF GENDER VIOLENCE

Conventional IR theories long considered the state to be the main provider of security for citizens during both peace and war. Starting from the 1990s and onwards, however, feminist scholars begun to question the state's ability to guarantee safety and analyse its gendered and gendering capacities based on the oppression and discrimination women experienced at the hands of states.[3] In groundbreaking works, Cynthia Enloe (1990) and Ann Tickner (1992) among others demonstrated how the state's inability to provide security for non-combatants derives from its gendered construction (see also Peterson 1992; Wilcox 2011). Rather than providing security, states' military capacity operates to legitimise a social order that valorises violence and threatens women's security (Tickner 1997). These insights generated analyses that challenged conventional notions of the state as the framework within which security should be defined. Specifically, feminist scholars pointed to the masculine structures and assumptions that gender state institutions and the discourses that emanate from them (Youngs 2004). States have enforced women's subordination by reflecting, creating and legitimising particular forms of gender relations (and their inherent inequalities) through laws, policies and practices (Waylen 1998). For example, Laura Shepherd (2005, 385) shows how discourses of violence against women are inherently gendered as they rest upon 'unstated and unquestioned' beliefs about gender and perceptions of what it means to be a victim or a perpetrator. Analysing gender discourses within the *Declaration on the Elimination of Violence against All Women*, Shepherd finds that women are cast as passive victims of violence whereas men are portrayed as aggressors that are in control, which aligns with dominant discourses and reproduces ideas of a 'natural' gender order. As states ratify the treaty and incorporate it into domestic legal frameworks, they reproduce dominant gender discourses.

States uphold gendered systems not only via structures and institutions such as the military but also through treaties and policies. Theorising the link between reproductive autonomy, policy and state violence, Bejarano Celaya and Acedo Ung (2014) proceed from the notion that the state, as the keeper of social order, uses violence to keep women in a subordinate position vis-à-vis men. Gender violence, in this case in the form of restrictive reproductive rights policies, operates to control women and keep them enclosed in the private sphere of the home. Legal frameworks that address women's bodies, such as abortion policies, thus constitute a space for the projection of state power and control and as such, a form of violence that maintains state dominance (Waylen 1998). Drawing on Galtung's conceptualisations of violence, the state's gendering power and capacity to maintain structures that subordinate women in themselves constitute forms of cultural and indirect violence, manifested through unequal and repressive structures but also via laws and policies that limit women's bodily autonomy. As Confortini (2006, 355) notes, gender relations are 'implicated in the very creation of violence. Violence is made possible by the existence of gendered power relations, and these structures in turn rely on violence for their reproduction'.

I start from the premise that the state must be understood as a power structure that seeks to maintain the gender relations that underpin its dominance. Building on previous feminist scholarship, I make three theoretical propositions with the purpose of advancing our understanding of state-perpetrated violence. First, to make visible the various forms that state-sanctioned violence can take, the state must be disaggregated to make visible the many different actors and instances involved.[4] Rather than a homogenous entity, the state comprises a collection of actors and institutions at varying governance levels that produce and reproduce inherently gendered discourses, policies and practices. Many of these constitute, or build on, existing forms of cultural and structural violence that the state enforces by authorising direct violence – for example, in the form of incarcerations. As my analysis demonstrates, the authorisation of state violence does not necessarily take place at the national level. Rather, state agents are placed at different governance levels and within a plethora of institutions that range from the legislature to the public health system and the judiciary. Second, because of the various actors and institutions involved in producing, reproducing and enforcing gender through discourses, policies and practices, the resulting violence can take many forms. The state has the power to maintain structural forms of violence such as economic inequality and discrimination but can also perpetrate cultural violence by shaping social values and beliefs that subordinate certain groups. It reproduces these types of violence through the judicial system, which sanctions direct violence. Thus, states have the capacity to perpetrate multiple types of violence simultaneously. Third, these forms of state-perpetrated violence intersect to target vulnerable groups. In a system that subordinates women, such groups commonly include individuals marginalised by their location at the intersection of gender, race/ethnicity and socioeconomic class.

ABORTION POLICY REFORM AND INCARCERATIONS: GENDERED LEGAL STRUCTURES

We are facing a serious violation of human rights, cruel, degrading treatment and torture, and inquisitorial and accusatory practices in which power and criminal law as well as women's ignorance and economic poverty are abused to create an authentic witch hunt. (Cruz Sánchez 2011, 182)[5]

The case of women incarcerated for alleged illegal abortions and aggravated homicide first received media attention in Mexico as well as internationally in 2010, when news broke of the indigenous women sentenced to up to thirty years in prison in the state of Guanajuato. The story of the nine women who were released after months of litigation work on behalf of a local NGO, *Centro Las Libres*, quickly turned into a nation-wide scandal.[6] Although authorities in the state, located just northwest of Mexico City, denied that any women were incarcerated for abortion-related crimes, *Las Libres* had begun to investigate cases in 2009, finding a total of 130 women sentenced for illegal abortions and nine sentenced with the maximum penalty of thirty years in prison for aggravated homicide (Cruz Sánchez 2011).

The case of the nine women unleashed a public debate that revolved around the injustice of the verdicts. Media condemned the long sentences, pointing to the marginalised situation of the imprisoned women, all of whom were young women of indigenous descent residing in poverty-ridden rural zones.

Several of the women did not speak Spanish at the time of their verdicts and, as I return to, did not receive translation services. All of the women were detained, prosecuted and imprisoned after seeking medical assistance for obstetric emergencies at public hospitals (Amuchástegui, Flores and Aldaz 2015; Cruz Sánchez 2016). The perception that these processes explicitly targeted marginalised women caused public outrage and *Las Libres* quickly became the symbol of the injustice of criminal procedures related to abortion in Mexico.

Incarcerations for alleged illegal abortions were largely unknown in Mexico prior to 2010. The Guanajuato scandal, however, became a catalyser for attention to abortion-related crimes and new cases quickly emerged from the state of Nuevo León in the north to Yucatán in the south (GIRE 2015). The number of criminal proceedings appeared to have increased in the aftermath of the wave of constitutional 'right-to-life' reforms that swept the Mexican states from 2008 and onwards as a conservative response to Mexico City's legalisation of abortion the previous year (Lopreite 2014).[7] In Guanajuato, as well as in other states that approved identical bills, the local constitution was amended to include a clause that lays out the state's responsibility to 'protect life from the moment of conception'. Although these amendments do not alter the penal codes that govern abortion, but rather create a complex legal dilemma of coexistence between the two, they are commonly interpreted to outlaw abortion (GIRE representative, Mexico City, interviewed May 6, 2016).

Consistent with this claim, the number of initiated criminal proceedings increased following the enactment of reforms across Mexico. Merely a month after the state of Baja California passed a 'right-to-life' reform, a twenty-year-old woman was arrested for having induced an abortion more than two years prior (Maier 2010). In the southeastern state of Yucatán, the number of abortion-related criminal processes more than tripled after the enactment of an identical reform in 2009. While thirty abortion-related criminal proceedings took place in the state between 1872 and 2009 – a time period of 137 years – the public ministry initiated eight procedures between 2009 and 2015 alone (Legal coordinator, Unidad de Atención Sicológica, Sexológica y Educativa para el Crecimiento Personal, UNASSE, Yucatán, interviewed 14 September 2015). Across the Mexican states, recent numbers suggest that authorities opened 426 criminal investigations related to abortion in the first nine months of 2018 alone (Gutiérrez González 2018). Moreover, judges in several states have interpreted constitutional reforms to grant embryos the same legal protections as full-grown adults, encouraging prosecutions for aggravated homicide rather than illegal abortions – crimes that carry significantly higher punishment with up to thirty years in prison (GIRE 2015; Toribio 2017). Table 7.1 shows the number of reports, trials and sentences for

Table 7.1. Reports, trials and sentences of abortion-related crimes per state

State	Reports	Trials	Sentences
Aguascalientes	6	1	1
Baja California	75	0	0
Baja California Sur	7	0	0
Campeche	3	0	No info
Chiapas	No info	2	0
Chihuahua	25	5	1
Coahuila	4	0	0
Colima	1	No info	No info
Durango	4	3	0
Guanajuato	50	1	1
Guerrero	0	1	3
Hidalgo	1	7	1
Jalisco	24	3	No info
México	No info	No info	No info
Mexico City	183	12	6
Michoacán	26	3	1
Morelos	4	2	3
Nayarit	1	2	No info
Nuevo León	45	0	0
Oaxaca	2	1	0
Puebla	9	7	1
Querétaro	11	2	0
Quintana Roo	81	1	No info
San Luís Potosí	6	4	3
Sinaloa	12	1	3
Sonora	8	2	1
Tabasco	2	2	0
Tamaulipas	26	4	1
Tlaxcala	5	0	0
Veracruz	57	7	1
Yucatán	3	2	1
Zacatecas	1	0	0
All states total	482	68	28

Source: GIRE 2015.

abortion-related crimes across the Mexican states from August 2012 through December 2013.[8]

Mexico's restrictive abortion policies circumscribe women's rights to decide over their own bodies. 'Right-to-life' reforms that in some states also give the foetus personhood status have exacerbated this lack of bodily autonomy by creating a perception that abortion is illegal under all circumstances. These deeply gendered legal structures must be understood in relation to the role of the state in constructing and controlling women's bodies. While building on layers of structural and cultural forms of violence, these policies, in turn, sanction direct violence in the form of incarcerations for abortion-related crimes. The motivation behind the enforcement of criminalising policies must be considered in relation to the implications for other realms, in particular the medical.

THE MEDICAL SPHERE: LEGAL UNCERTAINTY AND MANDATORY REPORTING

> You realize that the criminalization of women for abortion and aggravated homicide concern the way in which the state looks at you, treats you, threatens you – that the officials are the state. (Feminist activist and scholar, Guanajuato, interviewed 15 November 2016)

The enactment of 'right-to-life' amendments across the Mexican states produced a climate of confusion and fear regarding the legal status of abortion. In contrast to the penal code reforms in El Salvador and Nicaragua that completely outlawed abortion, Mexico's constitutional amendments have legal implications that remain largely unknown. As such, the reforms have caused widespread confusion among citizens and medical personnel concerning the circumstances under which abortion is legal or not. Many now believe that abortion is illegal under all circumstances. As a representative at *Grupo de Información en Reproducción Elegida* (Information Group on Chosen Reproduction; GIRE), Mexico's largest reproductive rights NGO, explains: 'Women, health care professionals, law enforcement – no one knows whether or not abortion is legal. And then you read in the newspaper that abortion is prohibited and you believe that it is true' (GIRE representative, Mexico City, interviewed 6 May 2016).

Unsure of abortion's legal status and obliged to report suspected criminal cases, doctors, nurses and social workers have begun to denounce women to a greater extent (GIRE 2015). As elsewhere in the region, health professionals in Mexico have a legal obligation to report patients suspected of illegal abortions to the police to not be considered accomplices (CIMAC Noticias 2017).[9] Indeed, experts at GIRE find that 'all they [medical personnel] know is that if a woman comes in with what can be considered an induced abortion, they will report it to avoid being prosecuted themselves' (GIRE representative, Mexico City, interviewed May 6, 2016). Consequently, public hospitals have converted into 'pipelines to prison for poor women who suffer miscarriages' (Driver 2017). Important to note here is that public hospitals report the bulk of alleged illegal abortions, which has implications for a particular group of women – those who cannot afford private health care. Indeed, in Guanajuato, medical personnel in public hospitals denounced the majority of the marginalised women reported and prosecuted for abortion or aggravated homicide (Cruz Sánchez 2011). As a politician in the local congress explains: 'Doctors and nurses are obliged to report cases and create a protocol, but it is supposed to enhance women's rights – not criminalise them. It shows the repressive nature of the state – a state that persecutes women' (Local politician, Guanajuato, interviewed 25 November 2015).

The 'right-to-life' amendments that a majority of Mexican states adopted between 2008 and 2015 resulted in widespread confusion regarding abortion's legal status. Unsure of its legality but obliged to report suspected abortion-related crimes, medical personnel have become agents of the state who report women and contribute to growing incarceration rates (see also Harman, this volume). These denunciations disproportionally target marginalised women who for economic reasons seek assistance at public hospitals rather than private clinics, and make visible the multiple forms of structural and cultural violence at play. Laws and policies that limit women's bodily autonomy in the field of sexual and reproductive health constitute forms of cultural violence (cf. Tanyag, this volume). Unclear legal frameworks that encourage the practice of reporting alleged illegal abortions, in turn, create new structures of inequality by transforming public hospitals into unsafe places for already marginalised women – a two-folded type of structural violence. Combined, structural and cultural violence legitimise and authorise direct violence in the form of incarcerations, which show their interrelated, almost circular, nature and highlight the state's central role as a perpetrator through its various actors and institutions.

FLAWED LEGAL PROCESSES: MULTIPLE FORMS OF STRUCTURAL VIOLENCE

Grave due process and human rights violations characterise the processes that result in sentences for abortion-related crimes in Mexico. While systematic data is largely lacking, available documentation suggests that many cases exhibit similar features, such as process violations that include a striking lack of evidence to establish criminal culpability (Toribio 2017). The story of Guadalupe in the state of Querétaro is illustrative: one month after receiving obstetric care at a public hospital, Guadalupe received a phone call from a police officer informing her that a criminal investigation had been initiated against her and that she was required to testify before the Public Ministry. Guadalupe had not been notified that hospital staff had reported her to the police, nor had she received the required formal summons. As the proceedings continued, it became evident that no evidence existed that indicated that Guadalupe had, in fact, attempted an illegal abortion. Furthermore, the case was built on the testimony of a doctor who acknowledged that he did not remember Guadalupe. A year later, due to the lack of evidence, authorities closed the investigation (GIRE 2015, 106). Although these irregularities constitute due process violations, they nevertheless appear common in criminal proceedings related to abortion. In several states, doctors and police officers have forced women to confess to having illegally induced abortions as a condition for receiving medical care, or while still under the effects of anaesthesia (GIRE representative, Mexico City, interviewed 6 May 2016; Montalvo 2013). These confessions – in legal terms self-incrimination – also constitute obvious cases of due process violations. Nevertheless, they have been used to determine culpability without additional corroborating evidence (GIRE 2015).

Beyond due process violations, a lack of evidence that binds women to their alleged crimes has characterised abortion-related proceedings. To distinguish between self-induced, illegal abortions and spontaneous miscarriages can be a difficult task for a trained medical doctor, and much more so for police officers or prosecutors without medical education (Carbajal 2016; journalist and feminist activist, Hidalgo, interviewed 18 February 2016). Yet state authorities have initiated criminal investigations against women regardless of whether or not evidence indicates an induced or spontaneous abortion (Toribio 2017). In most cases, mere assumptions have sustained the alleged crimes. In 2012, Hilda López de la Cruz in the state of San Luis Potosí was sentenced to one year in prison for an illegal abortion. The evidence that the State Attorney General's Office presented could not, however, verify her culpability as the required medical examinations were never carried out. Moreover, health personnel at the local public hospital conditioned her care on confessing to having ingested a pill to induce an abortion. No evidence could, however, validate that a pill provoked the abortion, and Hilda was sentenced to prison based solely on medical personnel's accusations (GIRE 2015). Similarly, in the case of *Las Libres* in Guanajuato, no evidence linked the alleged crimes to the sentenced women as the prosecutors failed to establish intention (Cruz Sánchez 2011). As I return to next, the prosecuted women's perceived transgression of expectations related to motherhood and sexuality motivated and legitimated these processes.

Law enforcement officers moreover use widely discredited methods to determine women's culpability. Responding to a GIRE-distributed questionnaire, public ministries in twenty-one out of Mexico's thirty-one states responded that they use the 'float test' as evidence in cases of aggravated homicide. Formally known as the *pulmonary docimasia* technique, the test is based on the idea that if the lungs of a foetus float when placed in a water container, it was born alive. The medical community has, however, disregarded this test since it lacks a scientific basis – several factors may, in fact, cause the lungs to float at the moment of birth. Many states nevertheless continue to use the technique as evidence in criminal trials, and in particular to determine culpability for aggravated homicide (GIRE 2015; Martínez 2014).

Marginalised women with few resources to defend themselves against the state's sanctioning power are particularly vulnerable to flawed legal proceedings, which ultimately make them the main targets for prosecutions for abortion-related crimes. Adriana Manzanares Calletano in Guerrero did not speak Spanish at the moment of her verdict and was denied translation services. Adriana, an eighteen-year-old indigenous woman from a poor rural area, was sentenced to twenty-seven years in prison in 2006 for aggravated homicide without any evidence presented against her (GIRE 2015; Martínez 2014). As Verónica Cruz Sánchez argues: 'Had these women [incarcerated for abortion-related crimes] been rich, they never would have gone to prison' (Director of Las Libres, Guanajuato, interviewed 26 November 2015).

Due process violations, insufficient evidence to determine culpability and the use of outdated methods characterise abortion-related legal proceedings in Mexico. These flawed processes constitute forms of structural violence perpetrated by state actors – in this case public ministries and state-level attorney general's offices that form part of the judicial system. Structural violence, in turn, authorises direct violence in the form of incarcerations. These flawed legal processes interact with gender, class and race/ethnicity to target marginalised women who are unlikely to afford a private lawyer and have to rely on state-provided legal aid. As a result, they are overrepresented among those convicted for abortion-related crimes. Despite the difficulties of determining whether an abortion is illegally induced or in fact a spontaneous miscarriage, prosecutors across Mexico seem to prioritise investigating cases of alleged illegal abortions. With a hint of irony, GIRE investigator Isabel Fulda expressed her surprise at this determination in an interview with the newspaper *Excelsior*: 'It is quite impressive how, given our country's poorly functioning justice system, criminal processes are initiated very quickly in these cases' (Toribio 2017). In what follows, I use Galtung's concept of cultural violence to explain why state agents come to prioritise abortion-related crimes.

CULTURAL VIOLENCE: SOCIAL EXPECTATIONS OF MOTHERHOOD AND SEXUALITY

The Catholic Church's centuries-long dominance in Mexico has shaped ideas of women's roles in society as well as values concerning the family, reproduction and sexuality. Catholic beliefs gave way to ideas of motherhood as sacred and women as the symbol of the family in their roles as mothers, caregivers and wives (e.g. see Ortiz-Ortega 2007). As Smith-Oka notes in her study of indigenous motherhood in Mexico: 'Within the Mexican imagination, mothers are revered, often held up as paragons of virtue; they are the embodiment of the Virgin Mary – chaste, purse, devoted, and self-sacrificing' (2014, 152). Women's association with motherhood and almost exclusive responsibility as caregivers under the premise of their reproductive capacity have created the notion that motherhood is the destiny of any and all women, and women's status in society remains closely linked to maternity (Bejarano Celaya and Acedo Ung 2014, see also Sánchez Bringas et al. 2004). Against this cultural backdrop, women accused of inducing illegal abortions or killing their newborns 'voluntarily' lose their children and 'choose' to not become mothers. Not only do they leave expectations related to the behaviour of 'good' mothers unfulfilled, they also contradict deeply rooted beliefs that motherhood constitutes the goal for all women.[10] Journalistic accounts of cases of abortion-related crimes both reflect and reproduce these notions. In Guanajuato, where media closely followed the story of *Las Libres*, a local politician described it as follows: 'The case of these women was very exemplary. Media portrayed them as brutal aggressors, as hyenas' (Local politician, Guanajuato, interviewed 25 November 2015). Indeed, media labelled Hilda López de la Cruz as well as the other women prosecuted for aggravated homicide as bad mothers: 'They said I did not want my son. In 2012, I was arrested again and media said it was because I am a murderer' (Montalvo 2013).

Not only in Mexico are socially constructed ideas of 'good' and 'bad' motherhood central aspects of abortion-related criminal proceedings. Analysing the case of seventeen women incarcerated for aggravated homicide in El Salvador, Viterna and Guardado Bautista also find that judges often 'cite women's violations of social expectations of motherhood to justify their guilty verdicts' and the idea that these women, as mothers, should have done more to prevent the death of their foetuses is recurring (2014, 20). One verdict explicitly states that: 'she [the prosecuted woman] was in a pregnant state, and as a result, she had an obligation to take care of and protect the little one she carried in her belly' (ibid. 2014, 9). In Mexico, prosecutors and judges commonly deride women for lacking the proper maternal instinct (Strochlic 2016). In the verdict that sentenced her to sixteen years in prison, Dafne McPherson in Querétaro was found to have acted with 'insufficient maternal instinct to protect her recently born child'. The judge argued that it was not credible that Dafne was unaware of her pregnancy and compared her to an animal, declaring that 'not even a dog would do this' (La Silla Rota 2018).

The association between alleged abortion-related crimes and 'bad' motherhood is, in turn, linked to women's sexuality and ultimately, morality. Many of the prosecuted women were involved with men who were not their husbands and became pregnant following non-marital relations As Smith-Oka notes: 'For the state, good mothers follow the rules, have few children, and invest in them emotionally; they are also expected to live in a nuclear family' (2014, 133). Analysing the prosecutions of the nine women in Guanajuato, Verónica Cruz Sánchez, director of *Centro Las Libres*, found that 'it was not the abortion, nor the 'homicide' itself that was judged – it was the sexuality of these women. They had relations with men who were not their husbands'. Indeed, a central element in many cases is infidelity, often in the context of migration: 'The husbands of these women were in the U.S. or they were separated for other reasons. They became pregnant in their non-marital relations and hid the pregnancy because of the stigma. In prosecutors or judges' minds, the scenario is clear – if she hid the pregnancy, it means she intended to kill the child once born' (Director of Las Libres, Guanajuato, interviewed 26 November 2015).

In the previously mentioned case of Adriana Manzanares Calletano, she was eighteen years old and had two children when her husband left for the US. Later, she found a new partner and became pregnant. When she miscarried, her partner denounced her before the *ejido* commissioner and took her to the village centre where the rest of the community exercised tribal justice and threw stones at her.[11] The women of the village indicated that Adriana's crime was not losing the baby but rather being unfaithful to her emigrated husband. She was later charged with aggravated homicide (Martínez 2014). Sexual relations that do not conform to normative ideas of marriage and reproduction thus become elements that incriminate women accused for abortion-related crimes.

The punishment for such crimes also constitutes a way to maintain state-established social values related to maternity and sexuality. Long prison sentences have a symbolic value that sends a warning signal to women who do not conform to the strict confines of the female role. In Guanajuato, *Centro Las Libres'* legal coordinator explained that according to state authorities, women 'should marry and procreate and, moreover, not become pregnant with married men' (Legal coordinator, Las Libres, interviewed via Skype 16 November 2015). The severe punishment for crimes related to abortion – especially aggravated homicide – demonstrates what awaits women who transgress the boundaries set by prevailing gender roles. Similarly, responding to the question of why women in Guanajuato were punished with up to thirty years in prison, the General Attorney's gender coordinator replied: 'You [as a woman] have the responsibility for your sexuality, you have to guard and protect it. If you do something that goes against cultural traditions, I [the state] have to punish you – I will make you an example' (Gender coordinator, General Attorney's office, Guanajuato, interviewed 6 November 2015). The director of Guanajuato's Women's Institute concurred: '[Incarcerations] are a way to continue controlling [women] . . . . It is a form of spreading fear, of saying "having an abortion is bad, you will go to prison if you have one"'. (Director of the Women's Institute, Guanajuato, interviewed 13 November 2015).

Incarcerations for abortion-related crimes are intimately linked to gendered expectations of motherhood and female sexual behaviour. Far from mere enforcements of restrictive reproductive health policies, sentences for abortion-related crimes reflect deeply ingrained ideas of women's roles in society. Women who deviate from socio-cultural expectations are punished not only for alleged illegal abortions but also for exercising their sexuality outside of the institution of marriage. Sentences for abortion-related crimes thus show how gendered social expectations as a form of cultural violence intersect with structural inequality to motivate and legitimise direct violence in the shape of incarcerations. Marked as transgressors, the state controls and disciplines women who do not conform to normative ideals of motherhood and female sexuality. Incarcerations therefore serve to uphold dominant gender relations. Also in this regard are marginalised women disproportionally affected because they lack the resources and education required to dispute the state's sanctioning power. As Verónica Cruz Sánchez argues: 'They are the perfect women [to punish] given their condition of marginalization, subordination and poverty. Their punishment is a symbol to all' (Director of Las Libres, Guanajuato, interviewed 26 November 2015).

STATE VIOLENCE AS GENDER-BASED STRUCTURAL, CULTURAL AND DIRECT VIOLENCE

Incarcerations for abortion-related crimes have received growing international attention in the past few decades. In Latin America, where abortion policies remain among the most restrictive in the world, cases began to emerge in 2010 and onwards that revealed how women from Mexico to Argentina were imprisoned for up to thirty years for alleged illegal abortions or aggravated homicide. Although no reliable official statistics exist, evidence suggests that states in the region have begun to enforce criminalising policies to a greater degree than before. Why? This chapter examined the case of incarcerations for alleged illegal abortions and aggravated homicide using Galtung's typology of violence as an analytical tool. Departing from his conceptualisation however, it attributed direct, cultural and structural violence to a specific actor with distributive powers – the state. Focusing on the state made visible the interconnected nature of these violences, showing how the state's various actors, institutions and instances perpetrate multiple forms of gender violence simultaneously. These violences intersect to target marginalised women. In the case of incarcerations for abortion-related crimes, the unclear legal status of abortion prompt medical personnel to report suspected illegal cases of crimes to a greater extent than before. Once investigations open, due process violations, insufficient evidence and use of outdated methods have characterised criminal proceedings. Social expectations related to motherhood and female sexuality grounded in traditional gender roles also play a significant role in this process. Women prosecuted for abortion-related crimes are perceived to have transgressed the gendered boundaries that allow the state to control women and their bodies. These findings illustrate how intersecting forms of structural and cultural violence motivate and legitimise direct violence in the form of incarcerations.

Above all, this chapter illustrated how different forms of state-perpetrated violence intersect to target vulnerable groups – in particular marginalised women. In the case of Mexico, this group is primarily made up of young, indigenous women with scarce resources who originate in impoverished rural communities. These women make up the majority of prosecuted individuals and are also disproportionally affected by the restrictive abortion policies currently in place in Mexico and across the region. Regardless of whether or not these women suffer obstetric emergencies or resort to illegal methods because they cannot afford clandestine abortions at private clinics, they seek medical assistance at public hospitals where doctors, nurses or social workers report them to local authorities. Without access to adequate legal aid or even basic translation services – also a function of their location at the intersection of gender, race/ethnicity and class – marginalised women are more likely to be sentenced in flawed legal proceedings. Finally, gendered expectations concerning motherhood and sexuality also operate to target vulnerable groups. Marginalised women who live in rural areas where traditional gender roles are often upheld to a greater extent than in large cities are punished when they transgress the boundaries set by prevailing gender norms.

This chapter centred on the state's role in perpetrating violence related to reproductive health. It showed how the state comprises a collection of actors and institutions at varying governance levels – including medical personnel, police officers, lawyers and judges – that reinforce dominant gender relations via laws, policies and practices. The state-centred analysis advanced in this chapter is also broadly applicable to other forms of gender-based violence, such as domestic violence and transphobic killings. Future research should consider ways in which to systematically gather data to analyse the numbers, causes and consequences of abortion-related incarcerations not only within Mexico but also throughout Latin America.

NOTES

1. According to interview sources, no nation-wide official records exist of the number of women imprisoned for abortion-related crimes or aggravated homicide specifically. The only way of obtaining such data would be to gather records from all

prison facilities in Mexico, which requires extensive additional fieldwork – a task well beyond the scope of this chapter. I draw on data from the *Grupo de Información en Reproducción Elegida* [Information Group on Chosen Reproduction] (GIRE), which to my knowledge is the most reliable source and encompasses all Mexican states.

2. Mexico's federal structure allows each state jurisdiction over the penal codes that govern abortion policies across the country to remain highly restrictive. With the exception of Mexico City, the majority of subnational entities permit abortion only in the case of severe fetal deformation or when the mother's life is at risk (Lopreite 2014).

3. Not all feminist scholars, however, disregarded the state based on its gendered structures. Mona Harrington (1992), for example, argued that the state could function as a possible emancipatory agent for women.

4. For analyses of disaggregated approaches to the state, see, for example, Waylen (1998) and Bedford (2013).

5. Author's translation from Spanish.

6. *Centro Las Libres* defended seven out of the nine released women (Cruz Sánchez 2011).

7. Sources indicate that incarcerations for abortion-related crimes indeed took place prior to the enactment of constitutional reforms (see, for example, Cruz Sánchez 2011). The statistics are, however, highly unreliable and to the author's knowledge, there are no systematic studies of incarcerations prior to 2008.

8. To the author's knowledge, these numbers compiled by GIRE constitute the only existing state-by-state data on incarcerations for abortion-related crimes.

9. To the author's knowledge, there have been no cases of medical personnel incarcerated for not reporting a suspected case of illegal abortion in Mexico.

10. The case of women incarcerated for abortion-related crimes bears interesting parallels to women who transgress expectations of female behaviour through their violent behaviour. See, for example, Sjoberg (2016).

11. An ejido commissioner is a local leader responsible for an area of communal land used for agriculture.

REFERENCES

Agren, David. 2017. 'Mexico Baby Death Trial Reveals Growing Persecution of Women Who Miscarry'. *The Guardian*, 8 November 2017. https://www.theguardian.com/world/2017/nov/08/mexico-miscarriage-trial-perscution-women-abortion. Accessed 6 July 2018.

Amuchástegui, Ana, Edith Flores and Evelyn Aldaz. 2015. 'Disputa Social y Disputa Subjectiva. Religión, Género y Discursos Sociales en la Legalización del Aborto en México'. *Revista Estudios de Género. La Ventana* 41 (Enero-Junio): 153–195.

Bedford, Kate. 2013. 'Gender, Institutions, and Multilevel Governance'. In *The Oxford Handbook of Gender and Politics*, edited by Georgina Waylen, Karen Celis and Johanna Kantola, 627–54. New York: Oxford University Press.

Bejarano Celaya, Margarita and Leyla Guadalupe Acedo Ung. 2014. 'Cuerpo y Violencia: Regulación Del Aborto Como Dispositivo de Control a Las Mujeres'. *Región y Sociedad*, no. 4: 261–283.

Carbajal, Mariana. 2016. 'Un Patrón Para Criminalizar El Aborto Espontáneo'. *Pagina 12* (July 25). Accessed 7 July 2018. https://www.pagina12.com.ar/diario/sociedad/3-305116-2016-07-25.html.

Center for Reproductive Rights. 2015. *Abortion and Reproductive Rights in Latin America: Implications for Democracy*. New York.

CIMAC Noticias. 2017. 'Criminalización Del Aborto: Exclusión, Persecución y Cárcel Para Salvadoreñas', 21 February 2017. http://www.cimacnoticias.com.mx/noticia/criminalizaci-n-del-aborto-exclusi-n-persecuci-n-y-c-rcel-para-salvadore. Accessed 6 July 2018.

Cohen, Dara Kay. 2013. 'Explaining Rape during Civil War: Cross-National Evidence (1980–2009) '. *American Political Science Review* 107, no. 3: 461–477.

Confortini, Catia. 2006. 'Galtung, Violence, and Gender: The Case for a Peace Studies/Feminism Alliance'. *Peace & Change* 31, no. 3: 333–367.

Cruz Sánchez, Verónica. 2011. 'Fin a Una Década de Criminalización Por Aborto Contra Mujeres Pobres En Guanajuato'. *Debate Feminista* no. 43: 176–191.

Driver, Alice. 2017. 'What Women's Lives Are Like When Abortion Is a Crime'. *CNN*. 5 October 2017. http://edition.cnn.com/2017/10/05/opinions/united-states-el-salvador-abortion-prison-driver-opinion/index.html. Accessed 7 July 2018.

Eggers, Michele. 2018. 'The Criminalization of Women for Abortion in Chile'. In *Global Perspectives on Women's Sexual and Reproductive Health across the Lifecourse*, edited by Shonali Choudhoury, Jennifer Toller Erausquin and Mellissa Withers, 173–188. Berlin: Springer International Publishing.

Enloe, Cynthia. 1990. *Bananas, Beaches and Bases: Making Feminist Sense of International Politics*. Berkely: University of California Press.

Galtung, Johan. 1969. 'Violence, Peace and Peace Research'. *Journal of Peace Research* 6, no. 3:167–191.

Galtung, Johan. 1990. 'Cultural Violence'. *Journal of Peace Research* 27, no. 3: 291–305.

GIRE. 2015. 'Niñas y Mujeres Sin Justicia: Derechos Reproductivos En México'. México D.F. http://informe2015.gire.org.mx/#/inicio. Accessed 21 December 2018.

Gutiérrez González, Rodrigo. 2018. 'Se Dispara Criminalización Del Aborto Un 60%'. *La Silla Rota*. 23 October 2018. https://lasillarota.com/se-dispara-criminalizacion-del-aborto-un-60/253636. Accessed 20 December 2018.

Guttmacher Institute. 2012. 'In Brief: Facts on Abortion in Latin America and the Caribbean'. https://www.guttmacher.org/pubs/IB_AWW-Latin-America.pdf. Accessed 5 July 2018.

Harman, Sophie. 2019. 'Violence and the Paradox of Global Health'. In *Gender, Global Health and Violence: Feminist Perspectives on Peace and Disease*, edited by Tiina Vaittinen and Catia Confortini. London and New York: Rowman & Littlefield.

Harrington, Mona. 1992. 'What Exactly Is Wrong with the Liberal State as an Agent of Change?' In *Gendered States: Feminist (Re)Visions of International Relations*, edited by V. Peterson, 65–82. Boulder: Lynne Rienner.

Kane, Gillian, Beatriz Galli and Patty Skuster. 2014. 'When Abortion Is a Crime: The Threat to Vulnerable Women in Latin America'. Policy report. Chapel Hill: Ipas.

La Silla Rota. 2018. 'Tras Años de Prisión Por Aborto Fortuito, Dafne Podría Quedar Libre', 7 November 2018. https://lasillarota.com/estados/tras-3-anos-de-prision-por-aborto-fortuito-dafne-podria-quedar-libre-caso-dafne-aborto-queretaro/256388. Accessed 20 December 2018.

Lopreite, Debora. 2014. 'Explaining Policy Outcomes in Federal Contexts: The Politics of Reproductive Rights in Argentina and Mexico'. *Bulletin of Latin American Research* 33, no. 4: 389–404.

Maier, Elizabeth. 2010. 'El Aborto y La Disputa Cultural Contemporáea En México'. *La Aljaba* XIV: 11–30.

Martínez, Paris. 2014. 'Corte Analizará Caso de Indígena Presa Por Aborto'. *Animal Político*. 21 January 2014. http://www.animalpolitico.com/2014/01/suprema-corte-analizara-manana-caso-de-indigena-presa-por-aborto/. Accessed 5 July 2018.

Montalvo, Tania. 2013. 'Documentan 25 Casos de Mujeres Criminalizadas Por Intento de Aborto'. *Animal Político*, 28 August 2013. http://www.animalpolitico.com/2013/08/piden-atencion-medica-y-son-acusadas-de-aborto-hay-25-casos-como-el-de-hilda/. Accessed 6 July 2018.

Ortiz-Ortega, Adriana. 2007. 'Law and the Politics of Abortion'. In *Decoding Gender: Law and Practice in Contemporary Mexico*, edited by Helga Baitenmann, Victoria Chenaut and Ann Varley, 197–212. New Brunswick: Rutgers University Press.

Peterson, V.S. 1992. *Gendered States: Feminist (Re) Visions of International Relations Theory*. Boulder, Colorado: Lynne Rienner.

Sánchez Bringas, Àngeles, Sara Espinosa, Sara Espinosa Islas, Claudia Ezcurdia and Edna Torres. 2004. 'Nuevas Maternidades o La Desconstrucción de La Maternidad En México'. *Debate Feminista* 30 (October): 55–86.

Sanford, Victoria, Katerina Stefatos and Cecilia M. Salvi. 2016. *Gender Violence in Peace and War: States of Complicity*. New Brunswick: Rutgers University Press.

Shepherd, Laura. 2005. 'Loud Voices behind the Wall: Gender Violence and the Violent Reproduction of the International'. *Millennium: Journal of International Studies* 34, no. 2: 377–401.

Sjoberg, Laura. 2016. *Women as Wartime Rapists: Beyond Sensation and Stereotyping*. New York: New York University Press.

Smith-Oka, Vania. 2014. *Shaping the Motherhood of Indigenous Mexico*. Nashville: Vanderbilt University Press.

Strochlic, Nina. 2016. 'Where Women with Zika Fear Prison'. *National Geographic*, 29 October 2016. https://news.nationalgeographic.com/2016/10/zika-el-salvador-women/. Accessed 5 July 2018.

Tanyag, Maria. 2019. 'Replenishing Bodies and the Political Economy of SRHR in Crisis and Emergencies'. In *Gender, Global Health and Violence: Feminist Perspectives on Peace and Disease*, edited by Tiina Vaittinen and Catia Confortini. London and New York: Rowman & Littlefield.

Tickner, Ann J. 1992. *Gender in International Relations: Feminist Perspectives on Achieving International Security*. New York: Columbia University Press.

Tickner, Ann J. 1997. 'You Just Don't Understand: Troubled Engagements between Feminists and IR Theorists'. *International Studies Quarterly* 41, no. 4: 611–632.

Toribio, Laura. 2017. 'Las Criminalizan Hasta Sus Familiares Por Aborto'. *Excelsior*, 29 October 2017. http://www.excelsior.com.mx/nacional/2017/10/29/1197835. Accessed 7 July 2018.

Viterna, Jocelyn and Jose Santos Guardado Bautista. 2014. 'Independent Analysis of Systematic Gender Discrimination in the El Salvador Judicial Process against 17 Women Accused of the Aggravated Homicide of Their Newborns'. White Paper. Accessed 7 July 2019. https://scholar.harvard.edu/files/viterna/files/final_report_english_pdf.pdf. Accessed 7 September 2019.

Waylen, Georgina. 1998. 'Gender, Feminism and the State: An Overview'. In *Gender, Politics and the State*, edited by Vicky Randall and Georgina Waylen. London: Routledge.

Wilcox, Lauren. 2011. 'Beyond Sex/Gender: The Feminist Body of Security'. *Politics & Gender* 7, no. 4: 595–599.

Youngs, Gillian. 2004. 'Feminist International Relations: A Contradiction in Terms? Or: Why Women and Gender Are Essential to Understanding the World "We" Live In'. *International Affairs* 80, no. 1: 75–87.

Chapter 8

When Is It Torture? When Is It Rape? Discourses on Wartime Sexual Violence

Élise Féron

Sexual violence is, among all types of violence committed during wars and conflicts, one the most well known and studied. It is the central focus of several UN Security Council Resolutions (1820, but also 1888, 1889, 1960, 2106, 2013, among others), of thousands of policy reports and academic articles and of a plethora of humanitarian and health organisations working in conflict areas. Yet, deciding which acts can be qualified as sexual violence, or not, is apparently not as straightforward as it seems, especially when victims are male. When it comes to wartime sexual violence, it is indeed primarily images of women and girls being raped, sexually enslaved, being forced to bear children or to abort, which come to mind. But what about men who endure forced nudity, beatings of the genitals, cigarette burns, forced marriage or forced circumcision?[1]

Cases of sexual violence against men and boys have been recorded in many conflicts and wars, both ancient and contemporary. Various factors have, however, contributed to keep them largely hidden from view. Literature usually focuses on different types of violence civilian and combatant men are victims of, such as killing, maiming, as well as imprisonment and torture. Of course, such types of violence can, and indeed do often, include sexual violence, but this is almost never discussed. In contrast, accounts of physical violence endured by women during conflicts or by imprisoned women disproportionately put the stress on sexual victimisation and especially on rape, overlooking their other experiences of violence (Baaz Ericsson and Stern 2013; Tanyag, this volume).

Difficulties associated to data collection explain the current lack of awareness on wartime sexual violence against men, as male survivors almost never report those episodes of violence. It is true that both male and female survivors of (wartime) sexual violence tend to underreport it, but there are clear indications that men report these cases even less than women and girls do (Sivakumaran 2007). Underreporting seems particularly high in societies where sexuality is a strong taboo (UNHCR 2017, 3). Another reason explaining the low visibility of the sexual victimisation of men is that because its patterns differ from what we know of conflict-related sexual violence against women, men's experiences of wartime sexual violence are not perceived as such. The narrative on 'rape as a weapon of war' has set gendered norms for sexual violence in conflicts, and the ways men are sexually brutalised during wars do not always fit neatly within these established categories. A comparison of statistics available on sexual violence in detention settings suggests that men are less likely than women to be targeted by rape, but are more likely to be victims of sexual mutilation, and of other forms of sexual torture like beatings of the genitals.

Against this backdrop, this chapter focuses on how conflict-related sexual violence is understood and qualified, and looks at the global health consequences of the differentiated framing of wartime sexual violence when victims are male, and when victims are female. From an empirical standpoint, this chapter relies upon the WHO's definition of sexual violence as: 'any sexual act, attempt to obtain a sexual act, unwanted sexual comments or advances, or acts to traffic, or otherwise directed, against a person's sexuality using coercion, by any person regardless of their relationship to the victim, in any setting' (Krug et al. 2002, 149). Sexual violence thus includes, but is not limited to, rape, sexual torture, sexual mutilation, sexual humiliation and sexual slavery, committed by armed actors on or off-duty, but also sometimes by non-combatant strangers.

This chapter notably builds on fieldwork data collected in two contrasted cases, the Great Lakes Region of Africa (2009–2014) and Northern Ireland (2005–2014). The choice to collect data in the Great Lakes region of Africa reflects the role the Congo and the rest of the region play in structuring and framing our current understanding of sexual violence in conflict zones, just like Bosnia did in the 1990s. Referred to as the 'rape capital of the world' by Margot Wallstrom, the UN's special representative on sexual violence in conflict in 2010 after her return from the country, the Democratic Republic of the Congo (DRC) and more specifically the conflicts raging in the North and South Kivu are often associated to images of war savagery and to human rights violations. However, cases of wartime sexual violence have been documented in many other regions of the world, and the use of sexual torture against prisoners, for instance, has been recorded in many conflicts displaying different characteristics than the current conflicts in the Congo. In order to account, at least partially, for these differences in context, I have also used data collected during interviews conducted in Northern Ireland, with (former) members of paramilitary groups who had been imprisoned. During the

Northern Irish 'Troubles', which spanned from the late 1960s to the signing of the Belfast/ Good Friday Peace Agreement in 1998, sexual torture was indeed used by members of official security forces such as the police and the military, as well as by paramilitary groups. My fieldwork data also includes interviews with various local NGO leaders, doctors, surgeons and psychiatrists in the Great Lakes Region of Africa as well as in Europe. Finally, I have included, for the purposes of this chapter, well-documented examples from other conflict areas, such as Bosnia-Herzegovina, El Salvador, Peru, Uganda, as well as some others on which evidence exists but is more scattered, like Syria. These examples demonstrate that the cases of the DRC and Northern Ireland are far from being isolated and anecdotal (Féron 2018).

Building on these data, the chapter examines the entanglements of violence (Confortini and Vaittinen, this volume) that result from the performative effect of wartime sexual violence against men, from direct and physical, to epistemic (Spivak 1988), and to cultural and structural (Galtung 1969). The chapter first briefly looks at how wartime sexual violence, especially when committed against men, is coded by global health and humanitarian organisations, and then prosecuted by judicial institutions. It shows how the sexual brutalisation of men is most of the time classified under the more general category of 'torture', whereas when women are targeted, it is considered and prosecuted as sexual violence. This differentiated treatment of direct forms of physical violence, embedded in deeply gendered understandings of violence, in turn, leads to clear forms of epistemic violence. The second section analyses the consequences of this epistemic violence for both male and female sexual violence survivors. It looks more specifically at how the coding depoliticises wartime sexual violence against women, and at how it feeds narratives associating men with agency, and women with vulnerability, thus generating further cultural and epistemic violence, and a strengthening of gendered understandings of violence. The final section describes the consequences of these narratives in terms of sexual violence survivors' access to support programmes, and shows how global health framings of wartime sexual violence generate structural violence against male survivors, by failing to question and challenge dominant gendered understandings of sexual violence.

HOW IS WARTIME SEXUAL VIOLENCE AGAINST MEN CODED AND PROSECUTED?

In order to fully capture the extent to which wartime sexual violence is framed differently when victims are male and when victims are female, it is useful to look at how it is defined by global health and humanitarian organisations, and by judicial institutions. According to a study conducted by Del Zotto and Jones, at the beginning of the 2000 decade out of more than 4000 non-governmental groups tackling conflict-related sexual violence, 'only 3% mention the experiences of males at all in their programs and informational literature. About one quarter of the groups explicitly deny that male-on-male violence is a serious problem' (Del Zotto and Jones 2002). And even when it is documented and reported as such, it appears that the wartime sexual brutalisation of men is usually not coded as sexual violence, but as torture or beatings (see Cohen et al. 2013; Kapur and Muddell 2016; Manivannan 2014, 643), especially when the violence has been committed in detention. This is true even in the humanitarian sector: 'If we consider the [sexual] torture of people as GBV, then we will have too many. We consider detained people as tortured and people outside of detention as GBV' (SGBV Officer, Jordan, quoted in UNHCR 2017, 64). The problem, of course, is that men are more likely to be detained than women, especially in conflict zones. Furthermore, legal definitions of sexual violence are not always gender-inclusive. A survey conducted in 2014 by Dolan (2014, 6) showed that out of 189 countries, a total of 63 countries, representing almost two-thirds of the world's population, still recognised only female victims of rape. Even countries such as the DRC that have recently adopted more inclusive laws only prosecute cases of sexual violence against women, with disappointing results (Kippenberg 2005).

In addition, even in cases where men are not explicitly excluded from the category of potential victims of sexual violence, the fact that definitions often restrict sexual violence to specific forms of aggression like rape dramatically hampers prosecution by overlooking the most frequent kinds of wartime male sexual victimisation, such as partial or total castration, or traumas to the genitals. In Peru, for instance, in spite of a rather broad definition of sexual violence, the Truth and Reconciliation Commission, whose mandate was to investigate the violent political conflict that occurred in the country in the 1980s and 1990s, limited its investigations on sexual violence crimes to cases of rape, and therefore ignored most instances of sexual violence against men. Leiby (2012, 343) recorded and analysed the original testimonies of Peruvian survivors of sexual violence and found out that 29 per cent of sexual violence victims were men, whereas the Truth Commission had found that only 2 per cent were men. In Colombian non-governmental and governmental databases too, episodes of conflict-related sexual violence against men, especially when committed by state security forces since the conflict began during the 1960s, have been registered as 'torture', thus hushing their sexual character (Quijano and Kelly 2012, 482).

There is also empirical evidence pointing at a strong gender bias in how the definition of rape is applied during national and local trials. In several court cases examined in Bosnia, and referring to the 1992–1995 war, different definitional elements have been used depending on the gender of the victim (OSCE 2015, 32). Different labels where used in cases of male sexual victimisation, such as in the Minić et al. case, where forced fellatio was qualified as an 'outrage upon [prisoners'] personal dignity' and as an 'inhuman treatment' by the Bijeljina District Court, when it had, in cases where victims had been female, been recognised as rape.

At a more general level, various international legal instruments allow the prosecution of acts of wartime sexual violence. In contrast with International Human Rights Law, which is mostly based on the CEDAW (Convention on the Elimination of all forms of Discrimination Against Women, entered into force in 1981), International Criminal Law and International Humanitarian Law offer numerous options for addressing cases of conflict-related sexual violence against men. International Criminal Law has notably been central in the work of the International Criminal Tribunal for the former Yugoslavia (ICTY), the International Criminal Tribunal for Rwanda (ICTR) and in the Rome statute of the International Criminal Court (ICC).

Over the years, these three institutions have built a wide-ranging and effective framework for the prosecution of such cases. They have notably relied on existing human rights treaties and conventions, regarding, for instance, freedom from torture and degrading treatment, rights to life, personal security and physical security and so on. The ICTR and the ICTY, in particular, were the first to consider that wartime rape, against both men and women, should be judged as a crime against humanity (Zawati 2007, 27). These tribunals have also spearheaded a more inclusive definition of wartime rape, and the Trial Chamber 1 of the ICTR even made a direct reference to male victims of rape in the 1998 Akayesu case (Obote-Odora 2005, 137). Although the Office of the Prosecutor of the ICTR eventually did not charge anyone with rape against men, this was, without doubt, a landmark ruling. It is, however, the ICTY that has proven to be the most progressive with regard to these issues, by pioneering an inclusive definition of sexual violence, and by actually prosecuting conflict-related sexual violence against men (Gorris 2015, 413). In its first decision issued in 1997 – significant also because it was the first international war crimes trial since Nuremberg and Tokyo – the ICTY found Duško Tadić, guilty of cruel treatment (violation of the laws and customs of war) and inhumane acts (crime against humanity) for the part he played in acts of sexual violence against men, in particular, male sexual assault and mutilation (King and Greening 2007, 1056).

These advances have been replicated by other courts and tribunals, such as the Special Court for Sierra Leone, set up in 2002 by the government of Sierra Leone and the United Nations, and put in charge of the prosecution of crimes that occurred during the civil war in Sierra Leone. In the *Prosecutor v. Sesay, Kallon and Gbao* case, for example, the Special Court for Sierra

Leone charged the accused of sexual offenses against both men and women with outrages upon personal dignity as war crimes, and recognised that both men and women can be victims of rape. These developments have been synthesised in the Rome statute of the International Criminal Court, adopted in 1998 and entered into force in 2002. Its article 7(1)(g) notably establishes that sexual offenses such as sexual slavery, enforced prostitution and enforced sterilisation may henceforth be considered as crimes against humanity, whether they are committed against women or against men.

There are, however, discrepancies between these inclusive definitions of conflict-related sexual violence, and the way they are used and applied by international criminal tribunals (Sivakumaran 2010, 272). Wartime sexual violence against men is indeed often initially mentioned, but eventually characterised as torture or inhumane treatment and not as sexual violence, a labelling which seems to suggest that men are less likely to be sexually victimised. In the 2012 *ICC Prosecutor* v. *Kenyatta* case, for instance, crimes of forced circumcision and male sexual mutilation were classified under the category of 'other inhumane acts'.

In many other court cases, episodes of male sexual brutalisation are described and characterised as sexual violence, but not condemned as such, or not condemned at all. This is what happened in the ICTR cases of *Prosecutor* v. *Muhimana*, who was notably charged of rape as a crime against humanity, or the case of *Prosecutor v. Bagosora*, charged of crimes against humanity and notably rape and other inhumane acts, as well as of war crimes, among which outrages upon personal dignity. At the beginning of both trials, cases of male sexual brutalisation had been mentioned and characterised as sexual violence, but in the end, the findings of the ICTR referred only to sexual violence against women, and not against men (Sivakumaran 2010, 274). The ICTR has recognised that both men and women can be victims of rape and sexual violence, but it has never charged anyone with committing rape or sexual assault against men, in spite of supporting empirical evidence. Cases examined at the Special Court of Sierra Leone have followed a similar trend, whereby episodes of sexual violence against men are noted, but not prosecuted as such (Oosterveld 2011, 71). Judgements at the ICTY have often been as disappointing: 'At the ICTY, only sixteen out of seventy-seven sexual violence indictments included charges of sexual violence involving male victims, of which seven led to convictions. An additional three cases that strongly indicated sexual violence against only male victims did not even lead to indictments for sex crimes' (Manivannan 2014, 663).

What this brief overview suggests is that, up to now, international criminal tribunals' punishments for wartime sexual violence against men are less severe than punishments for wartime sexual violence against women, or qualified as torture rather than as sexual violence. This trend can be understood as a consequence of the gendered framing of wartime sexual violence, which is assumed to affect mostly, if not only, women and girls.

Vulnerable Women, Agentic Men and the Depoliticisation of Sexual Violence against Women

The ways in which wartime sexual violence is understood, coded and prosecuted are crucial and have diverging consequences for both male and female survivors. In conflict zones, 'torture' has a strong political connotation (Peters 1996), especially when it is inflicted upon prisoners. Torture is used to extract confessions or to break opponents' spirits. Surviving, and not breaking under torture is often seen as a badge of honour for the communities to which the survivors belong. This stands in stark contrast with how sexual violence is connoted in political and media discourses. Sexual violence, too, is associated with the gendered notions of honour, but only because it brings shame to its survivors. In addition, the assumed motives behind sexual violence, like lust, excitement and frenzy, are most of the time seen as non-political. Admittedly, the 'rape as a weapon of war' thesis challenges these narratives (Kirby 2012), but it remains that torture is overwhelmingly considered as a (condemnable but almost unavoidable) part of war, whereas sexual violence is seen as just one if its (likewise condemnable but almost unavoidable) corollaries.

Labelling rapes, beatings of the genitals, sexual mutilations and so on, either as sexual violence or as torture is therefore tremendously important for both male and female survivors, and for their potential access to support programmes. As we have seen, male sexual victimisation is most of the time hidden behind accounts of 'torture', whereas when it is committed against women, it is acknowledged as sexual violence. Such a trend is hardly surprising, since international narratives on women and conflicts always put the stress on sexual violence. This is especially true of cases of rape, which tend to epitomise women's experiences of war, and to obscure other types of conflict-related physical violence they are victims of (Ericsson Baaz and Stern 2013). More specifically, when violence is exerted on female prisoners, narratives and court judgements tend to primarily focus on the sexual component of torture, even when sexual abuse constituted only a small part of the suffering the female prisoner has had to go through (MacDonald 1991).

In the previously quoted examples of ICTY trials for instance, most cases of sexual violence against women have been accompanied by other severe forms of physical and psychological violence, most of which have not been condemned as such, as if the charge of sexual violence was enough to cover these. These representations result in what could be called the 'biologisation' of women's wartime experience, that is, the belief that what matters about/to women in conflicts is their reproductive and sexual health (see, however,

Tanyag, this volume). Against this backdrop, it is well documented (see, for instance, Watts and Zimmerman 2002) that women – along with all other sections of war-affected populations – suffer from all sorts of plights during conflict times, including non-sexual violence like beatings, but also displacement, increased poverty, forced enrollment and so on. All this, as Tanyag's chapter in this volume suggests, has negative consequences on the sexual and reproductive health rights (SRHR) during conflicts, and in their aftermath. Yet, international discourses on women and security build first and foremost on this association between women and sexual violence, as if the other crimes committed against women were, by definition, of a lesser importance.

Further, according to several UNSC Resolutions, and especially Resolution 1820, sexual violence against women is assumed to be violence that is 'worse than death' (Seto 2013, 67). Sexual violence against women sits at the top of the hierarchy of crimes committed during conflicts and in post-conflict times, 'even appearing to take precedence over other forms of violence frequently equated with death in their severity' (ibid.). Resolution 1820, for instance, stipulates the 'evacuation of women and children under imminent threat of sexual violence to safety', and urges national institutions to provide 'sustainable assistance' to victims. Although there are other provisions and rules, in the Geneva Convention, for example, protecting civilians and, in particular, women and children and removing them from the vicinity of military objectives, this specific focus on sexual violence calls for attention. What is particularly worrying about this discourse is that it builds upon, and reinforces, an extremely patriarchal narrative that has always portrayed rape as the worst offense that can ever be done to women, and, by extension, to their male relatives. This is reminiscent of the Geneva Convention (1949), in which sexual violence is perceived and understood via patriarchal notions about the role of women in society. Art. 27 of the Geneva Convention states, for instance, that 'women shall be protected against any attack on their honour, in particular against rape, enforced prostitution, or any form of indecent assault'.

It is very clear here that sexual violence against women is seen and understood from the perspective of men, and fits into a patriarchal perspective. As Sharon Marcus (1992, 387) argues, 'In its efforts to convey the horror and iniquity of rape, such a view often concurs with masculinist culture in its designation of rape as a fate worse than, or tantamount to, death; the apocalyptic tone which it adopts and the metaphysical status which it assigns to rape implies that rape can only be feared or legally repaired, not fought'.

Conversely, when it comes to gender-based and sexual violence, international conventions and documents position men outside of the victims category, either because they are implicitly considered as perpetrators or because sexual violence against men is assumed to be triggered by different motives. In annual reports of the Secretary General of the United Nations on conflict-related sexual violence, for instance, cases of wartime sexual violence against men are most of the time related to political motives, for instance, to the use of torture in order to extract confessions. Similarly, in media narratives on the use of torture in detention settings, the sexual torture of male detainees is seldom mentioned at all.[2] Electric shocks applied to the male genitals, acid poured, cigarette burns, rape, forced rape of other prisoners and other types of sexual torture are euphemistically veiled under tales of beatings and abuse, thus overlooking their sexual and gendered meanings. As shown by Ross (2002), this type of framing builds an association between violence against men and race, politics or class, whereas violence against women is constantly associated to sexuality, and depoliticised. This is in line with how male survivors tell their own stories, almost always avoiding any direct reference to sex or to sexuality (Féron 2017).

In Northern Ireland, for example, former prisoners interviewed by Feldman (1991, 128, 158) disclosed almost offhandedly how they were sexually tortured: 'They don't say a word, they just beat you rabbit punches, squeezing the testicles, anything at all. Just general brutality. . . . It was very clear then strip searching wasn't a method for finding anything: it was an opportunity for them to do whatever they were going to do on you'. Similarly, the Northern Irish paramilitaries I have spoken with inscribed their experiences of sexual violence in detention within a larger narrative on their political struggle:

> They [interrogators] would beat me down there [gesturing at his groin], because they had tried everything else, and they couldn't break me, see? So they tried that too, trying to break me, but of course that didn't work. (Jim, interviewed in Belfast, 17 February 2006)[3]

For some of them, it was an almost natural part of prison experience, an additional vindication of their wish to bring down this abusive system:

> And yes of course like many others I was abused, you know, that is part of what you go through in there. But in a way that made our resolve stronger, because this is wrong, just like the whole system is wrong. It made us more determined to do whatever we can to bring it to an end. (Kieran, interviewed in Belfast, 5 November 2005)

The metaphorical concept of 'emasculation' plays a central role in male survivors' discourses, as something to be feared, resisted or avoided, but also in international narratives about the use of torture in detention settings. As noted by Ross (2002, 307–311), the concept of emasculation draws attention towards the political consequences of the sexual brutalisation of men (loss of agency, destabilisation, diminished status, etc.), while obscuring the materiality of sexual violence against men as practice. It mostly works as a *metaphor*. By contrast, narratives on sexual violence against women shed light on its *practicality* by detailing practices such as rape, sexual slavery, forced pregnancy and so on, while partially or totally veiling their political and metaphoric functions, even in the case of the 'weapon of war' thesis, as demonstrated by Buss (2009).

Most discourses on wartime sexual violence, especially at the international and humanitarian level (Féron 2017), present women as vulnerable and passive, whereas men are seen either as perpetrators or as potential allies in the fight against female sexual victimisation. Overlooking men's vulnerability to sexual violence, therefore, only strengthens the patriarchal trope associating women to vulnerability and passivity, and men to power and agency. It also means that sexual violence against women is understood as a crucial local and global health issue, whereas sexual violence against men is not. Women's health issues, especially in conflict areas, are equated with sexual and reproductive health ones, whereas men's health issues are most of the time assumed to be battle related, and non-sexual in nature. This, in turn, structures global health responses in conflict zones, and triggers other forms of structural, psychological, symbolic and epistemic violence.

CONSEQUENCES ON ACCESS TO SUPPORT PROGRAMMES FOR MALE SURVIVORS

In 2002, in its 'World Report', the WHO mentioned sexual violence against men and boys as a 'largely neglected' problem (Krug et al. 2002, 154). However, to date, in discourses and practices of health and humanitarian organisations active in conflict zones, the assumption is that it is first and foremost women and girls who are victims of wartime sexual violence, and this has dramatic consequences for male survivors. They are too ashamed to ask for help, and many prefer to bear the suffering on their own – thus still attempting to follow the script according to which they are strong and invulnerable – with sometimes fatal consequences. In the DRC as well as in Burundi, the medical personnel I have spoken with believes that male victims of sexual violence will not ask for medical help unless they really have no other choice. It means that those who come for treatment often have severe health issues like festering wounds or serious haemorrhage, and they cannot always be saved (see also Gettleman 2009). Many male survivors also experience what they see as shameful and unmanning sequels, such as physical impotence, or urinary or faecal incontinence (Refugee Law Project 2014, 8). They are reluctant to report even the most severe physical symptoms, because they think that it would further underscore their loss of (masculine) status. Male survivors therefore pledge to endure the pain on their own:

> I am still in pain, yes, some parts of me still hurt. But I don't want to . . . I can't really speak about it. So I have to live with it, and pray that it goes away. (Jean-Paul, interviewed in Goma, North Kivu, DRC, 1 May 2009)

Speaking about their pain to anyone, especially to their own relatives, often seems out of the question:

> I hurt, a lot. I cannot eat what I want, and even sitting is painful. But it won't change anything to speak about it. I don't want my family to know that I am suffering. This isn't proper. (Jacques, interviewed in Bujumbura, Burundi, 21 April 2013)

Because men are expected to suffer in silence, their pain becomes unspeakable. As a result they are locked in solitude and deprived of a much needed support. Here – in the gendered unspeakability of the experiences of direct, physical, sexual violence – emerges a form of epistemic violence, which, in turn, has structural consequences in the health services available to the victims.

The way wartime sexual violence is understood to happen means that there are very few facilities for providing support to male survivors. Most health and humanitarian organisations offering support to survivors of sexual violence in war zones focus exclusively on female victims. Their brochures, leaflets or posters almost never make any mention of male survivors, and most of their names even directly refer to support offered to women, which is likely to scare male survivors away. Such invisibility and writing out of male victims in the support programmes makes it even more difficult for male survivors to overcome their shame and ask these organisations for help, even when their injuries are life threatening (Personal communication, International Rescue Committee, Bujumbura, 21 April 2013). Their shame is related to the feeling, mentioned by most of the male survivors with whom I spoke in the Congo or in Burundi, of having been 'turned into women' or 'homosexualised'.

In order to fully understand what is going on in these examples, it is important here to remember that wartime sexual violence plays on the plasticity of gender norms and roles, and that feminisation is often used in social and political relations to produce and justify domination (cf. Lukić and Lotherington, this volume). Feminisation can be understood as a domination strategy that can be enforced both on female and male bodies (Hooper 2001, 71). Operating through gendered and sexualised stigmas (see Harman, this volume), it works as an ordering principle between hegemonic, dominant and subjugated masculinities, but also between masculinities and femininities, and between femininities. Among all the ways in which conflict actors can enforce the feminisation and subjugation of their 'enemies', sexual violence against both men and women appears to be particularly effective. Sexual violence enacts the victim's feminisation/subjugation, while simultaneously entailing the perpetrator's masculinisation/empowerment (Jones 2006, 459). This explains why it is almost impossible for male survivors to report such acts, since complaining would underscore their feminised status by recognising the violation, and by accepting the position of victim that women hold in narratives about sexual violence, symbolically and in practice:

> I don't need help. I don't want to speak about it. . . . [In response to my mentioning clinics and some local and international NGOs helping survivors of sexual violence]: They are treating only women over there. They do a good job, but this is not a place for me. (Aimable, interviewed in Bubanza Province, Burundi, 18 April 2010)

In an interesting illustration of how different forms of violence can intersect, the fact that male survivors are reluctant to speak about the direct physical violence that they have experienced maintains the level of reporting, and thus of awareness, at very low levels (epistemic violence). In turn, this hampers the provision of adequate support, which generates structural violence against male survivors: 'Some male survivors do not want the person they have confided in to share the information further, making referrals for additional service provisions problematic' (Refugee Law Project 2013, 26). Accurate and detailed data on cases of conflict-related violence against men, as well as on prevalence rates, are thus almost impossible to collect. This feeds the impression that there are very few, if any, male survivors. It is therefore not surprising that women are always presented as constituting the 'vast majority' of victims (an extremely plausible assumption, but based on reports, not on 'actual' cases), thereby relegating wartime sexual violence against men to the domain of the anecdotal.

The consequences of these discourses and representations are staggering for male survivors, because they directly hinder the setting up of targeted support facilities and programmes, and render them quasi-invisible in global health and humanitarian discourses, as Grey and Shepherd (2012, 122) put it:

> The absent presence of masculinity and the silencing effects of the logic of 'the vast majority' in scholarly literature on war-time rape denies the materiality of the violated male body. For us, this is problematic, as without envisioning the violated male body we can neither hope to prevent its violation nor seek redress for violence committed against it.

Since statistics are often indeed used for programming purposes, this is what can be described as a 'chicken and egg situation' (UN 2013, 16). There is a very clear intersection of different forms of violence here (physical, epistemic and structural), which feed each other and render the provision of care to male survivors very difficult to organise, not to mention speak about.

Beyond the issue of reporting, the provision of adequate support to male survivors is hampered by the lack of training and of preparation of medical staff and healthcare professionals, who expect to take care of female patients only. A good example of how epistemic violence operates in the everyday of health care is provided by the fact that almost no training regarding the detection, identification and treatment of injuries related to sexual violence against men is offered to medical staff and healthcare professionals (Interview, Caritas International, Goma, North Kivu, DRC, 3 May 2009). Even in the most affected conflict areas, the level of awareness among medical doctors is very low. In some areas where the prevalence of wartime sexual violence against men is well documented, such as in the rural areas of Eastern Congo, there seems to be almost no understanding that men can be victims of that type of violence, and more particularly that they can be raped. During a visit to a rural hospital in South Kivu, for instance, one of the doctors I spoke to seemed surprised when I mentioned sexual violence against men, and confused it with cases where men have to watch their female family members being raped. Surprisingly in a region where the prevalence of male sexual victimisation is so high, he said he had not heard about men being raped or castrated (Interview, FOMULAC Hospital, Katana, South Kivu, DRC, 29 April 2012).

Such obliviousness, added to the victim's shame, explains that the medical staff often misjudge the effects of sexual violence on men, and confuse it with other types of violence they are more knowledgeable on. The situation is, however, different in hospitals located in large cities. In the Panzi hospital of Bukavu (South Kivu), for instance, the doctors I met were all familiar with sexual violence against men, and all could list several cases that they recently had to deal with. In general, however, mirroring what happens at the judicial level, healthcare professionals frequently use categories such as torture or beatings for describing sexual violence against men, which conceal its sexual dimension and ignore its profound consequences on victims' gender identities and social positioning. By repeatedly veiling the sexual and gender dimensions of sexual violence against men, medical and humanitarian staff therefore overlook the fact that the gendered nature of these acts is likely to deeply influence the male victims' capacities for recovery.

In addition, most male survivors who report what happened to them are referred to gynaecology departments, because this is where services for survivors of SGBV are usually located. Beyond the obvious psychological and relational problems that this might create for both male and female survivors, it is important to underscore the fact that the medical staff working in these departments has usually not benefited from a proper training and preparation for taking care of the physical sequels associated with sexual violence against men, let alone its psychological consequences. This shows how gendered assumptions – and silences – in the practices of support to survivors (epistemic violence) can hinder health professionals to see anatomical differences in injury, and to help people heal – thus generating further structural, but also eventually physical violence. This is what one of the Burundian male survivors I have met experienced when he looked for help in one of the local clinics in Bujumbura:

> I think they believed me, yes, they could see what had been done to me. But they did not know what to do with me. I think they did not know how to help me. (Didace, interviewed in Bujumbura, 22 May 2014)

The medical staff often assumes that, apart from fistulas and unwanted pregnancies following rape, male survivors' needs are comparable to those of female victims, which is incorrect (UN 2013, 15). The fact that most staff working in facilities or departments offering support to victims of sexual violence are female constitutes another problem, since most male survivors are reluctant to speak to female service providers (UNHCR 2017, 43). This is sometimes interpreted as an indication of the need to set up separate units to accommodate them (Le Pape 2012, 4). Until now, most facilities that are located in conflict areas and that provide support to male victims offer joint services for both men and women. This appears to be the consequence of a lack of resources, rather than of an intentional choice: 'We try to do as much as we can with what we have, and we don't have much' (Chief Doctor, Interview, Panzi Hospital, Bukavu, South Kivu, DRC, 30 April 2012).

More generally, and beyond the issue of which qualifications – torture or sexual violence – are used, the programmes that are currently implemented by health organisations usually fall short of considering the context in which these acts are committed. As shown in this chapter, the sexual brutalisation of both men and women occurs alongside other types of violence, which are often all interrelated. Programmes and organisations that exclusively provide support to victims of sexual violence tend to overlook other types of violence that occur during conflicts, which constitute a continuum to which sexual violence belongs. These organisations thus run the real risk of coming up with unsuitable answers. Wartime sexual violence does not occur in a vacuum, and cannot be understood or fought without taking into account the context in which it has developed as a practice, for instance, whether sexual violence is used as a way to extract confessions in detention, whether it is perpetrated by roaming armed groups over deprived and helpless populations and so on. This is crucial for survivors themselves, as they often struggle to understand why they have been abused (cf. DeLaet, Golden and Laveta, this volume).

Contextualising sexual violence is, however, complicated because when women are victims, it becomes an all-encompassing category, as if, as we have seen, it was all that mattered about what happens to women during war. For male victims of wartime violence, the reverse happens: everything *but* their experience of sexual violence matters among all that they have been through. This means that neither male nor female survivors can own their experience of sexual violence: men because it is silenced, or because it is presented as an abnormality, and women because it becomes larger than them – it is categorised, standardised and 'relocated to a place (the imaginary body of a colossus) where it is no longer recognizable or interpretable' (Scarry 1985, 71). By impeding the recounting of specific experiences that do not match with pre-existing paradigms, the standardisation of sexual violence against women silences individual narratives. On the other hand, male victims' stories are dismissed, discredited, minimised or negated within grand narratives about war. For both male and female survivors, gendered epistemic violence hinders the possibilities of contextualising the individual experience – it becomes an impossible task.

ADDRESSING SEXUAL VIOLENCE AGAINST MEN AS PATRIARCHAL VIOLENCE

Wartime sexual violence is not a corollary of war. Whether perpetrated against male prisoners, and called 'torture', or against women and girls and called a 'weapon of war', it is fundamentally interwoven with greater military, political, economic and social struggles. The frequency and characteristics of sexual violence are directly connected to the way gender, ethnic, religious, caste, socioeconomic and other hierarchies intersect and produce structural violence. As such, it does not happen by chance, or as a result of a lack of military discipline. Wartime sexual violence is entrenched in the patriarchal system that upholds conflict dynamics, and one of its consequences is precisely to reassert a violent and heteronormative patriarchal order.

There is a pressing need to take critical feminist studies seriously, and to recognise that the performative effect of sexual violence, as gendering and enforcing domination, is more important than the victims' or even the perpetrators' sex. What is significant is not so much the fact that the victim is a man or a woman, but the meaning conveyed by sexual violence, that is a super/subordination relation that is also connected to larger matrixes of power and violence. This is crucial for both research and policy purposes, in particular because it affects the way survivors can handle what befell them (see also DeLaet, Golden and Laveta, this volume). When offering support to survivors, due attention has to be paid not just to the sexual or gendered aspects of sexual brutalisation, but also to the way it is intertwined with other structural, cultural or physical kinds of violence. The fact that survivors often belong to socially dominated groups – which also partly explains why women are more likely to be targeted for sexual violence – is a major impediment to their recovery. In other words, in order to offer proper support to both male and female survivors of wartime sexual violence, global health institutions should be aware of the performative effect of sexual violence, and in particular of the way in which the gendered understandings of sexual violence generate further cultural, structural and even physical violence for survivors. This notably requires global health professionals to understand and recognise how their own practices and assumptions participate in, and actually reinforce, this performative effect.

One of the ways to achieve this is to stop analysing and addressing sexual violence as a stand-alone type of violence perpetrated during wars, and instead to interpret it carefully within the frame of other oppositions and struggles that occur during conflicts, for instance, between different ethnic, caste, class or religious groups, between different ideologies and so forth. This is particularly important in light of how survivors experience sexual violence. Male and female survivors' narratives suggest that being sexually assaulted is not necessarily what they would describe as their most painful or most daunting experience of the conflict, and they almost always refer to other kinds of suffering they have been through, such as losing relatives or seeing them being hurt or killed, losing livelihoods or being displaced. It is important to understand that survivors have a better chance to cope with the experience of sexual violence if they are able to relate it to other kinds of violence they are victims of, whether structural or physical, as in the example of militants who are sexually brutalised because of their political opinions.

What this means concretely is that when we question and challenge the epistemic violence contained in discourses about wartime sexual violence, and when we connect the use of sexual brutalisation to other experiences of political, social and economic violence, we create spaces in which survivors can resist, and build resilience to the practice and effects of sexual violence. In addition, helping to make sexual violence against *all* human beings speakable would help to reduce the stigma attached to it. Eventually, this could also make sexual brutalisation itself a less effective instrument of dehumanisation, hence reducing the occurrence of this type of gendered violence altogether. Reinventing a way to speak about, and to address, conflict-related sexual violence, is therefore a major feminist task.

NOTES

1. This is not to suggest, of course, that men cannot be raped or sexually enslaved, or that women are not victims of forced nudity or beatings of the genitals. As we will see, there is, in fact, a great overlap in types of conflict-related sexual violence affecting men and women.

2. There are, of course, exceptions, like the Guantánamo/Abu Ghraib cases, but I would argue that the media focus on the sexual torture of Iraqi prisoners by female officers was not primarily produced by the sexual nature of these acts, but by the gender of their perpetrators. And, needless to say, the other (non-sexual) dimensions of torture used on Iraqi prisoners have been receiving ample media attention too. On Abu Ghraib, see Richter-Montpetit 2007.

3. The names of all interviewees are pseudonyms.

REFERENCES

Buss, Doris E. 2009. 'Rethinking "Rape as a Weapon of War"'. *Feminist Legal Studies* 17: 145–163.

Cohen, Dara Kay, Amelia Hoover Green and Elisabeth Jean Wood. 2013. 'Wartime Sexual Violence: Misconceptions, Implications, and Ways Forward'. *United States Institute of Peace*, Special Report 323 (February).

Confortini, Catia C. and Tiina Vaittinen. 2019. 'Introduction: Analysing Violences in Gendered Global Health'. In *Gender, Global Health and Violence: Feminist Perspectives on Peace and Disease*, edited by Tiina Vaittinen and Catia Confortini. London and New York: Rowman & Littlefield.

DeLaet, Debra L., Shannon Golden and Veronica Laveta. 2019. 'Therapeutic Justice for Survivors of Human Rights Violations and Wartime Violence'. In *Gender, Global Health and Violence: Feminist Perspectives on Peace and Disease*, edited by Tiina Vaittinen and Catia Confortini. London and New York: Rowman & Littlefield.

Del Zotto, A. and Adam Jones. 2002. 'Male-on-Male Sexual Violence in Wartime: Human Rights' Last Taboo?' Paper presented to the Annual Convention of the International Studies Association (ISA), New Orleans, LA, March 23–27. http://adamjones.freeservers.com/malerape.htm. Accessed 27 August 2019.

Dolan, Chris. 2014. 'Into the Mainstream: Addressing Sexual Violence against Men and Boys in Conflict', A briefing paper prepared for the workshop held at the Overseas Development Institute, London, May 14.

Eriksson Baaz, Maria and Maria Stern. 2013. *Sexual Violence as a Weapon of War? Perceptions, Prescriptions, Problem in the Congo and Beyond*. London: Zed Books.

Feldman, Allen. 1991. *Formations of Violence: The Narrative of the Body and Political Terror in Northern Ireland*. Chicago: The University of Chicago Press.

Féron, Élise. 2017. 'Wartime Sexual Violence against Men: Why so Oblivious?' *European Review of International Studies* 4, no. 1: 60–74.

Féron, Élise. 2018. *Wartime Sexual Violence against Men: Masculinities and Power in Conflict Zones*. Lanham: Rowman & Littlefield.

Galtung, Johan. 1969. 'Violence, Peace and Peace Research'. *Journal of Peace Research* 6, no. 3: 167–191.

Gettleman, Jeffrey. 2009. 'Symbol of Unhealed Congo: Male Rape Victims'. *New York Times*, 5 August 2009.

Gorris, Ellen Anna Philo. 2015. 'Invisible Victims? Where Are Male Victims of Conflict-Related Sexual Violence in International Law and Policy?' *European Journal of Women's Studies* 22, no. 4: 412–427.

Grey, Rosemary and Laura J. Shepherd. 2012. ' "Stop Rape Now?": Masculinity, Responsibility, and Conflict-Related Sexual Violence'. *Men and Masculinities* 16, no. 1: 115–135.

Harman, Sophie. 2019. 'Violence and the Paradox of Global Health'. In *Gender, Global Health and Violence: Feminist Perspectives on Peace and Disease*, edited by Tiina Vaittinen and Catia Confortini. London and New York: Rowman & Littlefield.

Hooper, Charlotte. 2001. *Manly States: Masculinities, International Relations, and Gender Politics*. New York: Columbia University Press.

Jones, Adam. 2006. 'Straight as a Rule: Heteronormativity, Gendercide, and the Non-combatant Male'. *Men and Masculinities* 8, no. 4: 451–469.

Kapur, Amrita and Kelli Muddell. 2016. *When No One Calls It Rape. Addressing Sexual Violence against Men and Boys in Transitional Contexts*. New York: International Center for Transitional Justice.

Kippenberg, Juliane. 2005. 'Seeking Justice: The Prosecution of Sexual Violence in the Congo War'. *Human Rights Watch*, March 17.

Kirby, Paul. 2012. 'How Is Rape a Weapon of War? Feminist International Relations, Modes of Critical Explanation and the Study of Wartime Sexual Violence'. *European Journal of International Relations* 19, no. 4: 797–821.

Krug, Etienne G., Linda L. Dahlberg,, Mercy Dahlberg, Zwi James A., Anthony B. and Lozano Rafael, eds. 2002. *World Report on Violence and Health*, Geneva: World Health Organization.

Le Pape, Marc. 2012. 'Suite à "Viols en temps de guerre: les hommes aussi"'. Paris: Centre de Réflexion sur l'Action et les Savoirs Humanitaires, Papers, January 23.

Leiby, Michele. 2012. 'The Promise and Peril of Primary Documents: Documenting Wartime Sexual Violence in El Salvador and Peru'. In *Understanding and Proving International Sex Crimes*, edited by Morten Bergsmo, Alf Butenschø Skre and Elisabeth J. Wood, 315–366. Beijing: Torkel Opsahl Academic EPublisher.

Lewis, Dustin A. (2009). 'Unrecognised Victims: Sexual Violence against Men in Conflict Settings under International Law'. *Wisconsin International Law Journal* 27, no. 1: 1–49.

Lukić, Dragana and Ann Therese Lotherington. 2019. 'Fighting Symbolic Violence through Artistic Encounters: Searching for Feminist Answers to the Question of Life and Death with Dementia'. In *Gender, Global Health and Violence: Feminist Perspectives on Peace and Disease*, edited by Tiina Vaittinen and Catia Confortini. London and New York: Rowman & Littlefield.

MacDonald, Eileen. 1991. *Shoot the Women First*. New York: Random House.
Manivannan, Anjali. 2014. 'Seeking Justice for Male Victims of Sexual Violence in Armed Conflict'. *International Law and Politics* 46: 635–679.
Marcus, Sharon. 1992. 'Fighting Bodies, Fighting Words: A Theory and Politics of Rape Prevention'. In *Feminists Theorise the Political*, edited by Judith Butler and Joan W. Scott, 385–403. New York: Routledge.
Obote-Odora, Alex. 2005. 'Rape and Sexual Violence in International Law: ICTR Contribution'. *New England Journal of International and Comparative Law* 12, no. 1: 135–159.
Oosterveld, Valerie. 2011. 'The Gender Jurisprudence of the Special Court for Sierra Leone: Progress in the Revolutionary United Front Judgments'. *Cornell International Law Journals* 44: 49–74.
OSCE. 2015. 'Combating Impunity for Conflict-Related Sexual Violence in Bosnia and Herzegovina: Progress and Challenges. An analysis of criminal proceedings before the courts of the Federation of Bosnia and Herzegovina, Republika Srpska and Brčko District BiH between 2004 and 2014'. Vienna: OSCE, July 13.
Peters, Edward. 1996. *Torture*. Philadelphia: University of Pennsylvania Press.
Quijano, Alejandra Azuero and Kelly Jocelyn. 2012. 'A Tale of Two Conflicts: an Unexpected Reading of Sexual Violence in Conflict through the Cases of Colombia and Democratic Republic of the Congo'. In *Understanding and Proving International Sex Crimes*, edited by Morten Bergsmo, Alf Butenschø Skre and Elisabeth J. Wood, 437–493. Beijing: Torkel Opsahl Academic EPublisher.
Refugee Law Project. 2013. *Report on the 1st South-South Institute on Sexual Violence against Men and Boys in Conflict and Displacement*. Kampala: Refugee Law Project, April 8–12. http://refugeelawproject.org/files/others/SSI_2013_report.pdf.
Refugee Law Project. 2014. 'Male Survivors of Sexual Violence in Kampala Demand for Better Services'. Kampala: Refugee Law Project. Accessed 27 August 2019.
Richter-Montpetit, Melanie. 2007. 'Empire, Desire and Violence: A Queer Transnational Feminist Reading of the Prisoner "Abuse" in Abu Ghraib and the Question of "Gender Equality"'. *International Feminist Journal of Politics* 9, no. 1: 38–59.
Ross, Marlon B. 2002. 'Race, Rape, Castration: Feminist Theories of Sexual Violence and Masculine Strategies of Black Protest'. In *Masculinity Studies and Feminist Theory. New Directions*, edited by Judith Kegan Gardiner, 305–343. New York: Columbia University Press.
Scarry, Elaine. 1985. *The Body in Pain: The Making and Unmaking of the World*. Oxford: Oxford University Press.
Seto, Donna. 2013. *No Place for a War Baby: The Global Politics of Children Born of Wartime Sexual Violence*. Farnham: Ashgate.
Sivakumaran, Sandesh. 2007. 'Sexual Violence against Men in Armed Conflict'. *European Journal of International Law* 18, no. 2: 253–276.
Sivakumaran, Sandesh. 2010. 'Lost in Translation: UN Responses to Sexual Violence against Men and Boys in Situations of Armed Conflict'. *International Review of the Red Cross* 92, no. 877 (March): 259–277.
Spivak, Gayatri Chakravorty. 1988. *Can the Subaltern Speak?* Basingstoke: Macmillan.

Stemple, Lara. 2009. 'Male Rape and Human Rights'. *Hastings Law Journal* 60: 605–645.

Tanyag, Maria. 2019. 'Replenishing Bodies and the Political Economy of SRHR in Crisis and Emergencies'. In *Gender, Global Health and Violence: Feminist Perspectives on Peace and Disease*, edited by Tiina Vaittinen and Catia Confortini. London and New York: Rowman & Littlefield.

UN. 2013. 'Report of Workshop on Sexual Violence against Men and Boys in Conflict Situations'. New York: United Nations, Special Representative of the Secretary General on Sexual Violence in Conflict, July 25–26.

UNHCR. 2017. '"We Kept It in Our Heart", Sexual Violence against Men and Boys in the Syria Crisis'. Geneva: UNHCR.

Watts, Charlotte and Cathy Zimmerman. 2002. 'Violence against Women: Global Scope and Magnitude'. *The Lancet* 359 (April 6): 1232–1237.

Zawati, Hilmi M. 2007. 'Impunity or Immunity: Wartime Male Rape and Sexual Torture as a Crime against Humanity'. *Torture* 17, no. 1: 2–47.

Part III

TOWARDS PEACE AND JUSTICE IN GLOBAL HEALTH

Chapter 9

Therapeutic Justice for Survivors of Human Rights Violations and Wartime Violence

Debra L. DeLaet, Shannon Golden, and Veronica Laveta

This chapter explores how the concept of therapeutic justice can contribute to transitional justice by integrating a focus on individual healing for survivors of human rights abuses and wartime violence. In an effort to facilitate healing, therapeutic justice prioritises the needs, preferences, and agency of individual survivors. A therapeutic lens calls attention to the ways in which participation in justice initiatives affects survivors' psychological health and wellbeing.

We build on therapeutic jurisprudence in the field of criminology and mental health law (Wexler 1990). Therapeutic jurisprudence is concerned with the intended and unintended ways in which legal rules, processes, and the actions of legal actors impact the psychological wellbeing of the people they touch. This understanding is used to advocate for policies or interventions that promote therapeutic outcomes and prevent anti-therapeutic impacts. Therapeutic jurisprudence has generally focused on domestic legal responses to crime; we extend the concept to national and transnational transitional justice initiatives. Unlike much of the scholarship on therapeutic jurisprudence, we place the justice needs of survivors, rather than those of alleged criminals or perpetrators, at the centre of our analysis.

Similar to how restorative justice addresses past wrongs through restoring relationships and retributive justice addresses wrongs through fair punishments, therapeutic justice identifies remedies for past violations in healing for individual survivors. Diverse practices or mechanisms can contribute to achieving a particular type of justice. Therapeutic justice is most likely to be achieved through mechanisms explicitly designed to prioritise survivors' healing. Any justice practice or mechanism could be designed with a therapeutic approach to maximise the likelihood that survivors will experience therapeutic justice. An activity is therapeutic if it helps survivors in their healing process by having a beneficial effect on the mind or body. Healing refers to processes of recovery that relieve distress and suffering and that restore health. A broad range of activities, beyond medical or psychosocial interventions, are potentially therapeutic.

We argue that several key principles distinguish therapeutic justice. First, therapeutic justice requires that survivors have the opportunity to define their notions of justice and to shape the justice initiatives in which they participate. Second, survivors should have a range of choices for participation in justice-related processes. Third, therapeutic justice requires that survivors have consistent, supportive relationships and interactions intended to facilitate their healing throughout a justice-related process. Finally, the necessary characteristic of therapeutic justice is that healing is defined by survivors themselves and that the justice processes contribute to fulfilling their healing goals; this is the defining characteristic of therapeutic justice. Survivors' definitions of healing might include psychological elements, including a reduction in symptoms or distress, increase in functioning, or an ability to move forward or make meaning. They might also include socioeconomic elements, including the pursuit of reparations or other forms of support. It might further include political or legal elements, such as participating in the trials of alleged perpetrators or in truth commissions.

This chapter explores the intersection of gender, global health, and violence in several ways. First, we examine how pursuing therapeutic justice strengthens the response to the trauma suffered by survivors of direct physical and psychological violence experienced in the context of war and human rights abuses. Second, we posit that transitional justice mechanisms that are not attentive to therapeutic justice may perpetrate psychological and structural violence to the extent that survivors experience re-traumatisation, exploitation, and other forms of harm through participation in these mechanisms. Third, we argue that therapeutic justice has the potential to promote individual healing that disrupts social cycles of violence. Trauma rehabilitation, for example, may reduce family violence. Further, healing can reduce the fear of the other that perpetuates patterns of intergroup violence.

We develop a case study of the Center for Victims of Torture (CVT), a non-governmental organisation that provides rehabilitation services to torture survivors in the US and multiple international sites.[1] We present CVT's efforts to integrate its therapeutic and advocacy work.[2] The organisation is exploring opportunities for survivors to shape processes, define justice agendas, determine individual and collective justice goals, and inform remedies for structural violence. These practices emphasise the healing of survivors rather than seeing survivors and their stories as primarily instrumental for broader advocacy goals. CVT's work with torture survivors provides a lens to explore challenges and potential benefits of pursuing therapeutic justice for survivors of violence.

TRANSITIONAL JUSTICE AND TRAUMA

Participation in transitional justice initiatives that do not incorporate therapeutic dimensions can harm survivors of human rights violations and wartime violence. Survivors who participate in justice initiatives may experience retraumatisation, stigmatisation, social marginalisation, and other forms of harm due to their participation in transitional justice processes; assuming individual benefit from participation thus may reproduce violence (Byrne 2004; Doak 2011; Ellison and Munro 2017; Hamber 2001; Herman 1992; Jackson 2003; Kagee 2006; Kesserling 2017; Martín-Beristain et al. 2010; Porter 2016).

We rely primarily on two literatures to inform our conceptualisation of therapeutic justice. First, we explore feminist analyses of gender-based violence (GBV) that suggest ways in which therapeutic approaches may mitigate the risk of harm for survivors. Notably, the insights from these feminist analyses apply to all survivors of wartime violence and human rights abuses, not only survivors of GBV. Second, we consider insights from vulnerability studies on how non-therapeutic approaches to transitional justice may increase vulnerability and exposure to psychological violence by failing to hear the voice and agency of the survivors.

Invisibility and Silence in Addressing Gender-Based Violence

Feminist scholarship on transitional justice demonstrates the limitations of justice initiatives that do not prioritise the needs and preferences of survivors. Early post-conflict justice initiatives often failed to recognise GBV (Bell and O'Rourke 2007). International legal norms now explicitly condemn GBV, and wartime rape is recognised as a violation of international law that has been prosecuted in the International Criminal Tribunal for the Former Yugoslavia, the International Criminal Tribunal for Rwanda, and the International Criminal Court.

Despite notable progress in raising the visibility of these crimes and the willingness of courts to prosecute, addressing GBV remains a persistent challenge in transitional justice initiatives. Survivors of sexual violence often remain silent rather than seeking recourse via transitional justice. Gender norms that create stigma for survivors of sexual violence contribute to the reluctance of survivors to discuss their victimisation in public settings, including trials or truth commissions (Byrne 2004; DeLaet and Mills 2018; Kesserling 2017; Mertus 2004; Porter 2016). Constructions of femininity that emphasise the importance of sexual purity and modesty invoke feelings of shame that hinder survivors' willingness to discuss sexual violence publicly.

Additionally, constructions of masculinity that emphasise male dominance and invulnerability make men who have survived sexual violence resistant to participate in justice initiatives that involve public testimony (DeLaet 2008; Féron, this volume). Further, rape survivors may be punished by their families or communities for adultery, including extreme forms of punishment including being killed or banished from their communities. The risk of facing these forms of violence is a barrier for survivors reporting the violence they have experienced as well as for participating in justice initiatives. Children born of wartime rape, likewise, are often rejected, ostracised, or even killed by their families and communities (Carpenter 2007).

Furthermore, survivors are sometimes used instrumentally in trials and truth commissions. Participation in these processes can lead to the retraumatisation and stigmatisation of survivors of GBV. Rather than contributing to the healing of survivors, testimony before trials and truth commissions may actively hinder healing or contribute to new forms of harm (Kagee 2006; Kesserling 2017; Porter 2016). Beyond feelings of shame associated with stigma, survivors of GBV who testify publicly in trials or before truth commissions can face social rejection, abuse, and violence from families and communities. In such cases, trials and truth commissions that instrumentalise the testimony and trauma of survivors in ways that are harmful can be seen as perpetrating new forms of psychological violence against survivors, undermining both peace and justice (for stigma as violence, see also Harman, this volume).

Feminist scholarship on GBV suggests that justice initiatives that place the needs and preferences of survivors at the forefront will be more likely to challenge or circumvent the gendered barriers to justice and peace. It is important to stress that these feminist insights are applicable for all survivors of wartime violence and human rights atrocities, who face risks of retraumatisation and other harms through participation in justice initiatives that do not prioritise their preferences and needs. By offering a survivor-centred framework that strives for therapeutic justice, we point to the importance of approaches that empower and make space for survivors to exert agency through shaping initiatives and practices that contribute directly to their healing.

Vulnerability

Vulnerability has often been treated as a given condition in global politics, in which marginalised populations are conceptualised as inherently vulnerable and in need of aid and support from powerful, advantaged, and 'invulnerable' actors (Clark 2013; Goodin 1985; Fineman 2008). Indeed, some populations are more susceptible to harm from violence, inequity, and social marginalisation due to structural inequities in the global system. However, institutional responses to global violence that privilege voices and perspectives of actors that already dominate influential political institutions and economic resources risk reinforcing rather than challenging the vulnerability experienced by marginalised populations (Clark 2013; Gilson 2014).

The risk that institutionalised notions of vulnerability at the global level may actually (re)constitute structural inequities is especially pronounced in regard to gender (Gilson 2014; Luna 2009). Women commonly serve as the ultimate signifiers of vulnerability, with 'innocent women and children' being central to national security and humanitarian policies of states and international organisations (Carpenter 2006). Often, states mobilise the concept of vulnerable women as a strategic rationalisation for self-interested, security-oriented policies rather than for humanitarian reasons. For example, the Bush administration relied heavily on constructions of vulnerable and innocent womanhood in Afghanistan to mobilise public support for the US invasion of Iraq (Sheperd 2006). Even when states or international organisations draw on the concept of vulnerable women to legitimate humanitarian considerations, the outcomes may reinforce gendered inequities in global politics.

Feminist ethics of care also resonate with insights from recent scholarship on vulnerability. According to a feminist ethics of care, ethical responses to global violence need to prioritise lived, embodied experiences of carers and value moral reasoning that emphasises relationality, interdependence, and care for others (Cohn 2014; Vaittinen 2015). A feminist ethics of care approach asserts that 'the vulnerable' need to have voice and agency and to drive structural change rather than being acted upon by the privileged and powerful (Robinson 2011; cf. Vaittinen, this volume).

These insights illuminate the potential value of therapeutic justice. When transitional justice initiatives are designed without significant input from survivors, they risk hardening rather than mitigating the vulnerability of survivors. In contrast, by placing survivors' healing at the centre of justice-seeking, therapeutic justice may alter the dynamics of initiatives that reinforce vulnerability by treating survivors as passive victims rather than critical agents of change. Although therapeutic justice has the potential to disrupt patterns that assume and reinforce vulnerability, it is important to critically consider vulnerability dynamics. In our conceptualisation of therapeutic justice, the key is to centre survivor preferences and needs regarding the justice initiatives in which they participate, to provide survivors with a range of choices, and to provide consistent support focused on healing.

Bringing Survivors In:
Trauma, Healing, and Therapeutic Justice

We propose therapeutic justice as a form of justice that emphasises the health and wellbeing of individual survivors, placing survivors at the centre and prioritising their healing and rehabilitation in the aftermath of violence.

This framework stresses the importance of fostering emotional repair for victims who have been traumatised (Doak 2011). More broadly, we argue that a therapeutic approach to transitional justice involves applying a healing lens to existing mechanisms (trials, truth commissions, and others), as well as imagining new therapeutic mechanisms to add to the transitional justice toolkit.

By contributing to the healing and rehabilitation of survivors, therapeutic justice may help to generate socio-cultural transformation in ways that contribute to peacebuilding. This conceptualisation of therapeutic justice complements Lambourne's (2009) call for a model of transformative justice that is holistic, transdisciplinary, and participatory. Individuals who have made progress towards their healing goals may be better able to participate in other justice processes, including restorative practices aimed at social repair, which may disrupt cycles of violence by contributing to reconciliation among groups that have been divided by violent conflict (Lundy and McGovern 2008; Silove 2013).

A range of methods and practices might contribute to therapeutic justice for survivors. Trauma therapy (at both the individual and group level) that facilitates healing and is connected to justice-related goals of survivors can be a mechanism of therapeutic justice (Herman 1992). Testimony therapy and narrative exposure therapy are examples of therapeutic interventions that explicitly attempt to connect a therapeutic process with testimony to amplify survivor voices in justice-related processes. The provision of direct services and reparations to survivors also might contribute to therapeutic justice. Community-based social rituals that support the needs and preferences of survivors also could contribute to therapeutic justice as conceptualised in this chapter (Martín-Beristain et al. 2010; Park 2010). Storytelling that provides survivors with opportunities to exercise agency in telling their own stories can be a powerful mechanism for pursuing therapeutic justice, as can other artistic forms that are practiced in the service of healing and self-expression for survivors (Baines and Stewart 2011; Porter 2016).

Although methods and practices that take place at the level of individuals and communities provide a robust setting for focusing on survivors, national or transnational justice processes, including trials and truth commissions, also can integrate therapeutic dimensions (Doak 2011). Recognising that a multiplicity of methods and institutions may best serve the goals of transitional justice (Roht-Arriaza and Mariezcurrena 2006), we argue that the core principles of therapeutic justice might be integrated in all transitional justice initiatives. In the case of trials, offering jurors evidence-based guidance about post-traumatic stress disorder and its effects on legal testimony, allowing victims to testify via videotape without having to confront the accused, and developing protections against unduly aggressive cross-examinations can make it more likely that trials serve therapeutic purposes for survivors (Ashworth 2004; Ellison and Munro 2017; Jackson 2003).

Although all transitional justice processes can integrate therapeutic dimensions, survivor preferences for participating in a range of justice initiatives will vary. Survivors are not homogenous; their unique experiences, needs, and preferences mean that therapeutic justice is not a one-size-fits-all model of justice. Some survivors focus on their own rehabilitation and healing as a path to justice. Others feel a deep need to see perpetrators punished as a form of justice and derive therapeutic benefit from participating in trials. Similarly, some survivors may find rehabilitation and healing by giving testimony in truth commissions. Thus, all survivors should have access to a full range of options. A critical element that distinguishes therapeutic justice is the facilitation of opportunities for survivors to express agency regarding if, when, and how they participate in justice initiatives to aid in their own healing.

Despite this complexity and variation, therapeutic justice offers a unifying approach that places survivors at the centre of transitional justice processes. One of our key arguments is that all approaches will be more likely to contribute to a comprehensive vision of justice and peacebuilding in the aftermath of human rights violations and wartime violence by addressing the needs and perspectives of survivors and by considering the therapeutic implications of the practices and processes that constitute a particular justice initiative. Indeed, the broadest implication of our argument is that all transitional justice mechanisms should include the goal of facilitating therapeutic justice for survivors. Therapeutic justice should not just be relegated to a separate sphere, whereby healing is pursued through community-based processes, such as reconciliation rituals or memorialisation. Rather, a comprehensive sense of justice requires that therapeutic justice is core objective of all transitional justice mechanisms.

THE CENTER FOR VICTIMS OF TORTURE AND THE INTEGRATION OF JUSTICE AND HEALING

The work of CVT with survivors of torture illustrates key elements of a survivor-centred therapeutic approach to transitional justice that may help mitigate the risks of re-traumatising or re-constituting vulnerability of survivors of human rights violations and wartime violence. This example offers insights into: (1) the complexity of implementation of the tandem pursuits of justice and healing for survivors; (2) one example of a therapeutic justice mechanism emerging from practice; and (3) practical suggestions of what could be integrated into other transitional justice mechanisms to develop a therapeutic approach.

CVT is a mid-sized international NGO founded in the 1980s to provide rehabilitation services to torture survivors in Minnesota, US, with a scope that now includes trauma rehabilitation services in nine international sites. For CVT, trauma rehabilitation includes interdisciplinary modalities to promote the mental health of survivors. CVT provides combinations of individual and group psychotherapy, physiotherapy, and social work services at established clinics in the United States, Kenya, Ethiopia, Uganda, and Jordan, primarily serving refugees, asylum seekers, or internally displaced persons. CVT works with refugees living in urban centres and in refugee camps and settlements, as well as with survivors living in post-war societies where the violence was perpetrated. CVT clients in international sites consistently show statistically and clinically meaningful improvements in post-traumatic stress, depression, anxiety, and somatic symptoms, and improvements in behavioural functioning.

The remainder of the chapter applies theoretical insights previously discussed to explore the development of the concept of therapeutic justice within one organisation and insights into how to build a therapeutic approach to advocacy or transitional justice work. The CVT case study demonstrates the critical role that non-state actors can play in promoting human rights and equity in transitional justice initiatives (DeLaet 2018). Additionally, the case study illustrates insights from the study of vulnerability, feminist peace research, and feminist ethics of care that emphasise the importance of hearing the voice and agency of persons from marginalised populations in transitional justice initiatives. We begin with a brief overview of CVT's mission and its programming around trauma rehabilitation and anti-torture advocacy. Second, we describe CVT's clinical model in greater detail, illustrating one approach to help survivors realise their right to rehabilitation. Third, we discuss CVT's early phase of integrating clinical and documentation work, which can be characterised as 'trauma-sensitive documentation'. Fourth, we discuss CVT's middle phase of integration, which involved moving towards 'survivor-centred documentation'. Finally, we describe a new CVT initiative, which builds on the earlier phases to develop an intervention model of 'therapeutic documentation'.

CVT's Mission:
Trauma Rehabilitation and Anti-Torture Advocacy

Both trauma rehabilitation and anti-torture advocacy are central to the two-pronged mission of CVT, which is to heal the wounds of torture and to end torture worldwide. CVT provides therapeutic services to survivors and engages in advocacy against torture, approaching these as two sides of the same coin, within a human-rights framework. For organisations engaged in this type of work, there are often tensions in implementing these two components cohesively (Birrell and Freyd 2006; Denborough 2005; Steel, Steel and Silove 2009). CVT, thus, is a microcosm of the broader structural, pragmatic, and theoretical challenges in the integration of healing and justice work.

CVT views its advocacy and trauma rehabilitation work as integrally connected. Nevertheless, it has faced illustrative tensions in balancing competing objectives of and approaches to these components of its mission. Some stem directly from the different levels of intended impact, as are often apparent in transitional justice work. Trauma rehabilitation is focused on individual-level positive change, whereas advocacy campaigns or transitional justice mechanisms are more typically focused on communal, national, or transnational social goods. Ideally, these areas of focus are complementary, but it is also possible for their goals to be in tension with each other.

Organisationally, CVT has had compelling reasons to maintain some distinctions between advocacy and justice activities and clinical work. For example, in the United States, CVT's legitimacy has been partially linked to its maintaining a reputation as a specialised clinical or health provider, rather than a human rights organisation. This reputational management has allowed clinical staff to more effectively advocate for survivors. Outside of the United States, CVT has also maintained some distance between its human rights advocacy work and its role as a humanitarian service provider, a decision that has allowed CVT to operate in contexts that may be closed to more overtly activist organisations.

On a practical level, CVT has separated its advocacy and trauma rehabilitation work due to the professional skills and training required in each sector. Professionals with expertise in mental health have primary responsibility for CVT's clinical work on trauma rehabilitation while lawyers have led most advocacy and justice-related initiatives. Although clinical activities inform advocacy, this work has generally been distinct from therapeutic programming. Relatedly, most of CVT's advocacy work has been conducted from a Washington, D.C., office, whereas the clinical work is conducted in Minnesota offices and global sites. Historically, these logistical arrangements have contributed to the functional segmentation of human rights advocacy and trauma rehabilitation.

There are conceptual and normative challenges to integrating health and justice frameworks. Some argue that trauma rehabilitation can be seen as contributing to justice for survivors. However, proponents of a justice-oriented approach argue that the individual healing process can contribute to justice through realising torture survivors' right to rehabilitation, but that it may not be sufficient to address their justice-related needs or priorities (e.g. Silove 2013). From this perspective, not offering survivors an opportunity to pursue justice discounts survivors' agency and may not allow full realisation of their healing goals. On the other hand, most clinical staff at CVT are rooted in a health and medical lens, and clinical training programmes typically do not include attention to justice issues. Some staff perceive the differentiation between the two spheres as appropriate, not only for structural and pragmatic reasons, but perceiving that concern for justice is an agenda not typically shared by survivors. On the other hand, some clinical staff have been actively engaged in justice work, perceiving that survivors do bring up justice concerns in counselling, and thus identify a need for integrating healing and justice.

The historical silos of CVT's justice and healing initiatives parallel a broader separation between mental health organisations and documentation or advocacy organisations (Moon 2012). This challenge is common for organisations interested in combining healing and justice work. The compartmentalisation of distinct components of the CVT mission reflects broader socio-political limitations of approaches that treat human rights as distinct from health. When human rights and health are treated independently, human rights can be seen as falling rigidly within the purview of the law and health as exclusively within the realm of health professionals (Sirkin et al. 1999). This dichotomous treatment can limit the fulfilment of both human rights and health-oriented goals, and limits the conceptions of justice that can be achieved for survivors.

The challenges related to the segmentation of advocacy, justice, and healing in CVT's work also demonstrate insights from socio-legal scholarship that highlight the limitations of formal law in efforts to advance rights and justice (Constable 2005; Merry 2009). In this regard, state institutions and the laws are seen as the appropriate spaces to seek the implementation of human rights as legal entitlements, whereas health-oriented rights are contested more frequently in non-state sites (cf. Finley, this volume). In an effort to strategically work across this divide, CVT frames its trauma rehabilitation work as working to fulfil survivors' right to rehabilitation, bringing a human rights framework to underpin its health-related work.

In its current efforts to effectively pursue integration, CVT views therapeutic justice as a conceptual bridge that can be used to link advocacy and healing goals in service of both human rights and health. This move towards deeper integration is building an inclusive, survivor-centred, therapeutically oriented approach to justice that fosters participation and agency among highly vulnerable survivors that are often excluded or marginalised in transitional justice processes.

CVT's Clinical Model:
Claiming the Right to Rehabilitation

CVT's international direct services to survivors of torture, war violence, and other gross human rights violations seek to achieve 'as much rehabilitation as possible', consistent with the right to rehabilitation established by Article 14 of the United Nations Convention against Torture (UNCAT). CVT works with refugees in some of the largest camps and settlements in the world, as well as in large urban centres hosting large refugee populations, with survivors coming from Syria, Iraq, Somalia, Eritrea, South Sudan, Ethiopia, Uganda, DRC, Rwanda, Burundi, and other countries.

In humanitarian contexts, the trauma rehabilitation needs of millions of survivors, many of whom have undergone multiple traumatic events, overwhelms the availability of services. CVT provides time-limited, ten-week group interventions, with the possibility of individual therapy for particularly high-need or high-risk situations. CVT promotes rehabilitation through an interdisciplinary approach to improve the mental health of survivors, or 'clients' within CVT's therapeutic context. CVT sees restored or improved functioning as critical for survivors to reclaim their agency and dignity. After receiving services, the goal is for survivors to be better prepared to take steps to advocate for themselves and their families, to meet basic needs, and to participate in justice related activities, if they so choose. This increased functioning can also better prepare them to confront current injustices that they are facing in a host country.

The group intervention model is structured to empower survivors to see themselves as agents in their own healing. The design of the group seeks to disrupt power structures that can be replicated in therapy – with an 'expert' serving 'vulnerable' clients – by locating much of the therapeutic benefit in the group process and the support they give to one another, thereby challenging a static notion of vulnerability, a notion which, as shown earlier, feminists have contested (see also Vaittinen, this volume). The group therapy process is intended to reinforce and build on the strengths of the participants and to give them the opportunity to offer something to others, rather than participating as passive 'victims' or recipients of assistance. Group members share coping strategies that have worked for them, which inspires and motivates others. Group members are encouraged to share contact information to support one another in between sessions and after the conclusion of the group sessions.

For many survivors, the opportunity to share a part of their trauma story can be particularly empowering. In addition to processing their own trauma, group members also serve as supportive witnesses to others as they share their traumatic experiences. At the end of group, survivors regularly recount that the support they receive from others during these critical sessions helped reduce their shame over what happened to them and relieved their emotional burden. Survivors have reported feeling enormous relief at being able to speak the unspeakable (Herman 1992) in front of supportive witnesses, contributing to the realisation they are not alone. Survivors can experience the power of naming what happened to them, thereby potentially diminishing shame as well as supporting others who are suffering. Group members often reflect on the importance of having the support of others throughout counselling; some find that telling their story in a group contributes to shared memory and helps ensure that the violence they endured will not be forgotten (Center for Victims of Torture 2015).

Despite the potential therapeutic benefits of sharing their stories through group counselling, the process includes risks. Anytime a survivor revisits a traumatic experience of violence, there is a risk of re-traumatisation (Denborough 2005; Hamber 2001; Herman 1992; Van Dijk, Schoutrop and Spinhoven 2003). Exposure to past traumatic material before a survivor is adequately prepared can increase intrusive symptoms and avoidance, exacerbating the problem. Although these risks cannot be completely eliminated, CVT takes these complexities seriously and takes many steps to mitigate risk, including prioritising relationship-building between clients, group members, and facilitators; helping clients develop coping and containment strategies; giving clients choices about whether, how, and when to share their stories; and providing extensive training and supervision for counsellors.

For survivors of complex trauma from torture, GBV, and other human rights violations, narrating what happened to them without adequate preparation in a therapeutic context is likely to produce strong negative repercussions. To minimise this risk, CVT's clinical model is designed with the intention of empowering survivors in their own healing goals and processes. The CVT model reflects key insights from the study of vulnerability and feminist ethics of care that place the embodied experiences of populations who have suffered from violence at the centre of the analysis and call for survivors to have voice and agency in responding to experiences of violence (Cohn 2014; Fineman 2008; Gilson 2014; Robinson 2011; Vaittinen 2015). In this way, experiencing dignity, agency, and healing during trauma rehabilitation services can contribute to therapeutic justice, as survivors are empowered to claim their right to rehabilitation.

Healing and Justice: From Silos to Integration

CVT has sought to meet the deep-rooted challenges of integrating healing and justice initiatives by developing opportunities for more substantive engagement between its trauma rehabilitation and advocacy activities. This has been pursued most fruitfully through documentation, which has progressed through three phases. The first phase pursued documentation in a way that was sensitive to the trauma of survivors. The second phase deepened awareness of how to put survivors in a more central role during the documentation process. In the third, ongoing phase, CVT has begun to conceptualise documentation processes specifically designed to have a positive therapeutic impact on individual survivors, with a pilot therapeutic documentation model focused on integrating healing and justice.

Phase 1: Trauma-Sensitive Documentation

CVT's efforts to more overtly connect its clinical therapy and its anti-torture advocacy began with a documentation project initiated in 2013. At this time, a lawyer from CVT's Washington, D.C., office began visits to CVT's Jordan programme to conduct in-depth interviews. Counsellors would refer former clients to the lawyer for a single interview about their experiences; there were no structured follow-up sessions unless the survivor presented as distressed or requested it. In addition, questions were added to the standard clinical intake assessment to collect data on human rights violations perpetrated against clients.

CVT project managers hoped the qualitative and quantitative data from this effort could be used for human rights documentation for criminal trials or other legal mechanisms. Over time, it became clear that the rigour of evidence collection possible in these interviews would not meet the standards for criminal prosecutions. This disconnect in expectations and outcomes highlights the tangible challenges in meaningfully integrating therapeutic and justice work, particularly more formal legal documentation.

In CVT's case, these challenges are related to several factors. First, as a health provider, CVT attracts survivors who are most distressed or have most severe symptoms. Offering them documentation opportunities is positive because it reaches torture survivors who may have otherwise had little hope of engaging with any kind of transitional justice, thus helping to provide them access to exercise their fundamental rights. On the other hand, their ability to provide detailed, coherent testimony is often derailed by traumatic memories, and they are very vulnerable to re-traumatisation. Second, survivors have often been ignored, dismissed, or blamed for what happened to them. The therapeutic alliance established during rehabilitation services requires staff to consistently and explicitly believe and support survivors. Conducting documentation in this context can make it difficult to highlight contradictions in survivor narratives or to ask probing questions that can be seen as adversarial, which is often necessary to establish the legal evidentiary standard. Third, similarly to other humanitarian service providers, CVT operates in contexts in which many torturers are still in power and protected; agents of oppressive states or groups are still tracking people within the countries where CVT works. There is a real fear of the consequences of providing detailed narratives. Finally, CVT staff are primarily trained in counselling, not in documentation for legal processes. Without personnel who have expertise in both areas, it is challenging to fully integrate therapeutic work and legal justice work.

Instead of being used as formal legal documentation, the interview and assessment data were compiled into reports used for advocacy on a range of issues identified by survivors in the reports (CVT 2015). These reports furthered efforts to advance advocacy based upon the concerns of survivors, not only regarding human rights violations experienced in countries of origin but also ongoing injustices in displacement.

At this stage, CVT's documentation was more consistent with approaches found in transitional justice mechanisms which are sensitive to trauma and utilise a do no harm approach. The 'do no harm' framework in medical ethics highlights the obligations of physicians and health professionals to prioritise a patient's wellbeing and to avoid doing harm with any interventions. Such a framework signals the importance of exercising caution when performing health interventions or procedures (Wessells 2009).

In this trauma-sensitive, do-no-harm approach, CVT advocacy staff only conducted documentation interviews after the clients completed a mental health and/or physical therapy programme with six-month follow-up care. Additionally, interviews began with detailed informed consent processes that outlined different uses of survivors' information. Held in CVT's clinical space, survivors were interviewed in a place that already was likely to feel safe to them, and where support was available from counsellors, if necessary. The interviewer was informed about how to notice and respond to signs of distress during an interview.

However, despite some advocacy priorities emerging from the interviews, survivors did not have particularly direct opportunities for engagement or agency within the process. CVT also found these efforts to be insufficient to achieve therapeutic value from the documentation process for most survivors. There was little space to integrate survivors' goals for the process or to involve them in the utilisation of the data. This case can illustrate how well-intentioned researchers, organisations, or justice mechanisms can still prioritise pursuit of a collective good over the more challenging work of integrating individual healing into the process. Building upon lessons learned in this experience, CVT continued to develop its approach to integrating individual healing into its documentation work.

Phase 2: Survivor-Centred Documentation

Reflecting on these challenges, CVT re-evaluated its approach to documentation and advocacy. The organisation found new energy and synergies for deepening integration work with opportunities for more cross-departmental engagement, as clinical, research, and policy staff members held discussions about how to make the CVT interview process more survivor-centred. CVT renamed the documentation activities the Transitional Justice Initiative, with the aim to further a survivor-centred approach to transitional justice. Moving beyond trauma-sensitivity, a survivor-centred approach refers to transitional justice that is shaped by survivors' priorities, promotes survivors' decision-making, and deeply considers how the activity will affect survivors (Nyseth Brehm and Golden 2017).

In this stage, documentation interviews continued to utilise trauma-sensitive practices, such as completing trauma rehabilitation services prior to documentation, having counsellors available, and conducting interviews in CVT clinical space. To refine the documentation approach in this next phase, CVT staff revised the informed consent process, better clarifying the purpose of the interviews as well as the risks and potential benefits of participation. In an effort to increase the survivor-centred emphasis of documentation interviews, the process moved from one interview to two to allow survivors to build trust with the interviewer, facilitating more in-depth interviews. The process also integrated an opportunity for survivors to review, correct, and retract information they had disclosed. A clinical advisor observed interviews and provided debriefing and coaching to the interviewer to improve the interview process to be more responsive to survivors' experiences and needs. This initiative also included structured follow-up to check in after interviews, to help mitigate any negative consequences survivors experienced. Finally, there were two series of interviews, with the second focused on Iraqi disappearances, emerging directly from Iraqi survivors voicing their concerns about this issue.

These steps moved CVT substantially towards a more survivor-centred approach to its documentation work. Even within this, however, there was recognition that there were opportunities for continued growth and deepening of the survivor-centred approach. Discussions continued about how to develop the work in a way that was driven even more by survivors, and which also integrated healing objectives. At this time, CVT was engaging in organisation-wide discussions about building a human rights framework for its work. There were additions of members of the executive team coming from a human rights background, including an incoming executive director from Amnesty International. These discussions included working with a consultant from Justice Rapid Response who facilitated a meeting on how to take this integrated work forward. During this time, CVT staff also collaborated on an article on survivor-centred approaches to transitional justice that focused on the use of trauma survivors' testimony in trials and truth commissions (Soueid, Willhoite and Sovcik 2017). Although the article focused narrowly on witness testimony for criminal prosecution, it laid out therapeutic principles to be considered in any justice-related activity. CVT deepened its commitment to the integration of healing and documentation by putting goals in its new strategic plan to create survivor-centred documentation opportunities within all CVT direct service sites, to provide survivors the opportunity to record their experiences for multiple purposes of their choice. Therapeutic documentation emerged as one way in which that commitment could be realised.

Phase 3: Therapeutic Documentation

Within the organisational context of CVT's increasing interest in pursuing justice-related programming and the larger context of a dramatic proliferation of civil society organisations documenting human rights violations in Syria, CVT launched a new project focused on Syrian survivors of torture. The objectives of the project include: (1) to build relationships between organisations doing clinical work and organisations doing human rights documentation; (2) to develop an innovative approach that reimagines principles and practices from both domains; and (3) to offer survivors the opportunity to participate in therapeutic documentation. It is CVT's first programme to explicitly integrate healing and justice services, pursued largely through the development of a therapeutic documentation model.

Therapeutic documentation is an approach that provides survivors a range of options to record their stories and to decide how their information is used, from individual uses to external uses such as advocacy or formal justice mechanisms. It is a process-oriented approach; to maximise the healing potential for the survivor every step of the process must follow therapeutic principles. CVT's therapeutic documentation model is one example of a therapeutic practice or mechanism that could be used in transitional justice processes to help survivors address the past and move towards a positive future.

CVT's therapeutic documentation model was originally envisioned as being implemented by a network of specialised documentation/advocacy and clinical/rehabilitation organisations. The project's goal is to promote positive collaboration and to develop new processes and content that integrates both trauma rehabilitation and human rights documentation approaches. The hypothesis of the project is that survivors may find therapeutic benefit from telling and recording their stories and from the uses of those stories if the process is designed to maximise healing. Furthermore, therapeutic documentation could provide documentation organisations with a rich repository of survivor stories that can contribute to justice through a variety of mechanisms. Alone, trauma rehabilitation may provide healing for individuals. In the context of transitional justice initiatives, documentation efforts may provide a sense of justice. Building a network of mental health and documentation organisations was envisioned as the first step to developing a new intervention integrating both healing and justice components, implemented in partnerships across sectors.

However, the project experienced challenges in building an integrated network able to collaborate on developing and piloting a new approach. Structural and contextual challenges, as well as divergent goals and approaches, resulted in a more long-range and incremental approach to network development. These challenges came from within both sectors.

First, as discussed throughout this chapter, formal documentation is sometimes done in a way that creates re-traumatisation; views individual survivors as an instrumental means to a collective good; and can engage survivors in a way that is disempowering, deepens their vulnerabilities, or is even exploitative. Although many documentation organisations are committed to do-no-harm principles, due to the pressing need from criminal justice mechanisms, lack of training on trauma-sensitive interviewing, and pressure from donors to produce a certain number of recorded stories, interviewers can inadvertently cause harm. This dilemma is particularly pronounced in regard to survivors of sexual violence (DeLaet and Mills 2018; Fineman and Zinsstag 2013; Franke 2006; Mertus 2004; Ross 2003), and harm to survivors of sexual violence through documentation efforts has been identified as a significant problem by some organisations working with Syrians. Documentation organisations may pressure survivors who are not ready or wanting to tell their stories. This pressure may have a double damaging effect – the survivor can be re-traumatised and then often will not seek mental health services they may need, due to fear of being pressured to tell their story. Mental health organisations can be hesitant to encourage clients to participate in documentation.

On the other side, organisations doing trauma rehabilitation face critiques that they pursue healing for individuals without routinely offering opportunities to survivors who want or need another step in their healing (Ibrahim 2013; Silove 2013). As a pathway to justice, some survivors might need an institutional response to the broader context or individual(s) who contributed to or caused the violence against them. This critique is not surprising, as clinical work focuses on individual- and family-level change, and it tends to focus advocacy efforts on increasing awareness about mental health and the need for services.

The two sectors, with their divergent goals, lack of knowledge about the other sector, and well-founded critiques of one another can face barriers in working together. With these challenges, CVT's network integration objective shifted to a longer timeline. Plans for the therapeutic documentation intervention shifted back to within CVT itself, developing a mini-network internally in which advocacy/policy, media/communications, clinical, and research departments each developed a component of the approach.

As a first step to develop a model for therapeutic documentation that was trauma-sensitive and survivor-centred, CVT conducted a series of interviews with Syrian survivors who had received CVT trauma rehabilitation services in Jordan. The goal was to understand survivors' perspectives on healing, justice, and documentation. As survivors defined what 'justice' meant to them, it was clear how deeply these ideas are shaped by context, suggesting that survivor-centred documentation to further justice priorities should be responsive to how survivors' needs change over time and place. In 2017, with the war in Syria ongoing, survivors living in refuge in Jordan most commonly described justice as: (1) equality and fairness, in giving each person the same treatment, having freedom from discrimination, and having equality and protection under the law; (2) morality and doing right, or upholding an ethical distinction between right and wrong, at both individual and collective levels; and (3) rights and responsibilities, built on respect for the humanity of all people, which necessitates limits on acceptable behaviours. Survivors' conception of justice resonates with ethics of care principles that prioritise relationality, interdependence, and care for others (Cohn 2014; Vaittinen 2015). From the information gathered, CVT recognised that documentation to further survivors' sense of justice must have opportunities to utilise information and engage survivors in advocating for freedom and protections for refugees in Jordan, as well as for them to tell their stories within a broader lens of morality and truth-telling.

In these interviews, most survivors expressed a desire to have their experiences documented in some form. Despite this, almost all also expressed fear of reprisals by parties within Syria if their stories were to be made public. There was also substantial variation in their specific documentation preferences. Some preferred documentation for community archiving or memorialisation, others for media, advocacy, research, or accountability purposes, and still others for their own personal use. From this, CVT recognised that 'documentation' could be broadly conceived, referring to any way by which survivors' experiences are recorded. These interviews also led to the concept of documentation 'pathways', offering options for the types of documentation interviews and opportunities to use information, with survivors choosing the option(s) they desired from among the pathways.

CVT's therapeutic documentation approach is in its pilot phase, with the intention to refine the model and develop a scaled-up approach to implement the model within an integrated network. The pilot phase offers six pathways, and each participant can select one or more to fit their own goals. Pilot pathways include: (1) a communications pathway for those interested in raising awareness about torture and its effects, or about rehabilitation services, through online content or other media; (2) a policy pathway for survivors interested in documenting what happened to them as a way to advocate for increased resources for services or protections and support for other survivors of human rights violations; (3) an activism pathway to become directly involved in grassroots advocacy efforts for refugees or survivors of human rights abuses; (4) a creative expression pathway that allows survivors to document their experiences through artistic or creative media, such as poetry, memoir, painting, or drawing, rather than through documentation interviews; (5) a personal documentation pathway that allows survivors to document what happened to them for their own personal use, which might include documentation for asylum cases or other legal proceedings, or recording personal narratives for use in family histories or community archives; and, finally, (6) a pathway for formal legal documentation for those who would like the record to be available for potential use in a future criminal investigation or commission of inquiry. Because CVT does not have internal capacity to conduct interviews for formal legal documentation, participants who select this pathway are referred to an external documentation partner for trauma-sensitive documentation.

In the pilot of the therapeutic documentation model, CVT clients who completed rehabilitation services and attended a follow-up session were given information about the documentation opportunities. Those who expressed interest were contacted by a psychotherapist, who held an individual consultation to describe the pathways available. Survivors could express interest in participation at that time but were also encouraged to reflect upon the opportunities before making a decision. Pathways selected by survivors shape the nature of the interviews, the extent to which documentation is shared publicly, the outputs or usages of the documentation material, and the opportunities for survivors' continued engagement.

Survivor consent and agency are an essential component of the process. After being given time to reflect on documentation options, survivors have a second meeting focused on consent, reviewing potential documentation pathways, and discussing questions. At this time, the survivor can decide to participate in documentation. Consent is respected as an ongoing process; at each point of interaction, staff reinforce the message that the participant can choose if and how to continue. Giving survivors multiple options for participation, including ones with relatively low risks, keeps documentation from being an all or nothing proposition. Rather, survivors can decide what level of risk they want to take (if any) and weigh the risks and benefits. They can also decide to participate in options in the future when they feel more comfortable doing so (e.g. less fearful of reprisals or having more of an understanding of the documentation process).

The second stage of therapeutic documentation is a documentation interview. The interview content is customised to produce the types of information relevant to the selected pathway(s) and may be conducted over multiple sessions. Carried out by psychotherapists with interviewing training, the documentation interview itself is designed to have a therapeutic effect and deepen the healing process.

The final stage of therapeutic documentation is the utilisation of the information to further the survivors' justice and healing goals. Each pathway offers opportunities for outputs and includes mechanisms for survivors' continued engagement in these processes; some are short-term utilisations of the documentation, while others are orientated towards longer-term goals. By following therapeutic principles in all stages of the process from initial therapy through documentation processes and continued engagement, the goal is to provide survivors opportunities to further their individual healing and at the same time contribute to individual and collective justice goals.

During the pilot, most participants initially chose individual use or creative expression pathways. Still, many expressed interest in other pathways and indicated they may be interested in participating in other pathways in the future. After understanding the levels of de-identification available to them as well as having their questions answered about the pathways and terminology (e.g. advocacy), participants were more interested in media and advocacy options. Hesitation to participate in formal documentation often was due to fear that there could be spies in Jordan who would turn them in or that if they ever returned to Syria, they would be targeted for having spoken out. Some who were interested in formal documentation preferred to be referred to a European mechanism partly due to these concerns. Ultimately, about 60 per cent selected creative expression, 45 per cent individual use, 30 per cent communications, 30 per cent activism, 15 per cent policy, and 10 per cent formal documentation.

Regardless of survivors' choice of pathways, including those who did not choose a pathway, all expressed appreciation for the consultation. Many mentioned their trust in CVT as a key factor in their interest in finding out more about documentation. One lesson learned from the pilot thus far is that therapeutic documentation has the potential to promote broader participation in documentation and to elevate the voices of survivors who are rarely heard.

There are several key elements in this model of therapeutic documentation. First, it prioritises survivor agency, affording multiple opportunities to make decisions throughout the process. Second, it focuses on multiple levels, with potential individual and communal benefits, but prioritising individual benefits. Third, it is oriented towards facilitating healing, or having therapeutic value, for survivors at each stage of the process. The decision-making process, the documentation process, and the pathway or use of the information are all designed to have direct therapeutic value to the survivor. Therapeutic documentation does not see survivors as instrumental towards achieving broader human rights objectives; rather, CVT provides survivors with opportunities to shape processes, define justice agendas, determine individual and collective healing goals, and inform remedies for personal and structural violence. Conducted within an organisation that has already built rapport through provision of trauma rehabilitation services helps ensure survivors have caring and trusting relationships to help them work through the processes with safety and emotional stability.

A final point to highlight is that the development of this model is based on assumptions about what may contribute to healing for survivors. In actuality, there is little rigorous research evidence establishing therapeutic value in documentation of human rights abuses. However, clinical observations of cases in which survivors are offered supportive means to tell or record what happened to them suggests that therapeutic documentation offers potential opportunities for healing. In its pilot stage, this model of therapeutic documentation builds upon clinical observations and expressed desires of survivors themselves to document their stories. Research is needed to refine the model and to identify which causal mechanisms contributed to positive or negative outcomes for survivors. As a contribution to filling this gap, CVT is collecting data throughout implementation of the pathways to allow evaluation of the conditions under which documentation may be therapeutic for survivors. Survivors have opportunities to reflect on the documentation interview and the outputs or uses of their information, including sharing which steps of the process contributed to or detracted from their own experiences of healing and justice.

THE ROLE OF THERAPEUTIC JUSTICE IN COMPREHENSIVE VISIONS OF JUSTICE

Therapeutic justice seeks to remedy past wrongs through prioritising healing for individual survivors. This is a survivor-centred justice framework, in which individual survivors' needs are prioritised and their agency and voice are essential, particularly expressed through defining their own healing processes and goals. Therapeutic justice can and should be prioritised in all transitional justice mechanisms; developing a therapeutic approach is possible, moving beyond do-no-harm goals.

Our case study, however, illuminates the significant pragmatic, conceptual, and normative challenges to integrating healing and justice work. This discussion provided practical insights into the progressive development of a therapeutic approach to justice work, particularly distinguishing between practices that are trauma-sensitive, survivor-centred, and, ultimately, therapeutic. The case study also described one example of a new model or mechanism that was specifically designed to pursue therapeutic justice for survivors.

Therapeutic justice may be particularly likely to produce positive outcomes at the intersection of gender, violence, and global health. It offers potential advantages for responding to trauma suffered by survivors of direct physical and psychological violence from war and human rights abuses. Therapeutic justice may mitigate the risks of harm, including re-traumatisation, stigmatisation, social marginalisation, and others, which survivors can experience when they participate in transitional justice mechanisms that do not incorporate therapeutic dimensions. Because of its emphasis on survivors' agency, therapeutic justice may help minimise the risk that transitional justice initiatives construct or reproduce vulnerabilities – thus perpetrating psychological and structural violence – among populations that have survived war violence or human rights abuses. Therapeutic justice can also expand participation to those who tend to not be reached by existing mechanisms. Finally, therapeutic justice may contribute to peacebuilding by facilitating the healing and rehabilitation of survivors, who will be more able to productively participate in other peace processes.

Therapeutic justice offers a unifying framework that places survivors at the centre of transitional justice processes. The broadest implication of our argument is that *all* transitional justice approaches will be *more likely* to contribute to a comprehensive vision of justice and peacebuilding by integrating therapeutic dimensions. Insights and practices from clinical organisations that provide rehabilitation services to survivors could help transitional justice mechanisms refine their approaches to be more likely to have therapeutic benefit for survivors, with a secondary effect of increased numbers of survivors interested in and able to participate.

NOTES

1. For more information about CVT's history, mission, programmes, activities, and sources of funding, visit www.cvt.org.

2. Veronica Laveta and Shannon Golden are staff at CVT and have contributed to this chapter as both researchers and practitioners.

REFERENCES

Ashworth, A. 2004. 'Victims' Rights, Defendants' Rights and Criminal Procedure'. In *Integrating a Victim Perspective within Criminal Justice: International Debates*, edited by A. Crawford and J. Goodey, 185–204. Aldershot: Ashgate Dartmouth.

Baines, Erin and Beth Stewart. 2011. ' "I Cannot Accept What I Have Not Done": Storytelling, Gender, and Transitional Justice'. *Journal of Human Rights Practice* 3, no. 3: 245–263.

Bell, Christine and Catherine O'Rourke. 2007. 'Does Feminism Need a Theory of Transitional Justice? An Introductory Essay'. *The International Journal of Transitional Justice* 1, no. 1: 23–44.

Birrell, Pamela J. and Jennifer J. Freyd. 2006. 'Betrayal Trauma: Relational Models of Harm and Healing'. *Journal of Trauma Practice* 5, no. 1: 49–63.

Byrne, Catherine C. 2004. 'Benefit or Burden: Victims' Reflections on TRC Participation'. *Peace and Conflict* 10, no. 3: 237–256.

Carpenter, R. Charli. 2006. *'Innocent Women and Children': Gender, Norms, and the Protection of Civilians*. New York: Routledge.

Carpenter, R. Charli. 2007. *Born of War: Protecting Children of Sexual Violence Survivors in Conflict Zones*. Bloomfield, CT: Kumarian Press.

Center for Victims of Torture. 2015. *Reclaiming Hope, Dignity, and Respect: Syrian and Iraqi Torture Survivors in Jordan*. Accessed 26 January 2019. http://www.cvt.org/sites/default/files/attachments/u11/downloads/ReclaimingHope_01042016.pdf.

Clark, Ian. 2013. *The Vulnerable in International Society*. Oxford: Oxford University Press.

Cohn, Carol. 2014. '"Maternal Thinking" and the Concept of "Vulnerability" in Security Paradigms, Policies, and Practices'. *Journal of International Political Theory* 10, no. 1: 46–69.

Constable, Marianne. 2005. *Just Silences: The Limits and Possibilities of Modern Law*. Princeton: Princeton University Press.

DeLaet, Debra L. 2018. 'Lost in Legation: The Gap between Rhetoric and Reality in International Human Rights Law Governing Women's Rights', *Global Discourse* 8, no. 3: 387–404.

DeLaet, Debra L. 2008. 'Gender, Sexual Violence and Justice in War-Torn Societies'. *Global Change, Peace & Security* 20, 3: 323–338.

DeLaet, Debra L. and Elizabeth Mills. 2018. 'Discursive Silence as a Global Response to Sexual Violence: From Title IX to Truth Commissions'. *Global Society* 32, 4: 496–519.

Denborough, David. 2005. 'A Framework for Receiving and Documenting Testimonies of Trauma'. *International Journal of Narrative Therapy and Community Work*, no. 3/4: 34–42.

Doak, Jonathan. 2011. 'The Therapeutic Dimension of Transitional Justice: Emotional Repair and Victim Satisfaction in International Trials and Truth Commissions'. *International Criminal Law Review* 11, no. 2: 263–298.

Ellison, L. and V.E. Munro. 2017. 'Taking Trauma Seriously: Critical Reflections on the Criminal Justice Process'. *International Journal of Evidence and Proof* 21, no. 3: 183–208.

Féron, Élise. 2019. 'When Is It Torture? When Is It Rape? Discourses on Wartime Sexual Violence'. In *Gender, Global Health and Violence: Feminist Perspectives on Peace and Disease*, edited by Tiina Vaittinen and Catia Confortini. London and New York: Rowman & Littlefield.

Fineman, Martha A. 2008. 'The Vulnerable Subject: Anchoring Equality in the Human Condition'. *Yale Journal of Law and Feminism* 20, no. 1: 1–23.

Fineman, Martha A. and Estelle Zinsstag, eds. 2013. *Feminist Perspectives on Transitional Justice: From International and Criminal to Alternative Forms of Justice*. Cambridge, UK: Intersentia.

Finley, Laura. 2019. 'Domestic Violence and Public Health: Beginning Steps for Creating More Just and Effective Community Responses'. In *Gender, Global Health and Violence: Feminist Perspectives on Peace and Disease*, edited by Tiina Vaittinen and Catia Confortini. London and New York: Rowman & Littlefield.

Franke, Katherine. 2006. 'Gendered Subjects of Transitional Justice'. *Columbia Journal of Gender & Law* 15, no. 3: 813–828.

Gilson, Erinn C. 2014. *The Ethics of Vulnerability: A Feminist Analysis of Social Life and Practice*. New York: Routledge Publishers.

Goodin, Robert E. 1985. *Protecting the Vulnerable: A Reanalysis of Our Social Responsibilities*. Chicago: University of Chicago Press.

Hamber, Brandon. 2001. 'Does the Truth Heal? A Psychological Perspective on the Political Strategies for Dealing with the Legacy of Political Violence'. In *Burying the Past: Making Peace and Doing Justice after Civil Conflict*, edited by Nigel Biggar, 155–176. Washington, D.C.: Georgetown University Press.

Harman, Sophie. 2019. 'Violence and the Paradox of Global Health'. In *Gender, Global Health and Violence: Feminist Perspectives on Peace and Disease*, edited by Tiina Vaittinen and Catia Confortini. London and New York: Rowman & Littlefield.

Herman, Judith Lewis. 1992. *Trauma and Recovery*. New York: Basic Books.

Kira, Ibrahim A. 2017. 'A Critical Outlook at Torture Definition, Structure, Dynamics, and Interventions'. *Peace and Conflict: Journal of Peace Psychology* 23, no. 3: 328–333.

Jackson J. 2003. 'Putting Victims at the Heart of Criminal Justice?' *Journal of Law and Society* 30, no. 2: 309–326.

Kagee, Ashraf. 2006. 'The Relationship between Statement-Giving at the South African Truth and Reconciliation Commission and Psychological Distress among Former Political Detainees'. *South African Journal of Psychology* 36: 880–894.

Kesserling, Rita. 2017. *Bodies of Truth: Law, Memory, and Emancipation in Post-Apartheid South Africa*. Palo Alto, CA: Stanford University Press.

Luna, Florencia. 2009. 'Elucidating the Concept of Vulnerability: Layers Not Labels'. *International Journal of Feminist Approaches to Bioethics* 2, no. 1: 121–139.

Lundy, Patricia and Mark McGovern. 2008. 'Whose Justice? Rethinking Transitional Justice from the Bottom Up'. *Journal of Law and Society* 35, no. 2: 265–292.

Martín-Beristain, Carlos, Darío Páez, Bernard Rimé and Patrick Kanyangara. 2010. 'Psychosocial Effects of Participation in Rituals of Transitional Justice: a Collective-level Analysis and Review of the Literature of the Effects of TRCs and Trials on Human Rights Violations in Latin America'. *Revista de Psicología Social* 25, no. 1: 47–60.

Meier, Benjamin Mason. 2014. 'An Agenda for Normative Policy Analysis in Global Health Governance'. In *Law and Global Health*, edited by Michael Freeman, Sarah Hawkes and Belinda Bennett, 593–608. London: Oxford University Press.

Merry, Sally Engle. 2009. *Gender Violence: A Cultural Perspective*. Hoboken, New Jersey: Wiley-Blackwell.

Mertus, Julie. 2004. 'Shouting from the Bottom of the Well: the Impact of International Trials for Wartime Rape on Women's Agency'. *International Feminist Journal of Politics* 6, no. 1: 110–128.

Moon, Claire. 2012. 'What One Sees and How One Files Seeing: Human Rights Reporting, Representation, and Action'. *Sociology* 46, no. 5: 876–890.

Nyseth Brehm, Hollie and Shannon Golden. 2017. 'Centering Survivors in Local Transitional Justice'. *Annual Review of Law and Social Science* 13: 101–121.

Park, Augustine S.J. 2010. 'Community-Based Restorative Transitional Justice in Sierra Leone'. *Contemporary Justice Review* 13, no. 1: 95–119.

Porter, Elisabeth. 2016. 'Gendered Narratives: Stories and Silences in Transitional Justice'. *Human Rights Review* 17, no. 1: 35–50.

Robinson, Fiona. 2011. 'Stop Talking and Listen: Discourse Ethics and Feminist Care Ethics in International Political Theory'. *Millennium: Journal of International Studies* 39, no. 3: 845–860.

Roht-Arriaza, Naomi and Javier Mariezzcurrena. 2006. *Transitional Justice in the Twenty-First Century: Beyond Truth versus Justice*. Cambridge: Cambridge University Press.

Ross, Fiona. 2003. *Bearing Witness: Women and the Truth and Reconciliation Commission in South Africa*. London: Pluto Press.

Sheperd, Laura J. 2006. 'Veiled References: Constructions of Gender in the Bush Administration Discourse on the Attacks on Afghanistan post-9/11'. *International Feminist Journal of Politics* 8, no. 1: 19–41.

Silove, Derrick. 2013. 'The ADAPT Model: a Conceptual Framework for Mental Health and Psychosocial Programming in Post Conflict Settings'. *Intervention* 11, no. 3: 237–248.

Sirkin, Susannah, Vincent Iacopino, Michael Grodin and Yael Danieli. 1999. 'The Role of Health Professionals in Promoting and Protecting Human Rights'. In *The Universal Declaration of Human Rights: 50 Years and Beyond*, edited by Yael Danieli, Elsa Stamatopoulou and Clarence Dias, 357–370. Boca Raton, Florida: CRC Press, Taylor & Francis.

Soueid, Marie, Ann Marie Willhoite and Annie E. Sovcik. 2017. 'The Survivor-Centered Approach to Transitional Justice: Why a Trauma-Informed Handling of Witness Testimony Is a Necessary Component'. *The George Washington International Law Review* 50, no. 1: 125–179.

Steel, Zachary, Catherine R. Bateman Steel and Derrick Silove. 2009. 'Human Rights and the Trauma Model: Genuine Partners or Uneasy Allies?' *Journal of Traumatic Stress* 22, no. 5: 358–365.

Vaittinen, Tiina. 2019. 'Exposed to Violence While Caring: From Caring Self-Protection to Global Health as Conflict Transformation'. In *Gender, Global Health and Violence: Feminist Perspectives on Peace and Disease*, edited by Tiina Vaittinen and Catia Confortini. London and New York: Rowman & Littlefield.

Vaittinen, Tiina. 2015. 'The Power of the Vulnerable Body: A New Political Understanding of Care'. *International Feminist Journal of Politics* 17, no. 1: 110–118.

Wessells, M. G. 2009. 'Do No Harm: Toward Contextually Appropriate Psychosocial Support in International Emergencies'. *American Psychologist* 64, no. 8: 842–854.

Wexler, David B. 1990. *Therapeutic Jurisprudence: the Law as a Therapeutic Agent*. Durham, North Carolina: Carolina Academic Press.

Chapter 10

Domestic Violence and Public Health: Beginning Steps for Creating More Just and Effective Community Responses

Laura Finley

The World Health Organisation (WHO) found in 2013 that nearly one-third of the world's women had endured physical or sexual intimate partner violence (WHO 2013). As much as 38 per cent of all murders of women around the globe are domestic violence related (WHO 2013). In the United States, one in four women and one in seven men are victims of domestic violence. It is estimated that every nine seconds a woman is physically assaulted by an intimate partner, and some 1300 people are killed each year by abusers in the United States alone (Chemaly 2012). Far more Americans – generally women – have been killed by their partners than in the wars in Iraq and Afghanistan combined. American women are twice as likely to suffer domestic violence as breast cancer, and homicide by a partner is the leading cause of death for African-American women ages fifteen to thirty-four (Chemaly 2012). In other countries, homicide rates are even higher. In Guatemala, two women are murdered each day by current or former partners. In Europe, domestic violence causes more deaths than cancer and traffic accidents combined (Chemaly 2012). According to a study by the WHO, women are at greater risk at home than in any other location (Garcia-Moreno et al. 2005). Domestic violence kills more women worldwide than civil wars (Parker 2014).

Although things have changed somewhat in recent years, the typical response to domestic violence, especially in the United States and the so-called global north, is to involve the criminal justice system. For decades, countries have looked to enact and enforce domestic violence legislation. The primary piece of federal legislation related to domestic violence in the United States is the Violence against Women Act (VAWA), which has continually prioritised legal and criminal justice responses (Weissman 2013). Yet this response is rife with limitations, not least of which is that it addresses only individual cases, not the broader issue of domestic violence. Such an individual approach ignores the community, institutional, and societal factors that promote abuse. As such, it cannot possibly result in any dramatic reductions in the scope or extent of the problem. Similarly, the shelter model that has been the predominant vehicle for providing safety for victims in the United States since the 1970s may serve as needed triage but cannot transform social norms nor address the gender inequalities that are the underlying causes of domestic violence.

Both the criminal justice approach and the shelter model originated in response to feminists' rejection of the medicalisation of abuse. Prior to the 1970s, such medicalisation was a feature of theories that saw domestic violence as a result of relationship dysfunction caused by defective personalities. Such a view blamed women and privatised abuse, thereby resulting in personalised responses rather than social change (Houston 2014). Feminists in the 1970s struggled with the degree to which the law should be involved in domestic violence cases. Liberal feminists felt that partnering with the state was essential to keep women safe, while radical feminists believed that the 'male' state was simply replacing one form of male control with another oppressor (Schechter 1980). Radical feminists emphasised consciousness raising. The idea behind it was that women were also raised in a society where men dominated and thus were not truly aware of the ways that were oppressed, because they took them as normal. Catherine MacKinnon (1983), for example, wrote that what women 'know' is from a male perspective that is presented as truth, thereby prohibiting women from seeing 'male violence for what it is: patriarchal force that reinforces a larger system of male domination' (Houston 2014, 237). Consciousness raising, then, involved opportunities for women to listen to one another and for lived experiences with male violence to be shared. This did not necessarily connect well with a criminal justice response to domestic violence.

Eventually the liberal side prevailed, and the emphasis was put on ensuring better police response to domestic violence. Other debates between these two types of feminists focused on prostitution and pornography, and the degree to which these were matters requiring state intervention (Stansell 2010). Even more contentious was support for mandatory criminal intervention, a debate that continues to resonate today. Some feminists, for instance, argue such intervention can do more harm than good, especially for poor women and women of colour (Coker 2000). The contemporary domestic violence movement has, in many ways, given up a good portion of its feminist principles, or least followed a liberal feminist emphasis on legal and political rights rather than broader societal change. Both the criminal justice approach and the shelter model are often not feminist or at least not in a critical sense. Critical feminists today seek to reclaim the radical emphasis. One way to do this is through a feminist public health model that recognises domestic violence as a violation of human rights.

The 1993 United Nations Declaration on the Elimination of All Forms of Violence against Women recognised violence against women as a human rights issue, and declared that it is both a result of and an obstacle to gender equality. In 1995, the Beijing Platform for Action on the Fourth World Conference on Women called broadly for the elimination of all violence directed at women and girls but also issued a series of specific recommendations. These include the collection of data and research on domestic violence and other forms of violence against women as well as studies regarding the effectiveness of prevention and assistance programmes. Further, the Platform called for additional measures of the costs of violence against women in various sectors, noting that in all countries but especially in the global south, scarce resources are being drained when domestic violence and other forms of gender-based violence are allowed to continue. This was an important attempt to show that not only is ending GBV a moral issue, but also one of public concern with dire economic and social consequences.

The 2000 Millennium Development Goals (MDGs) recognised that violence against women and girls adversely affects a country's development. Domestic violence affects not just individuals but entire communities. As Jacqui True (2012, 13) puts it:

> These costs include direct costs, as well as opportunity costs, of the failure to prevent violence for individual women; for governments, business and society; and for children or future generations . . . gender-based violence in public and private spheres prevents women from being able to access economic opportunities, livelihoods, and welfare benefits.

Abuse gets in the way of poverty reduction initiatives and instead increases the likelihood of inter-generational poverty. This is particularly true for women of colour, who are more likely to be victimised and also more likely to be in poverty in the United States. Because it is costly in terms of direct medical, criminal justice, social service, and mental health effects, domestic violence takes away from time and funding to ameliorate other social issues. Victims often suffer from financial abuse, and are controlled by abusers such that their work histories may be sporadic, at best (McLean and Bocinski 2017). As such, they are more likely to live in poverty and to be homeless. GBV is thus a site where complex entanglements of structural, inter-generational, and direct forms of violence come together.

The reduction of violence against women and girls was included as one of seven priority issues in the MDGs, with initial reduction goals set for 2015, and later reiterated in the Sustainable Development Goals with target year 2030. Although these goals have not necessarily been achieved, there has indeed been progress, and the fact that GBV was included is an important symbolic and practical step. In addition to the WHO, other international organisations such as the Inter-American Commission of Women of the Organization of American States have recognised domestic violence as a public health issue (Chelala 2016).

A feminist-informed public health approach to domestic violence is clearly needed in the United States and elsewhere. Here, the 'public' does not simply refer to state-funded health services. Rather, I propose in this chapter a public health approach to domestic violence that includes the state in terms of allocating funding and prioritising domestic violence legislatively. In the United States, for instance, the state is currently not doing nearly enough to address these issues. Yet the 'public', particularly in countries such as the United States, where publicly funded health services are limited, must also include actors beyond the state. The necliberal state is ill-equipped to challenge patriarchy as it benefits from the status quo, and other, non-state sectors must contribute in order to address comprehensively the root causes of abuse. The public in my feminist public health approach to domestic violence, then, also includes schools, corporations, non-profit organisations, social service providers, and healthcare professionals.

Such an approach emphasises that gender oppression is endemic and yet difficult to recognise because it is taken for granted as normal. It seeks to contest claims of gender neutrality and to reveal the self-interest of the dominant groups in society involving, mostly, males. It promotes social justice practices and platforms as the way to eliminate oppression based on gender and other interrelated factors. A critical feminist approach values the experiential knowledge of women and observes that women are differentially discriminated against based on their intersectional identities (MacKinnon 1983, 1991; Wing 2003). A public health approach to domestic violence, then, would include many groups and institutions. In essence, 'the public' should really include just that; all citizens. As people know more and challenge traditional gender role norms, they will be equipped to support others in their quest to engage in healthy relationships. Feminist activists and scholars are still essential to the consciousness-raising frame. Educators have a role in ensuring that we teach about abuse and its underlying factors, and even before, using radical techniques to challenge gender inequality and gender role stereotypes that contribute to abuse. Political leadership is critical to giving GBV priority legislatively and in shifting the nation's focus from one of domination and aggression to one that prioritises human needs. Corporate leadership can ensure not just that workplace policies are appropriate to address domestic violence but that women receive fair wages and supports. Social service agencies and groups that assist the poor and homeless must be enlisted to address the link between domestic violence and poverty. Health care and mental health professionals must play a role in the early detection of domestic violence. New studies have shown that when doctors are educated about abuse, they better identify both physical and behavioural signs, and therefore can help a victim medically as well as supporting her to receive other services. While there still is a role for law enforcement and domestic violence shelters in this model, these are only part of what is needed.

Understanding domestic violence from a feminist political economy approach can shed further light on a feminist public health model for domestic violence. True (2012, 20) provides a feminist political economy analytical framework for understanding violence against women and for developing policy and change programmes. Such a framework would recognise: (1) The gender division of labour within the family and household economy; (2) The contemporary global, macro-economy in which capitalist competition fuels the quest for cheap sources of labour, often women's labour and for deregulated investment conditions; and (3) The masculine protector and feminine-protected identities associated with war and militarism, and division of war front/home front associated with armed conflict and its aftermath. In a gendered public-private sphere, women are often relegated to invisible, unpaid labour that creates inequalities 'in household bargaining power between men and women'. And, 'while the neoliberal policy environment has led to the expansion of women's employment, it has also led to the intensification of their workload in the market and at home, and to the "feminization of poverty"' (True 2012, 31). That is, the marginalisation of women's work and minimisation of wage-earning potential contribute to women's poverty and dependence on male earners, which then exacerbates the difficulties women have in freeing themselves from abusers.

The protector-protected model parallels the abuser-victim model in domestic violence relationships. Further, True (2012) argues that state and state-sanctioned violence celebrate male aggression and that the security state prioritises violence abroad while deprioritising violence in the home. Monies spent on war – in the United States, approximately half of all federal taxes – cannot be used for addressing these root causes of GBV. Finally, 'the hegemonic western brand of masculinity today increasingly takes the form of a "transnational business masculinity" and is associated with autonomy, the capacity for reason and control, mobility, and power, whereas the hegemonic notion of femininity is associated with the absence or lack of these characteristics' (True 2012, 36). Efforts to challenge this 'brand' of masculinity must be part of a feminist-informed public health approach to domestic violence.

This chapter describes the problem of domestic violence, focusing on its social, economic, and health consequences. The emphasis is largely on the United States, although brief mention is made of other countries or regions. The public health approach in this chapter is defined as opposed to and going beyond approaches where responses are compartmentalised as issues of criminal justice and individual healing and responsibility, and builds on insights from feminist political economy analysis (cf. Tanyag, this volume). I draw attention to the limitations in viewing these issues as individual or criminal justice problems, and then begin to outline what a feminist-informed public health model for domestic violence would look like.

THE COSTS OF DOMESTIC VIOLENCE

Some (e.g. Bumiller 2008) have taken issue with the monetisation of crime, in general, and domestic violence, in particular. The idea is that monetising plays into a neoliberal agenda that continues to see issues only in terms of dollars and cents. While this critique is certainly not without merit, emphasising the economic costs of domestic violence is, I argue, still essential. Many public policy and public health decisions are made based on financial considerations, at least in part. Until that is not the case, monetising domestic violence remains critical in terms of keeping it on the agenda. As True (2012, 14) notes, 'Economic rationales . . . have been very successful at increasing awareness and government funding for antiviolence programmes, especially in developed countries'. They are, otherwise put, still an important piece of consciousness raising.

Studies have found the cost of domestic violence to be approximately $9.3 billion (Max, Rice, Finkelstein, Bardwell and Leadbetter 2004). Domestic violence is the most common cause of injury for women in the United States, ages 15 to 44. As such, victims use emergency healthcare services far more frequently – eight times – than do non-victims (Bonomi, Anderson, Thompson, and Rivara 2009). Women who have been abused may suffer from a variety of health consequences. They are 70 per cent more likely to have heart disease, 80 per cent more likely to have a stroke, and 60 per cent more likely to develop asthma during their lifetime. They are three times more likely to suffer from depression, four times more likely to commit suicide, and suffer from post-traumatic stress disorder at six times the rate of non-victims. Women experiencing physical abuse are also three times more likely to report having a sexually transmitted infection than non-abused women (Chelala 2016). Studies have found that these are not just short-term costs; rather, the increased healthcare costs for victims can persist for as long as fifteen years after the abuse (Pearl 2013). Further, according to a 2005 survey, some 64 per cent of domestic violence victims say the abuse has impacted their work. It is estimated that victims lose eight million paid days of work annually. Homicide by an intimate partner is the second leading cause of death for women in the workplace (Workplace Statistics 2016).

Data are clear that domestic violence is costly in other countries and regions as well. Walby's (2004) study of domestic violence in England

and Wales included three types of costs: (1) services, including criminal justice, health care, social services, housing, and civil legal assistance; (2) economic output losses, both for the victims and their families as well as for employers; and (3) human and emotional costs to the victim. It was found that, for one year, the cost to the criminal justice system was around £1 billion, which was at the time approximately one-quarter of the criminal justice system's annual budget for violent crime. Healthcare costs for physical injuries were estimated at £1.2 billion, with an addition £176 million for mental health care. Nearly £0.25 billion was spent annually on social services, and an estimated £0.16 billion was spent on housing for victims. Civil legal services cost an estimated £0.3 billion. Lost economic output tallied to as much as £2.7 billion. The biggest cost, however, was the cost of addressing the emotional toll that domestic violence takes on victims, which was measured at £17 billion. This included mental health services, counselling, and other related services. Altogether, the cost of domestic violence in England and Wales in 2004 totalled a staggering £23 billion annually (Walby 2004). The Home Office issued a statement reporting that in 2017, the social and economic costs of domestic violence topped £66 billion (Home Office 2019).

A similar study in 2003 found the cost of domestic violence in Spain to be the equivalent of US$2.9 billion, while Australia spends approximately AUD8 billion annually (Day, McKenna and Bowlus 2005). Another report from Australia predicted that, if nothing dramatic changes, the cost of domestic violence in that country will be AUD15.6 billion annually by 2021/2022 (Lomborg 2015). The Australian government estimated in 2009 that violence against women cost the country AUD13.6 billion annually, while the costs calculated in Fiji added up to the equivalent of US $300 million, or 7 per cent of GDP (True 2012, 13).

Although it included issues beyond just domestic violence, a conservative estimate found that GBV costs South Africa between R28.4 billion and R42.4 billion per year – or between 0.9 per cent and 1.3 per cent of GDP annually (KPMG n.d.). According to a study in India, a woman loses an average of at least five paid work days for each incident of intimate partner violence, while in Uganda, about 9 per cent of violent incidents forced women to lose time from paid work, amounting to approximately eleven days a year. In Nicaragua, 63 per cent of children of abused women had to repeat a school year and they left school on average four years earlier than other children (UNIFEM n.d.). The total cost of domestic violence has been estimated to be between $4.4 trillion and $8 trillion per year, or more than 5.2 per cent of global GDP (Lomborg 2015).

Although it is vitally important to analyse the costs of domestic violence, as True (2012, 14) notes, 'These economic rationales . . . will likely not help the most vulnerable women in the world in the short to medium term. The realisation of social and economic rights for these women is an immediate and essential condition for eliminating the prolonged and systemic violence they experience'.

LIMITATIONS OF CRIMINAL JUSTICE AND SHELTER-BASED APPROACHES TO DOMESTIC VIOLENCE

In the late 1960s and into the 1970s, domestic violence emerged as a prominent social issue, first in the UK and then in the United States. As was noted earlier, the movement emphasised getting victims to safety, followed by holding abusers accountable through the criminal justice system. As legislation was enacted to criminalise domestic violence, police were required to treat the issue far more seriously. Yet many still did not, owing to a lack of detailed training and the difficulty of these kinds of calls. Abusers are unpredictable and manipulative and victims often scared to talk, making the work challenging for law enforcement. Reports of officers demeaning victims or not taking them seriously persist today. This is likely due to a patriarchal culture that is very much mirrored within the policing subculture (Waldron 2015). Richard and Hagland (2015) did find that adoption of international human rights law, in particular, the Convention on the Elimination of All Forms of Discrimination against Women (CEDAW) resulted in stronger domestic laws and better protections for women. The US has signed but never ratified CEDAW. However, although legislation does seem to reduce fatal domestic violence, it is not clear whether it reduces less severe forms of abuse (Amin, Islam and Lopez 2016).

Another concern with policing practices stems from the Minneapolis Domestic Violence Experiment, which was conducted by Sherman and Berk and resulted in mandatory arrest policies being enacted across the US. Critics such as Ruttenberg (1993) and Coker (2001) note that mandatory arrest policies place victims in danger of retaliatory violence, and that they disempower victims who may not actually want their abuser arrested. In some cases in which it is difficult to determine who the aggressor is, police may make dual arrests, which then revictimise the party who was not at fault (Celik 2013). An unintended consequence of mandatory arrest policies has been an increase in the arrest of women for domestic violence. Although in some cases the female may be the abuser, in many others she is actually the victim but officers arrest both parties and attempt to let the court system figure it out. Some studies have found that victims are more likely to be killed if their abuser was arrested and incarcerated rather than being warned and returned to the home (Sherman and Harris 2014).

Given current and historical tensions between minority communities and law enforcement in the United States owing to a long list of dubious shootings and documented bias and harassment, many do not trust police and are less-than-cooperative. Further, incarceration of abusers can result in dramatic economic consequences for victims, especially for women of colour who often bear the burden of childcare, poverty, and lack of job skills (Crenshaw 1991). Even feminist movements have often struggled to adequately address the unique needs of women of colour (Crenshaw 1991).

If a perpetrator is arrested, many victims do not want to cooperate with the prosecution. Studies have shown that victim non-cooperation is the primary reason why domestic violence cases are dropped (Waldron 2015). Victims cite a variety of reasons why they do not wish to have the case prosecuted, including fear of retaliation, the trauma of rehashing abuse during a lengthy hearing, and lack of faith that legal interventions will change the abuser. Studies showing that 40 to 60 per cent of perpetrators of domestic violence re-offend within thirty months of incarceration do not exactly inspire confidence (Waldron 2015). Further, prosecutors often do not choose to move forward with a case. These are the primary reasons cited by those who assert that criminal justice responses are not always the most appropriate in domestic violence cases (Celik 2013). The failure to listen to what women want was a concern of the feminists who started the anti-domestic violence movement in the US and it remains one today.

Not only are there limitations to the criminal justice approach, but it is also a costly one. There are direct financial costs in terms of the number of police officers needed to respond to domestic violence situations and the prosecutors, defense attorneys, and judges employed in such cases, but there are other costs as well. The time and resources spent on criminal justice responses to the very preventable issues of domestic and dating violence take away from the time and resources that can be spent on other types of crime. Domestic violence calls are among the most dangerous for police officers, and in some cases, they pay with their lives. More than 20 per cent of the officers killed on duty in the United States between 2010 and 2014 were murdered responding to a domestic violence incident (Pyke 2015).

Yet another issue is the over-representation of police officers as abusers. One study found that law enforcement families endured abuse at rates four times those of the general public (Nedig, Russell and Sang 1992). Another study focusing only on older, more experienced officers found 28 per cent more domestic violence (Johnson 1991). Yet accusations against officers are often handled informally, and few who are found guilty suffer any serious sanction (Friedersdorf 2014). Domestic violence is significantly underreported as it is, and, in particular, when it involves law enforcement officers as perpetrators (Jeltsen and Liebelson n.d.). Friedersdorf (2014) comments that 'there is no more damaging perpetrator of domestic violence than a police officer, who harms his partner as profoundly as any abuser, and is then particularly ill-suited to helping victims of abuse in a culture where they are often afraid of coming forward'.

The case of Jessica Lenahan-Gonzales highlights not only the problems with relying on a criminal justice approach to domestic violence but also the need to see abuse as a human rights issue with public health consequences and solutions. In 1999, Jessica Lenahan-Gonzales' estranged husband, Simon Gonzales, took her three girls from their yard. This was a violation of a permanent restraining order requiring him to remain at least 100 yards from her and her children unless it was a scheduled visitation. After Jessica made multiple calls and visits to the police station, the police of Castle Rock, Colorado, still refused to enforce the restraining order. Simon Gonzales pulled up to the police station and opened fire in the early hours of the morning. It is unclear why. Police officers returned fire and, after confirming Gonzales to be dead, found that the three girls were as well. Jessica's legal case against the police reached the Supreme Court, which ruled 7-2 that Castle Rock and its police could not be sued for failing to enforce a restraining order. Jessica's attorneys brought the case before the Inter-American Commission on Human Rights (IACHR) in 2011. That body held that the US had failed to protect both Lenahan and her daughters from domestic violence and to provide equal protection before the law (Finley 2010a). The IACHR also determined that 'all States have a legal obligation to protect women from domestic violence', and this is 'a problem widely recognized by the international community as a serious human rights violation and an extreme form of discrimination' (Richards and Hagland 2015). Importantly, it was the pressure from feminist activists that encouraged international courts to see domestic violence as a human rights issue (Richards and Hagland 2015).

Although domestic violence shelters often do yeoman's work to assist victims in desperate need of housing, this model of assistance also fails to address the broader social issues underlying abuse. In the United States, these services are often overfull: a review of the National Census of Domestic Violence Services, which surveyed more than 2000 programmes, found that one in ten victims who ask for help in a twenty-four-hour period are turned away (Iyengar and Sabik 2009). And because non-profit organisations in the United States are increasingly influenced by neoliberal ideology, which emphasises free market solutions, deregulation, and sees social problems as individual issues requiring personal remedies, they are particularly ill-suited for social transformation. As Baines (2010, 14) explains, in many non-profit organisations that operate in the social service sector, the acceptance of neoliberal ideology and practice has 'supplanted discourses of collective care, economic equality, and social solidarity'. Organisations such as Incite! Women of Color against Violence (2007) have long-critiqued what they refer to as the non-profit industrial complex and, as such, have disavowed non-profit status. This is not to suggest that for-profit organisations are necessarily better equipped but instead to show the need for a public health approach. Likewise, feminist scholars maintain that focus has shifted from localised solutions to those that will sound most appealing to funders. Donors want to see a return on their investment, and thus blanket-style approaches to community problems that would require more nuanced and individualised approaches prevail, while creativity is often stifled through excessive bureaucracy and competition for those scarce resources (Finley and Esposito 2012). Funders do not want to 'take a chance' on something innovative, so domestic violence agencies often propose more of the same so as to receive their lot (Finley 2010b).

Bumiller (2008), Ferraro (1996), Pleck (1987), and others have argued that funders do not seem to appreciate feminist-based approaches and programmes that are perceived as too radical. As a result, the domestic violence movement has minimised the 'critique of women's position within the family, and the larger culture has been silenced by the rhetoric of "family values". As the battered women's movement has become institutionalized and bureaucratized, individual family pathology has been substituted for radical critiques of the status quo' (Ferraro 1996, 80). The result is a movement that provides services to victims but does not truly address the root causes of abuse and gender inequalities.

Berns (2004) notes that the current individual 'frame' for the domestic violence movement is 'empowerment-based'; that is, victims are told that they have been robbed of their power by their abusers and that service providers will help them take their power back. This mantra may be an improvement on the previous medicalised emphasis, which saw abuse as a clinical issue. Clinical or medicalised approaches emphasise diagnosis and treatment, and implicitly indicate that something is wrong with the victim. The empowerment frame still aims exclusively on the individual, not on social or systemic issues, and the onus for change lies squarely on the victim. Power here refers to making personal choices, not harnessing broader social or structural power to effect meaningful social change (Morgen and Bookman 1988). A more critical feminist conception of empowerment, however, involves an understanding of structural violence, that is, 'an understanding that powerlessness is a result of structural and institutional forces that allow for inequality in power and control over resources. Therefore, empowerment should be a process that aims to identify and change the distribution of power within a culture to achieve social justice' (Berns 2004, 154).

Consistent with this, Berns (2004, 3) comments that the current perception of empowerment as solely a personal issue 'may help build support for programs that help victims of domestic violence. However, it does little to develop public understanding of the social context of violence and may impede social change that could prevent violence'. In other words, focus on the individual hinders possibilities to recognise entanglements between intersectionally gendered structural violence and domestic violence, which, in turn, hinders adequate public health responses and policies to prevent domestic violence. Nancy Fraser (2009, 115–117) argues that the emancipatory purpose of feminism depends on our 'reconnecting struggles against personalized subjection to the critique of a capitalist system', and encourages feminists to 'think big' when it comes to our view on violence against women. The narrowly defined shelter version of empowerment is simply not 'big' enough, and minimises or even ignores the political economy of GBV (True 2012). As Brainard and Siplon (2004, 436) assert, 'The soul of the non-profit sector seems to be up for grabs'. That is, many non-profit organisations operate far more like cold and bureaucratic businesses than comprehensive, feminist-informed helping entities.

Another issue with reliance on non-profit shelters is that there is often an assumption that the people involved are benevolent do-gooders who are well informed about the issue. There is also the tendency to believe that doing something is always better than nothing, which can result in inappropriate programmes (Stein 2001). None of that can ever begin to transform a society into a less-violent one. Kivel (2007) argues that the neoliberal model of service and aide co-opts leaders from diverse communities who succumb to the allure of paid work and whose interests then shift to the continued maintenance of the system. As Thunder Hawk (2007, 105–106) explains,

> People in non-profits are not necessarily consciously thinking that they are 'selling out'. But just by trying to keep funding and pay everyone's salaries, they start to unconsciously limit their imagination of what they could do. In addition, the non-profit structure supports a paternalistic relationship in which non-profits from outside our communities fund their own handpicked organizers, rather than funding us to do the work ourselves.

A public health approach would begin to address the limitations of both the criminal justice and shelter models in the US and would reclaim the radical roots of the domestic violence movement. As noted earlier, as I envision it, a public health model would not omit either of those responses but would instead be more inclusive of other individuals and institutions. It would thus be more aligned with the political economy model outlined by True (2012) and, while not entirely rejecting the influence of neoliberalism (as this seems unlikely in a capitalist economy), the mix of government, non-profit, for-profit, and general public efforts would at least minimise it. The following section provides a brief history of the public health approach to violence in the United States, first generally and then specific to domestic violence.

A PUBLIC HEALTH APPROACH TO VIOLENCE

The idea that violence of any sort is a public health concern is relatively new in the United States. The country became significantly better at preventing and treating many infectious diseases, like tuberculosis, pneumonia, yellow fever, typhus, and more by the mid-twentieth century in part due to advances in our understanding of sanitation and immunisation. Simultaneously, homicide and suicide rose in the rankings of the most frequent causes of death. By the 1980s, it was clear that homicide and suicide were now among our biggest concerns, in particular, involving young people and people of colour. According to the US Center for Disease Control, suicide rates for people ages fifteen to twenty-four years nearly tripled between 1950 and 1990, while homicide rates for fifteen-to-nineteen-year-old males increased 154 per cent between 1985 and 1991. Among African-American males, the increase was even more dramatic (Dahlberg and Mercy 2009).

These statistics and the knowledge acquired from prevention efforts related to heart disease, cancer, and strokes highlighted the fact that prevention efforts must include not just individual behavioural change but also a different way of talking about the issues and of creating policies and programmes. Further, the medical advances noted earlier in text prompted calls for deeper understanding of the causes of violence and risk factors for both perpetrators and victims, at the individual, family, school, and community levels and, drawing on the epidemiological approach used in prior generations, a public health focus on violence.

In 1979, the US Surgeon General Julius B. Richmond issued a report documenting the public health advances made on fifteen areas and listed several to be prioritised in future. Control of stress and violent behaviour was identified as a priority. The report resulted in detailed objectives that were outlined in the document Promoting Health/Preventing Disease: Objectives for the Nation. Among others, the objectives included reducing child abuse incidents and fatalities, homicide rates among African-American youth, the number of privately owned handguns, and suicide rates.

The US trend in addressing violence as a public health issue is mirrored at the global level. In 1996, the World Health Assembly elevated the discussion of direct violence as a public health issue when it adopted Resolution WHA49.25, which declared violence 'a leading worldwide public health problem'. Further, the resolution required the WHO to begin public health activities that not only documented the scope and extent of personal violence and its effects but also assessed the effectiveness of prevention programmes, in particular those focused on women and children and community-based initiatives. Additionally, the WHO was tasked with helping to coordinate international cooperation towards the cessation of violence. Four years later, the WHO created the Department of Injuries and Violence Prevention to provide education about violence globally and to facilitate public health action. Its 2002 *World Report on Violence* provides guidance throughout the world in regard to a public health approach to violence.

To be clear, there are many legitimate criticisms of the WHO, including that it too emphasises medicalisation and is infused with neoliberal ideology. The WHO has been accused of overemphasising cost efficiency and depoliticising public health, as well as failing to address indirect violence (Schrecker 2016; cf. Nuño, this volume). Its approach is not really informed by feminist principles, either. But in terms of advancing a public health approach on a global scale, the WHO has certainly played some role.

Important to a public health approach to violence is that it is interdisciplinary and community-based. Scholars from Public Health, Sociology, Psychology, Gender Studies, Public Policy, Political Science – and indeed the transdisciplinary fields of Peace Research and Global Health – along with practitioners, advocates, and activists, should work together to engage in rigorous research that results in creative, effective, and collaborative initiatives. Currently, that is not necessarily happening in the United States. There are four basic steps involved in a public health approach, according to the WHO's model. First, it is imperative that systematic data collection advances basic knowledge about the scope, extent, characteristics, and consequences of violence at all levels (from local to international). The next step involves conducting research to identify the causes and correlates of violence, risk, and protective factors. This is followed by designing, implementing, monitoring, and evaluating various interventions, and then finally disseminating those results (WHO 2003). What is unclear is who is responsible for these steps. I contend that it must be state-funded and supported, at least in part. Further, while there is a role for non-profits and charities, the WHO model does not specify a role for healthcare professionals, educators, corporations, and, in particular, the general public. Missing in the WHO model is also the purposeful eliciting of women's voices. Further, the WHO model does not acknowledge the intersecting and multiple violences women experience, and the different ways in which the intersection of those violences affects them based on their identities and social positionings. Nor does it address the need for a systemic challenge to patriarchy (True 2012).

DOMESTIC VIOLENCE AS A PUBLIC HEALTH ISSUE

In the United States, the later 1970s saw the introduction of an ecological model to understand child abuse, which was later applied to domestic violence.

Such a model focuses on identifying the individual and contextual factors that result in abuse. It begins by identifying biological and personal history factors that shape abusers. In doing so, it looks at peer, intimate partner, and family relations that place an individual at risk for perpetrating abuse. This includes childhood exposure to abuse and peer support for violent behaviour, as well as head injuries and other traumas that increase the risk of perpetration. Again, while there is data to show that these are legitimate factors in some cases, the concern is that emphasising individual risk factors, especially those related to biology or medical issues, reinforces an individualistic approach to abuse and deemphasises or ignores the social and structural factors.

The ecological model does consider the community context of domestic violence, however, including how it is related to institutions including neighbourhoods, schools, and workplaces. For instance, the model recognises that high levels of residential mobility increase the risk for violence, as does a more heterogeneous population, high poverty levels, a shortage of institutional supports, and a more densely populated community. At the societal level, the ecological model considers those cultural norms and policies that create an acceptable climate for violence and those that make violence less likely. These include norms that imply that violence is an acceptable way to resolve conflict, the notion that violence is an individual choice rather than a preventable act, the belief in male superiority, and more. This is consistent with a feminist approach focusing on the role of hegemonic masculinity, how it is created socially, and how it is historically embedded into US institutions, in particular policing, and in policy and politics (Connell 1987; True 2012).

More recently, domestic violence advocates have begun to discuss the importance of primary prevention (Cornelius and Ressegie 2007; Finley 2015; Whitaker et al. 2006). In contrast to tertiary prevention, which focuses on the long-term care of victims, and secondary prevention, which provides more immediate care, primary prevention aims to prevent violence before it occurs. Similarly, attention has been focused on three types of interventions with perpetrators. Indicated interventions are addressed towards those who have already demonstrated violent behaviour. Selected interventions target those at increased risk for perpetration. More broadly, however, universal interventions reach the general population. These often include educational programmes in schools or media campaigns. The WHO has noted that policies and programmes designed to stop violence against women are often based on very little evidence-based information, with many studies focusing on identifying risk factors over preventive factors and funding largely for protection and prosecution, not prevention. The studies that do focus on prevention are often focused on the individual or family-level factors, not community, societal, or economic structural factors (True 2012). A feminist public health approach would include involvement of healthcare professionals, educators, and corporations. It would involve the voices of survivors as well as allies to the cause. It would pay attention to not just individual risk factors but to structural issues, including wage disparity between men and women, lack of affordable housing, and prioritisation of government funds for militarism instead of human services.

SKETCHING A FEMINIST PUBLIC HEALTH APPROACH TO DOMESTIC VIOLENCE

Far be it from exhaustive, it is possible to identify some key elements of a public health approach to domestic violence. Similar to True's suggestions (2012), these include increasing women's political representation, affording girls greater access to education, creative training, education, access to health care and reproductive services, media initiatives to challenge hegemonic masculinity, and community activism to address the structural issues cited earlier. It should involve school and community groups and deliberate efforts to include a diversity of women. Funding and support from the state is still essential, but monies can also come from the other involved institutions and from charitable donations. Rather than rely on just the state or just the non-profits, such a model involves many intersecting parts.

Rather than focusing on individual heroes (Finley 2015), a feminist public health approach would be collegial, not hierarchical, and address both the personal and social dimensions of abuse (Hasyim 2014). As Rojas (2007) explains and as this chapter has shown, complex problems of varying forms of violence are increasingly criminalised, medicalised, or non-profitised, all of which result in independent, non-collaborative, and overly simple responses, which do not challenge the interlocking forms of violence, of which domestic violence is one manifestation. Ultimately, understanding domestic violence as a public health issue is in its infancy, in the United States and elsewhere, and as such, efforts to raise awareness about the scope and extent of the problem, its costs, and the underlying socio-political-economic factors has to come first. As True (2012, 190) notes, 'The more an issue finds purchase in public consciousness, the more politicians will pay attention'.

While there is great concern in the United States that the administration of Donald Trump is a setback in terms of challenging any form of gender discrimination, there is much to be hopeful about. Studies have found that having more women in government has a positive effect on the number and type of legal protections related to GBV (Richards and Haglund 2015), and the 2018 elections saw a record number of women elected to Congress. Importantly, they include women of colour, lesbian women, and women with disabilities, although these groups are still significantly underrepresented in politics. The hope is, however, that these new legislators will take GBV more seriously as one component of a public health approach. The #MeToo movement has made sexual harassment and assault far more public in the United States in 2017 and 2018, and, importantly, is modelling the importance of women's stories and voices in a way that can hopefully benefit efforts to address domestic violence as well. I have argued elsewhere (Finley 2015) that in the United States a recent trend is 'hashtagising', or presuming that one is making a significant social difference by sharing a hashtag about a social issue. #MeToo, however, shows how hashtags can be part of a social change initiative, just never all there is to one.

In sum, this chapter has documented the horrifying global scope of domestic violence and its dire consequences. Further, it has made evident the need for a public health approach that goes far beyond individually focused criminal justice interventions or shelter spaces for victims. As Murray (2008) reminds us, it is past time that we use our outrage over domestic violence boldly and courageously, and that we work collaboratively and thoughtfully to contain the epidemic that is domestic violence.

REFERENCES

Alfred, Charlotte. 2014. 'These 20 Countries Have No Law against Domestic Violence'. *Huffington Post*, 10 March. http://www.huffingtonpost.com/2014/03/08/countries-no-domestic-violence-law_n_4918784.html?slideshow=true. Accessed 7 September 2019.

Baines, Donna. 2010. 'Neoliberal Restructuring, Activism/Participation, and Social Unionism in the Nonprofit Social Services'. *Nonprofit and Voluntary Sector Quarterly* 39, no.1: 10–28.

Bebbington, Anthony, Samuel Hickey and Diana Mitlin. 2008. *Can NGOs Make a Difference? The Challenge of Development Alternatives*. London: Zed Books.

Berns, Nancy. 2004. *Framing the Victim: Domestic Violence, Media, and Social Problems*. New York: Aldine de Gruyter.

Bonomi, Amy, Melissa L. Anderson, Frederick P. Rivara and Robert S. Thompson. 2009. 'Health Care Utilization and Costs Associated with Physical and Nonphysical-Only Intimate Partner Violence'. *Health Services Research* 44, no. 3:1052–1067.

Brainard, Lori and Patricia Siplon. 2004. 'Toward Nonprofit Organization Reform in the Voluntary Spirit: Lessons from the Internet'. *Nonprofit and Voluntary Sector Quarterly* 33, no. 1: 435–457.

Bumiller, Kristin. 2008. *In an Abusive State: How Neoliberalism Appropriated the Feminist Movement against Sexual Violence*. Durham: Duke University Press.

Çelik, Ahmet. 2013. 'An Analysis of Mandatory Arrest Policy on Domestic Violence'. *International Journal of Human Sciences* 10, no.1: 1503–1523.

Chelala, Cesar. 2016. 'The Public Health Impact of Domestic Violence'. *Counterpunch*, 12 February. http://www.counterpunch.org/2016/02/05/the-public-health-impact-of-domestic-violence/. Accessed 7 September 2019.

Chemaly, Soraya. 2012. '50 Actual Facts about Domestic Violence'. *Huffington Post*, 6 December. http://www.huffingtonpost.com/soraya-chemaly/50-actual-facts-about-dom_b_2193904.html. Accessed 7 September 2019.

Coker, Donna. 2000. 'Shifting Power for Battered Women: Law, Material Resources, and Poor Women of Color'. *UC Davis Law Review* 33, no. 1: 1009–1058.

Coker, Donna. 2001. 'Crime Control and Feminist Law Reform in Domestic Violence Law: A Critical Review'. *University of Miami Law School*. Accessed 4 March 2019. https://repository.law.miami.edu/cgi/viewcontent.cgi?article=1286&context=fac_articles.

Connell, R. W. 1987. *Gender & Power*. Stanford, CA: Stanford University Press.

Cornelius, Tara and Nicole Resseguie. 2007. 'Primary and Secondary Prevention Programs for Dating Violence: A Review of the Literature'. *Aggression and Violent Behaviour* 12, no. 3: 364–375.

Crenshaw, Kimberle. 1991. 'Mapping the Margins: Intersectionality, Identity Politics, and Violence against Women of Color'. *Stanford Law Review* 43, no. 6: 1241–1299.

Dahlberg, Linda and James Mercy. 2009. 'The History of Violence as a Public Health Issue'. *CDC*. Accessed 31 December 2018. http://www.cdc.gov/violenceprevention/pdf/history_violence-a.pdf.

Day, Tanis, Katherine McKenna and Audra Bowlus. 2005. 'The Economic Costs of Violence against Women: An Evaluation of the Literature'. *UN Women Watch*. Accessed 31 December 2018. http://www.un.org/womenwatch/daw/vaw/expert%20brief%20costs.pdf.

Ferarro, Kathleen. 1996, fall. 'The Dance of Dependency: A Genealogy of Domestic Violence Discourse'. *Hypatia* 11, no. 4: 77–92.

Finley, Laura. 2010a. *Examining Domestic Violence as a State Crime: Nonkilling Implications*. Global Nonkilling Working Paper #2.

Finley, Laura. 2010b. 'Where's the Peace in This Movement? A Domestic Violence Advocate's Reflections on the Movement'. *Contemporary Justice Review* 13, no.1: 57–69.

Finley, Laura. 2015. 'Do We Need New Heroes? Reflections on the Cult of Personality and Peace, Human Rights and Social Justice Movements'. *Peace Studies Journal* 8, no. 2: 17–33.

Finley, Laura and Luigi Esposito. 2012. 'Neoliberalism and the Non-Profit Industrial Complex: The Limits of a Market Approach to Service Delivery'. *Peace Studies Journal* 5, no.3: 4–26.

Fraser, Nancy. 2009. *Scales of Justice: Reimaging Political Space in a Globalizing World*. New York: Columbia University Press.

Friedersdorf, Colin. 2014. 'Police Have a Much Bigger Domestic Abuse Problem Than the NFL Does'. *The Atlantic*, 19 September. https://www.theatlantic.com/national/archive/2014/09/police-officers-who-hit-their-wives-or-girlfriends/380329/. Accessed 7 September 2019.

Garcia-Moreno, Claudia, et al. 2005. *WHO Multi-Country Study on Women's Health and Domestic Violence against Women*. Geneva: World Health Organization.

Hasyim, Nur. 2014. *How Far Can Men Go? A Study of the Men's Movement to End Violence against Women in Indonesia*. Wollongong: University of Wollongong.

Home Office. 2019. 'The Economic and Social Costs of Domestic Abuse'. Accessed 2 March 2019. https://assets.publishing.service.gov.uk/government/uploads/system/uploads/attachment_data/file/772180/horr107.pdf.

Incite! Women of Color against Violence. 2007. *The Revolution Will Not Be Funded*. Boston: South End Press.

Iyengar, R. and L Sabik. 2009. 'The Dangerous Shortage of Domestic Violence Services'. *Health Affairs* 28, no. 6: 1052–1065.

Jeltsen, Melissa and Dana Liebelson. 2017. 'The Super Predators'. *Huffington Post*, 21 June. https://highline.huffingtonpost.com/articles/en/police-domestic-violence/. Accessed 7 September 2019.

Johnson, Leanor. 1991. *On the Front Lines: Police Stress and Family Well-being*. Hearing before the Select Committee on Children, Youth, and Families House of Representatives: 102 Congress First Session May 20, 32–48. Washington DC: US Government Printing Office.

Khurana, Bharti et al. 2017. 'How Radiology Can Help Uncover Evidence of Domestic Abuse and Sexual Assault'. *Brigham and Women's Hospital*. https://bhartikhurana.bwh.harvard.edu/rsna-2017-how-radiology-can-help-uncover-evidence-of-domestic-abuse-sexual-assault/. Accessed 7 September 2019.

Lomborg, Bjorn. 2015, June 16. 'The Gigantic Cost of Domestic Violence: $8 Trillion a Year'. *Huffington Post*. https://www.huffpost.com/entry/domestic-violence-8-trillion-a-year_b_7078822. Accessed 7 September 2019.

MacKinnon, Catherine. 1991. 'Reflections on Sex Equality under the Law'. *The Yale Law Journal* 100, no.5:1281–1328.

MacKinnon, Catherine. 1983. 'Feminism, Marxism, Method and the State: Toward Feminist Jurisprudence'. *Signs* 7, no.1: 515–544.

Max, Wendy, Dorothy P. Rice, Eric Finkelstein, Robert A. Bardwell and Steven Leadbetter, 'The Economic Toll of Intimate Partner Violence against Women in the United States'. *Violence and Victims* 19, no. 3 (June 2004): 259–272.

McLean, Gladys and Sarah Bocinski. 2017. 'The Economic Cost of Intimate Partner Violence, Sexual Assault, and Stalking'. *Institute for Women's Policy Research*. https://iwpr.org/publications/economic-cost-intimate-partner-violence-sexual-assault-stalking/. Accessed 7 September 2019.

Morgen, Sarah and Ann Bookman. 1988. *Women and the Politics of Empowerment*. Philadelphia: Temple University Press.

Murray, Anne. 2008. *From Outrage to Courage: Women Taking Action for Health and Justice*. Monroe, ME: Common Courage.

Neidig, P., H. Russell and A. Seng. 1992. 'Interspousal Aggression in Law Enforcement Families: A Preliminary Investigation'. *Police Studies*, 15 no. 1: 30–38.

Nuño, Néstor M. 2019. 'Rethinking Global Health Priorities from the Margins: Health Access and Medical Care Claims among Indonesia's *Waria*'. In *Gender, Global Health and Violence: Feminist Perspectives on Peace and Disease*, edited by Tiina Vaittinen and Catia Confortini. London and New York: Rowman & Littlefield.

Parker, Clifton. 2014. 'Women and Children Bear Brunt of Domestic Violence, Stanford Scholar Says'. *Stanford Report*. http://news.stanford.edu/news/2014/september/domestic-violence-toll-092314.html. Accessed 7 September 2019.

Pearl, Robert. 2013. 'Domestic Violence: The Secret Killer That Costs $8.3 Billion Annually'. *Forbes*, 5 December. http://www.forbes.com/sites/robertpearl/2013/12/05/domestic-violence-the-secret-killer-that-costs-8-3-billion-annually/#2f1264 13c136. Accessed 7 September 2019.

Pleck, Emily. 1987. *Domestic Tyranny*. Cambridge: Oxford University Press.

Pyke, Alan. 2015. 'New Report on Police Deaths Comes with Grim Revelations'. *Think Progress*. https://thinkprogress.org/new-report-on-police-deaths-comes-with-grim-revelations-516b20b0dff7#.o9v1lcn45. Accessed 7 September 2019.

Richards, David and Jilliene Haglund. 2015. 'How Laws around the World Do and Do Not Protect Women from Violence'. *Washington Post*. Last modified 11 February 2015. www.washingtonpost.com%2Fnews%2Fmonkey-cage%2Fwp%2F2015%2F02%2F11%2Fhow-laws-around-the-world-do-and-do-not-protect-women-from-violence%2F&usg=AFQjCNEIxR02PGJ1GhjrbjS7mIlYEeTjDQ

Rojas, Clarissa. 2007. 'We Were Never Meant to Survive:' Fighting Violence against Women and the Fourth World War'. In *The Revolution Will Not Be Funded: Beyond the Non-profit Industrial Complex*, edited by Incite! Women of Color against Violence, 113–128. New York, NY: South End Press.

Ruttenberg, Maria. 1993. 'A Feminist Critique of Mandatory Arrest: An Analysis of Race and Gender in Domestic Violence Policy'. *Digital Commons*. Accessed 4 March 2019. https://digitalcommons.wcl.american.edu/cgi/viewcontent.cgi?referer=https://www.google.com/&httpsredir=1&article=1210&context=jgspl.

Schechter, Susan. 1982. *Women and Male Violence: The Visions and Struggles of the Battered Women's Movement*. Boston, MA: South End Press.

Schrecker, Ted. 2015. ' "Neoliberal Epidemics" and Public Health: Sometimes the World Is Less Complicated Than It Appears'. *Critical Public Health* 26, no. 5: 477–480.

Sherman, Lawrence and Richard Berk. 1984. 'The Specific Deterrent Effects of Arrest for Domestic Assault'. *American Sociological Review* 49, no. 2: 261–272.

Sherman, Lawrence and Heather Harris. 2014. 'Increased Death Rates of Domestic Violence Victims from Arresting vs. Warning Suspects in the Milwaukee Domestic Violence Experiment (MilDVE) '. *Journal of Experimental Criminology* 11, no. 1: 1–20.

Stansell, Christine. 2000. *The Feminist Promise: 1792 to the Present*. New York, NY: The Modern Library.

Tanyag, Maria. 2019. 'Replenishing Bodies and the Political Economy of SRHR in Crisis and Emergencies'. In *Gender, Global Health and Violence: Feminist Perspectives on Peace and Disease*, edited by Tiina Vaittinen and Catia Confortini. London and New York: Rowman & Littlefield.

Thunder Hawk, Madonna. 2007. 'Native Organizing before the Non-Profit Industrial Complex'. In *The Revolution Will Not Be Funded: Beyond the Non-Profit Industrial Complex*, edited by INCITE! Women of Color against Violence, 101–106. Boston, MA: South End.

True, Julie. 2012. *The Political Economy of Violence against Women*. New York: Oxford.

UNIFEM. n.d. 'The Facts: Violence against Women and the Millennium Development Goals'. Accessed 25 November 2016. http://www.endvawnow.org/uploads/browser/files/EVAW_FactSheet_KM_2010EN.pdf.

Walby, Sylvia. 2004. 'The Cost of Domestic Violence'. *England's Women and Equality Unit*. Accessed 25 November 2016. http://citeseerx.ist.psu.edu/viewdoc/download?doi=10.1.1.393.886&rep=rep1&type=pdf.

Waldron, Travis. 2015. 'Why Victims of Domestic Violence Don't Testify, Particularly against NFL Players. *Think Progress*. https://thinkprogress.org/why-victims-of-domestic-violence-dont-testify-particularly-against-nfl-players-e76fe2e39165#.v41nm3ffr. Accessed 7 September 2019.

Weissman, Deborah. 2013. 'Law, Social Movements and the Political Economy of Domestic Violence'. *Duke Journal of Gender, Law and Policy* 20, no. 1(Spring 2013): 221–254.

Whitaker, DJ et al. 2006. 'A Critical Review of Interventions for the Primary Prevention of Perpetration of Partner Violence'. *Aggression and Violent Behavior* 11, no. 2: 151–166.

WHO. 2003. 'Violence: A Global Public Health Problem'. Accessed 28 October 2016. http://www.who.int/violence_injury_prevention/violence/world_report/en/chap1.pdf.

WHO. 2013. 'Global and Regional Estimates of Violence against Women: Prevalence and Health Effects of Intimate Partner Violence and Non-Partner Sexual Violence. Accessed 31 December 2016. http://apps.who.int/iris/bitstream/10665/85239/1/9789241564625_eng.pdf.

Wing, Adrien. 2003. *Critical Race Feminism: A Reader*. New York, NY: NYU Press.

World Bank. 2016. 'Overview: Girls and Education'. Accessed 31 December 2016. http://www.worldbank.org/en/topic/girlseducation/overview#1.

Workplace Statistics. 2016. *Corporate Alliance to End Partner Violence*. Accessed 31 December 2016. http://www.caepv.org/getinfo/facts_stats.php?factsec=3.

Chapter 11

Exposed to Violence While Caring: From Caring Self-Protection to Global Health as Conflict Transformation

Tiina Vaittinen

As Sophie Harman notes in the concluding chapter, those with power to care may sometimes end up hurting their care-recipients: if not directly then indirectly, when carers reproduce gendered violences imbued in the structural, symbolic, cultural, and epistemic orders of global health. In this regard, global health forms a paradoxical political space where care not only coexists and overlaps with but sometimes also *includes* violence. In this chapter, I suggest that feminist global health should be understood as a field of conflict transformation that recognises what feminist peace researcher Berenice A. Carroll (1972, 22) denoted as the power of 'the so called "powerless", that is, of those who lack the power of dominance'. In global health, the so-called powerless include very often not only the care-recipients, but also the carers, who are vulnerable to violence too.

My argumentation in the chapter builds on the work of two feminist care and disability theorists, namely Christine Kelly (2017) and Stacy Clifford Simplican (2015), who show that care is not an antonym of violence. Rather, as previously argued by feminist care ethicists, care is about political relations where complex webs of power and domination are inherently present (Tronto 1993), as is the potential for violence and injustice (Robinson 1999, 128; 2011, 5; Vaittinen 2017). Thus, if global health is about caring, and given that the aim of our book is to rethink global health in more just ways, it is crucial that we recognise and respect the grey areas of violence *within* the material-discursive structures of health and social care. This is because romanticising care, or indeed global health, as something inherently 'good' risks depoliticising them – while making invisible their hurtful dimensions.

To provide an empirical account of the ways in which care includes violence, I draw on my ethnographic work on mundane peace and conflict in residential dementia care.[1] The research was conducted in winter 2017–2018 in a Finnish care home that follows a philosophy of good care. In addition to field notes from ethnographic participant observation, I utilise data from two focus group discussions, conducted with the nurses working in the home, one taped and transcribed verbatim, and the other recorded in my field diary only. All names mentioned in the analysis are pseudonyms.

My analysis in this chapter focuses on tabooed situations of intimate dementia care (e.g. continence care and showering), where nurses regularly experience physical violence committed by their vulnerable, yet aggressive, care-recipients. These situations – where the nurses can be hit, kicked, bitten, shoved, and yelled at – are an inherent part of dementia care. While it is true that adequate staffing and good working conditions help reduce this type of violence – as well as the violence of carers against their care-recipients (e.g. Banerjee et al. 2008) – some forms of dementia cause aggression and violent behaviour to the extent that the violence experienced by carers cannot be completely eradicated. It is violence that requires critical, destigmatising analysis.[2] For these purposes, I devise in this chapter the concept of *caring self-protection*, by examining the nurses' strategies of seeking to provide good care in the face of regular threats of violence in intimate dementia care.

Caring self-protection is a concept that emerges from my ethnographic observations. It consists of various inter-corporeal tactics and techniques that the nurses I observed utilise, to protect themselves from the physical violence they are exposed to while caring – while simultaneously ensuring they do not hurt the care-recipients, and that good care is provided regardless of the violent situation. Thus, their methods of caring self-protection are not only about protecting the self in a dyadic relationship with a singular, threatening, yet vulnerable other, but about something more complex that requires the nurses to disentangle various potentialities of violence simultaneously, while providing care. I argue that caring self-protection is best understood as inter-corporeal conflict transformation – and that lessons from these micro-level encounters can be useful for our thinking about global health.

With the exception of Sara Ruddick's (1990) work on maternal thinking and the work of other feminist care ethicists (e.g. Confortini and Ruane 2014; Robinson 1999; 2011; Robinson and Confortini 2014; Tronto 1993; Vaittinen et al. 2019), the feminised skills of low-paid or unpaid care workers are rarely utilised as a basis from which to extrapolate to other (often masculine) realms of expertise – such as conflict resolution theories and biomedical discourses of global health. Yet, towards the end of the chapter, I consider what it might mean if we conceptualised feminist global health as caring self-protection – that is, as ongoing, situated, inter-corporeal practices of conflict transformation.

THE EMPIRICAL CONTEXT

As Lukić and Lotherington show in this volume (see also Lukić 2019), symbolic violence towards people living with dementia is widely normalised today. The care home in which I conducted my fieldwork is, in this regard, an exceptional institution. Its practices concretely demonstrate Lukić and Lotherington's argument that valorising life with dementia as a life worth *enjoying* is possible – also in institutionalised settings. The practices of care in this home follow both person-centred and relation-centred principles of care (see Nolan et al. 2004). The care-recipients' personalities, unique lives, and relationships are placed in the centre of daily routines, and the duties of the staff are designed to flexibly respond to their needs and preferences, without letting the staff rota or biomedical understandings of geriatric health to order the rhythms of life. The staff spend time with the residents throughout the day – eating their meals and having their coffees *with* the residents, rather than on breaks in a separate staff area. In addition to providing basic care, they seek to ensure each resident some mundane pleasures they were accustomed to before moving to the home – be it a cold beer after their weekly sauna,[3] or wearing nice cloths every day. Collaborating with volunteers and charities, the staff organise special outings, such as taking a former biker for a motorbike ride, a group of residents to the movies or for an assisted swim in the lake on a hot summer day. Importantly, the staff and the administration appreciate that, as a shared home of different personalities, the home is a *living community* with different kinds of conflicts that can be solved only by appreciating the relational agency of everyone involved – regardless of how limited their cognitive capacities or means of self-expression are.

The understanding of conflicts as a natural part of human life was particularly helpful for my project, the goal of which was to learn about mundane events of peace and conflict in residential dementia care. Embarking upon my ethnography, I expected to observe conflicts that would involve some *indirect* forms of violence – such as structural and epistemic. I anticipated to see conflicts emerging from limited staffing resources, for instance, or from communication problems and inabilities of the non-demented to comprehend the epistemic realities of those who live with dementia (cf. Lindholm 2015). What I did not expect to see were situations of direct, physical violence. Yet, eventually, some of my central findings had to do with mundane fears of being hurt by fists that hit and teeth that bite. Only, those regularly exposed to such violence were not the frail residents, but their carers, the nurses, who in situations of intimate care risk getting hurt on a regular basis. In what follows, I draw on critical feminist care and disability theory as well as my empirical material to better comprehend these situations, and what should be learned from them.

CARERS' EXPOSURE TO VIOLENCE IN DEMENTIA CARE

> *Today was the day of showering for Maija, a resident known for aggressive behaviour during intimate care. As the nurses put on the plastic aprons and the white rubber boots, which they use to keep dry when showering the residents in their en-suite bathrooms, I asked them whether they felt anxious. Kirsti replied to me that yes, always, 'since you never know what comes next', referring to Maija's aggression, which tends to erupt in an instant.*
>
> *I have discussed the same several times with the other nurses, and there is a clear pattern in their responses: with a few residents (not everyone, this depends on the stage and kind of dementia), the nurses routinely face a threat of violence while providing intimate care. The nurses are used to it, it is part of their work and profession – but this does not mean that they would not fear getting hurt. Only some time ago, one of the nurses had her spectacles broken by Maija's fist. Today, to protect themselves as much as Maija, the nurses had given Maija a light sedative half an hour before the showering routines were to take place. When I asked, whether this usually works, Kirsti responded to me hesitantly: 'Well, you never know really'.*
>
> *What we know is that it is unpredictable, since those living with dementia live in an instant, as do their joys – and aggressions. And the nurses, they live* with *it. Skilfully so*. (Field Notes, 26 January 2018, my translation from Finnish)

This vignette relates to the kind of mundane situations of intimate care that I regularly observed when participating in the life of the care home. It is known that nurses working with people with dementia experience different degrees of violence on a regular basis. This violence, however, is not much spoken about, since it usually takes place in the tabooed and 'dirty' realm of intimate care – when changing incontinence pads full of excrement, for instance, when cleaning bed-ridden residents' genital areas from urine or faeces, or helping someone with toileting (for care as 'dirty work', see, for example, Isaksen 2002; Molinier 2011, 252–253). Even within the nursing profession, talking about the violence may be discouraged, because raising the issue in public risks resulting in victim blaming, where the nurses who experience violence are accused of having caused the violence by bad care (e.g. Banerjee et al. 2008; Focus Group Discussion, 9 October 2018).

For those not familiar with dementia care, it may be difficult to imagine that a frail and vulnerable elderly person could hurt their care-providers with direct, physical violence. As one of my nurse interlocutors in the care home noted, the popular imaginary of the elderly in care homes is one of cute grannies, 'who just sit in the rocking chair, knitting woolly socks!' (Field

Notes, 19 February 2018, my translation from Finnish). Or try a Google image search for 'elderly care', and you will get (feminised) images of old women (and some men), whose hands the good nurses hold, and whose rosy cheeks the carers caress. In the daily realities of the set of cognitive disorders denoted as dementia, however, the care-dependent persons are usually no longer capable of knitting socks, and the good care is not only about holding hands or caressing cheeks. Instead, it requires a much more complex set of embodied skills and practices.

The Finnish Social Policy scholar Silva Tedre (2004) has called for a better recognition and appreciation of such skills, arguing for a 'disgust-materialist' [*inhomaterialistinen*] approach to care. This is a perspective to care research, policies, and practices that puts the material necessities of bodily life (that are sometimes if not often 'disgusting') at the centre of attention (see also Isaksen 2002; Twigg 2000). The body here is not an abstraction, and relations of care do not simply hang out in the air. Instead, Tedre's 'body-political care manifesto' (*ruumispoliittinen hoivajulistus*) begins with concrete care encounters, where care *necessitates* the presence of at least two embodied persons 'in the same place at the same time' (Tedre 2004, 45, my translations from Finnish). Care encounters for Tedre thus go beyond the practices of holding hands or caressing cheeks. In disgust-materialist care, the bodies of care-participants 'come together' in an *obligatory proximity that is stronger than touch*' (Tedre 2004, 46, my translation and emphasis), and care turns into something much more than encounters. It is 'bodies being forcibly embraced by one another, sometimes as in a wrestling hold' (Tedre 2004, 47, my translation).

When bodies come in this close proximity with one another – regularly and necessarily – the risk of the bodies hurting each other is immanent. Particularly in intimate care, the provision of good care requires the carers to work closely not only with but also *on* the care-recipient's body, including on their most intimate body parts. The care-recipient may be naked, or partially naked, and good care requires not only that the intimate areas of this other person are touched, but that adequate *time is spent while touching* – for instance, that faeces are properly cleaned from genital areas to avoid urinary tract infections. Simultaneously, the care-recipient may not remember where they are, or who they are. Dementia may have taken them back to their childhood, away from the epistemic realities of the time and place where this intimate touching happens.

Depending on the kind and stage of their disease, people living with dementia may resist the practices of intimate care (cf. Featherstone, Northcott and Bridges 2019), also physically, defending themselves with their fists and teeth, for instance, and their mood may change from peaceful to aggressive in an instant. This is understandable. Just imagine yourself there, believing you are a child – *being* a child – or living through your adolescent years: a nurse, possibly of the opposite sex, wipes your genital areas with some wet cloth, in a room that smells of faeces, urine, and disinfectant. There may be two persons present in the room, working on your naked and aching body. They do it gently, providing *good care*, but you do not understand what is going on. What would you do, not knowing what these people do to you, and why, and where? Maybe you would defend yourself, with all the power left in your body: hit, kick, bite, shove, and yell. I think I would.

In such situations then, the nurses risk getting hurt. With some residents – depending on the kind and stage of the disease – this threat of violence may be present several times a day, whenever intimate care is given. Yet, the nurses do the washing, seeking to do it with care. They cannot disregard the needs of intimate hygiene, as doing so would count as bad care and neglect, that is, violence. I return to such impossible decisions between care and exposure to violence later on in the chapter. First, however, I will briefly engage with previous research on carers' exposure to violence.

ENTANGLEMENTS OF STRUCTURAL AND DIRECT VIOLENCE

The direct violence experienced by nurses in dementia care remains widely unaddressed in care policies, in Finland and beyond. In critical care research, however, nurses' and other personal care workers' exposure to violence has been recognised for some time. Over a decade ago, Albert Banerjee and his colleagues, for instance, conducted a comparative study on the violence experienced by professional carers in long-term care in Canada, Denmark, Finland, Norway, and Sweden (Banerjee et al. 2008). They found the experiences of violence to be regular (see also Åkeström 2002; Kelly 2010). The forms of violence involved slaps, punches, kicks, verbal abuse, racism, and even sexual abuse such as the carer having their cloths torn off by a care-recipient in a shower room. Banerjee et al. also showed how poor structural conditions of work contributed to increased risks of violence. For instance, in Canada, staffing shortages were considerably higher and chronic when compared to the Nordic countries, which contributed to the significantly higher levels of violence experienced by Canadian carers (cf. Kelly 2017, 105). Other structural factors adding to the risk of violence included lack of autonomy to organise one's own work (so that adequate time be reserved for each encounter); lack of appropriate training (to conditions such as dementia); and a 'culture of blame', where the violence was easily seen as resulting from bad care (Banerjee et al. 2008; see also Baines 2006).

In Finland, where my research was conducted, the structural conditions of long-term care work have generally worsened over the recent years, due to austerity measures and attempts to 'increase productivity' (i.e. produce the same 'amount' of care with less staff), and hence chronic shortages in staffing. A recent comparative study showed that the structural conditions of work in Finnish long-term care are today considerably worse than in the other Nordic countries (Kröger, van Aerschott and Puthenparambil 2018; also Erkkilä 2016; Rytkönen 2018). In institutionalised settings of care (e.g. residential care homes), 40 per cent of the respondents reported to experience violence or threats thereof on a weekly basis, the percentage having doubled over the past ten years. Carers' experiences of sexual abuse at work are more prevalent in Finland than in the other Nordic countries. The rapid commodification and marketisation of public care services (e.g. Karsio and Anttonen 2013; Vaittinen, Hoppania and Karsio 2018) in turn has effectively led to 'a task-based understanding of care that splinters care into unrealistic timed units that are simply impossible to carry out' (Kelly 2017, 105). As Hanna-Kaisa Hoppania and I have argued elsewhere (Hoppania and Vaittinen 2015), the necessarily embodied and relational nature of care fits poorly with the compartmentalised models of commodified care, which valorise documentation and quality measurement over situated and timely responses to the care-recipients' needs. Such design of care work is itself violent, since it not only makes it impossible to provide good care, but it practically forces the caregivers to make impossible choices as to which care 'tasks' (commodities) to attend to, and whose care needs to neglect, in order to make it through their daily rota.

Elsewhere Banerjee et al. (2012) have conceptualised poor working conditions in long-term care as structural violence (Galtung 1969), showing how it contributes to the direct violence that carers experience. This is relevant also in regard to wider structures of global health. Namely, as the chapters in this book demonstrate, the structures of healthcare provision are often not only violent in multiple ways, but the violence of these structures also allow for other forms of violence to emerge (e.g. Nuño; Reuterswärd; Oinas; Finley, this volume). In the case of dementia care, violent structures of work expose carers to direct violence – but they also cause cynicism and fatigue among carers, which increases their risk of violent, even sadistic behaviour towards their vulnerable care-recipients (Kelly 2017, 105; Kelly, F. 2010). Such entanglements of violence are reproduced by the kind of symbolic violence against persons with dementia that Lukić and Lotherington analyse (this volume). The violences are also easily hidden by self-stigmatisation among the carers, whose feminised work and professional skills remain undervalued in the masculine, biomedical, and increasingly neoliberal orders of health and social care across societies (for stigma as violence, see Harman, this volume). It is not, however, enough to merely look at how different forms of violence intertwine in care. Sometimes, it must be recognised that care itself includes violence.

WHEN CARE INCLUDES VIOLENCE

It is important to emphasise that reducing structural violence in working conditions decreases the direct violence experienced by both the carers and the cared for (Banerjee et al. 2008, 2012). Yet, due to the symptoms of aggression present in some forms of dementia and some other cognitive disabilities, the direct violence experienced by carers may never be fully eradicated, which brings us to the uncomfortable truth that care may also include violence. This perspective on care is not yet widely acknowledged. However, feminist disability scholars such as Stacy Clifford Simplican (2015) and Christine Kelly (2017) have begun to develop vocabularies by which violence in care becomes speakable, and hence better recognised.

Based on her research on the experiences of personal support workers in Canada, Kelly (2017) has argued that rather than understood as a realm of life that is external or opposed to care, violence should be conceptualised as part of care. Doing so, Kelly (2017, 98) argues, does not mean displacing compassion and empathy and other positive dimensions of caring; it merely serves as a starting point from which to transform the organisation of care in societies. Kelly's notion of care as inclusive of violence thus goes beyond the analyses that portray care as *influenced by* different forms of violence – as in my earlier discussion. She invites us to 'consider how oppression and violence may be embedded *within* the very concept of care' (Kelly 2017, 99, emphasis mine), yet 'without losing its transformative potential or undermining the need for care provision' (ibid., 109).

Kelly's account is thus very much in line with the ethos of feminist peace research, accustomed to working with violence in realms that the status quo would rather portray as peaceful (see Confortini and Vaittinen, this volume). Her challenge also resonates with the aims of our book, which seeks to point to the various ways in which global health includes gendered violence, while simultaneously seeking to respect and revitalise the transformative potential of global health to pave way for positive peace, that is, global social justice.

Kelly builds on Stacy Clifford Simplican's work, whose concept of *complex dependency* is helpful when trying to come to terms with the paradox of violence within care. This is a form of dependency, where 'individuals inhabit both intense vulnerability and aggressive power' (Kelly 2017, 99, citing Simplican 2015, 225). Both Simplican and Kelly maintain that such an understanding of relations of dependency allows a conception of care that is 'open to conflict' (Kelly 2017, 99; Simplican 2015, 224) – including conflicts that may turn violent. This, as I will later show in the chapter, is crucially important for a conception of care (and global health) that aims at feminist justice.

Simplican's account of complex dependency begins with the story of Trudy Steurnagel, who was brutally beaten to death by her care-dependent, autistic son in January 2009 (Connors 2009; Simplican 2014). Steurnagel, professor of Political Science at Kent State University, United States, was a single parent, whose son's autism had developed symptoms of severe aggression since puberty. The violence would erupt particularly from his frustration about being unable to express himself verbally. The violence was known in the community, yet Steurnagel was left to cope on her own. After several years of managing the outbursts, Steurnagel was found lying on her kitchen floor, with massive trauma to her head; broken ribs; a collapsed lung; a damaged eye socket; and bite marks on her face, arms, and upper legs. Eight days later she died.

Beware of the risk of adding to the stigma of cognitive disorders, Simplican argues it to be important to recognise the kinds of violent relationships of dependency that killed Trudy Steurnagel. She begins with a critical reading on Eva Kittay Feder's widely cited theorisation of dependency (e.g. Kittay 1999), criticising Kittay for building her theory only on loving experiences of care. This, Simplican argues, obscures 'the everyday struggles of carers and dependents' (Simplican 2015, 220), and in addition, it makes violent experiences of care and dependency unintelligible – and difficult to respond to in ways that would protect both the carers and the cared for. Whereas Kittay represents disabled dependents as permanently 'loving, vulnerable, and powerless' (Simplican 2015, 222), Simplican reminds us that disability is not a synonym for vulnerability, and that dependents can 'exercise power amid vulnerability' (ibid., 224) – sometimes violently so. Relationships of dependency are thus not dyadic, unidimensional relations of power, where the able-bodied (and able-minded) carers would under all circumstances have power over the cared for. Dependency relationships are much more *complex and fluid* than that, as should thus be our understanding of the relationships between care and violence.

Drawing on Judith Butler's (2004, 2005) notions of opacity in relations of vulnerability, Simplican underscores that carers can never fully comprehend the needs of the cared for. Therefore, it is pivotal to allow identities and relations of power to remain in flux, so that the dependent other has space to act from within the limits of one's own epistemic realities. The call for a notion of care that includes violence thus means recognising not only the potential of physical violence in care, but also the ways in which practices of care may involve epistemic violence against the care-dependent. As further elaborated in the course of this chapter, particularly when working with cognitive disabilities such as dementia, 'some selves lack the ability to narrate their own selves' (Simplican 2015, 226), with carers having to construct narratives for the care-dependent, without the words of the dependent persons themselves.

This can be seen as a situation of Spivakian epistemic violence, where the disabled person is the subaltern of care who 'cannot speak', given an imposed epistemic order (Spivak 1988; see also Confortini and Vaittinen, this volume), but also with limited individual abilities of verbal self-expression.

Here, then, different forms of violence – structural, direct, epistemic – become irreducibly entangled with relations of complex dependency. Vulnerability and exposure to violence become mutually shared conditions of being with the other, while involved in a corporeal care relation. This means that it is never only one or the other party in care – carer or the cared for – that is vulnerable to the other's violence. Both are – while simultaneously having to negotiate their embodied relatedness vis-à-vis the wider epistemic and material structures in which their relationship of care emerges, and remains in flux. In the following section, I elaborate these entanglements of violence further, returning to that ordinary morning in a care home, when I followed Maija's shower day.

VIOLENT REFUSALS OF CARE

As we reach Maija's room, the nurses gently wake up Maija, calling her name, calling her beautiful, introducing themselves by name. They walk her to the en suite bathroom, Maija using her walker. She usually sits in a wheelchair, so this assisted trip to the bathroom alone is tedious. Maija, drowsy still, paces peacefully, however, step by step, without resistance. In the bathroom, with Maija still standing, the nurses remove a large incontinence pad full of faeces from her, and assist her to sit on the toilet. Kirsti comes back to the bedroom to fetch chocolate, which the staff call 'magic chocolate'. The sweet treat in an aggressive resident's mouth has a calming effect, giving their senses something positive to dwell upon.

With magic chocolate in her mouth, Maija sits on the toilet. The nurses guide her to grab the bar on the wall, installed to provide support for the semi-mobile resident. 'Maija, please grab the bar for us, Maija, please do not hit us'. At this point, Petra closes the door to the bathroom. I lose my view.

I stay behind the door, however, and when the washing begins, I hear Maija's resistance start; the nurses talking to Maija in ways that seek to calm Maija down. I don't hear Maija speak. Kirsti talks to her in a friendly tone, repeatedly having to say: 'Maija, please don't hit us. We're only doing you good, Maija, only doing our work. Maija, now I must hold your hands. Maija, please do not try to hit us. Maija, we are only doing you good'. Maija changes her mode of resistance. 'Maija, please do not bite us. Maija, you are not allowed to bite. Maija, please, lift yourself up a little bit. We do need to wash you there, carefully, so you don't get infections. Maija, please. This is about taking care of your hygiene. Here, between women, we take care of this now'. I understand that they are washing the genital areas.

When the washing is almost over, Kirsti roots for Maija: 'We're almost there, Maija!' And then they are done. I hear the nurses pondering, whether to fetch the wheelchair – and then Petra notices that there is another poo coming. 'Well, wipe we must then', comments Kirsti, laconically. I take Maija's wheelchair to the bathroom door, moving her walker out of the way.

With the door ajar now, I see Maija sitting on the toilet, again, her orange cotton nightie half-way up the back. Kirsti stands in front of Maija, directing her hand to grab the bar on the wall. Petra stands next to them, ready to wipe. They fail to lift Maija's body upwards from the toilet so they could reach to the bottom properly. They ask me to help. I step in, asking for advice for how to lift. I stand to the left of Maija, put my left hand below her armpit, while supporting her from the back with the right hand. I try to caress her back gently with this hand, to calm her down, wondering whether I'm doing it right. We count to three, and on the third, we lift Maija to a half-standing position. Her legs do not hold, and she is very heavy to hold up, even though we are three. Petra does not lift, but she supports Maija from the back. She manages to wipe Maija's bottom once, with a moist disposable wash glove, after which she reaches beside me to put the soiled glove in the bin. I notice myself worrying that I get excrement in my clothes. Petra takes a fresh wash glove, wipes again, reaches beside me to put the dirty glove in the bin. And repeats this as many times as it takes to have Maija cleaned up.

I caress Maija on the shoulder. Mimicking Kirsti from the episode of showering, I tell her that we're almost done now, almost there. Maija looks at me, deep in the eye, as if smiling a tiny bit. I glance at her free hand, and see the fist: a tight, hard bundle of fingers, ready to swing. I realise that I would have no idea how to protect myself from a hit, and how to protect Maija and the nurses around her, while protecting my own body.

At the end, we assist Maija to the wheelchair. I step outside the bathroom, and hear Kirsti talking to Maija, while helping her to get ready for breakfast: 'Maija who, you ask? You are Maija. Your name is Maija'.
(Field Notes, 26 January 2018, my translation from Finnish)

This vignette describes the everyday practices of intimate care with a care-dependent person who, due to her dementia, tends to aggressively resist care. Here, Maija's physical violence entangles with the epistemic violence of the situation. The epistemic realities of the care-participants seem incompatible: the nurses know that the care-dependent person *must* be washed for her own wellbeing, yet the person herself, lacking comprehension of the reasons behind all that action on her body, violently refuses the operation. The carer lacks access to the reality in which the care-recipient perceives the washing as threatening, and conflict, even violence, seems inevitable. While in this particular care home resources are relatively good, structural pressures also affect the situation. The nurses' intimate care duties can be interrupted by the needs of other residents, by the doorbell, or various other events resulting from the fact that two to three staff nurses per shift per thirteen to fifteen residents can handle only so many embodied duties at each moment. Very often their working, caring bodies are needed at several places simultaneously, and they must prioritise and make choices between needs. Yet, with adequate time provided for the nurses to manage the situation, the conflicting epistemic realities can be peacefully negotiated so that direct violence is avoided, mitigated, and minimised.

In its longsome descriptiveness, the vignette demonstrates the multifaceted, embodied choreographies that the care-participants must perform, to get the washing done, needs met, and care tasks completed. These actions often involve, as Silva Tedre's disgust-materialist care approach would put it, forced embraces reminiscent of wrestling holds. With the threat of physical violence overshadowing the nurses' movements, and the epistemic barrier of dementia making the washing incomprehensibly threatening to the resistant care-receiver, the washing is, for both parties, 'forced care' (cf. Sointu 2018, 105). Yet, in these processes, care emerges with violence, in complex intertwinements of power, dependency, and respecting the other across epistemic barriers. It is the nurses' skills in working *with/in* these intertwinements that I call caring self-protection.

CARING SELF-PROTECTION

When observing the nurses in their work, I was in admiration of the wide range of inter-corporeal skills that they utilised to protect themselves, every day, usually without further reflection. When I asked, after such situations, where they had learned the techniques, they would often shrug: 'I don't know, I didn't even realise'. I was shocked to find out that they were not taught the skills *anywhere* – they just learn them on the job (see also Kelly 2017, 103, 105). This made me angry, thinking in comparison about any 'manly' job with a risk of being assaulted by clients while working – for example, jobs in the security business. Surely, skills of self-protection would be a central part of the training then? But when it is about (mostly female) nurses working in the feminised field of dementia care – oh well, carers, they'll manage, altruistically, naturally (cf. Bates 2006).[4]

My research participants agreed with these comparisons but said that there is such a thick veil of taboo around the violent behaviour of the frail elderly that the issue is difficult to discuss. Some expressed concern that discussing the violence in public would further stigmatise their work, as well as care homes as institutions. Elderly care already gains a lot of scandalous attention in the Finnish press; the fear was that talking about the violence would merely add to that negative image (Focus Group Discussion, 9 October 2018). As a peace researcher, then, the main finding of my project was not simply that violence against the nurses is a mundane part of their job, but that we need to find constructive, destigmatising ways of speaking about that violence, so it can be worked with and reduced.

Playing with the comparison between feminised carers as protectors and imageries of manly men in professions of security – protecting themselves, often violently, while protecting the citizens – I started to imagine the nurses at their mundane work of bedside care as the *Real Rambos of Dementia Care*. Here, the image refers of course to Sylvester Stallone's character Rambo, the militant action hero defending fiercely the 'free world' in a number of Hollywood productions. (Yes, the guy with the bandana in his head; sweaty biceps exposed while holding a massive gun.) For the Rambos of dementia care, the uniforms do not involve bandanas and bare biceps, and their weaponry mainly consists of working bodies, empathetic orientation, team skills, and cunning tricks to attract the sensory experiences of the care-recipient to positive rather than negative, aggression-triggering emotions. But *boy* (sic), aren't these Nurse-Rambos, too, ready to get dirty and take on whatever threats the day may throw at them. Day after day, battle after battle! Their skills of solving the situation are non-violent, while also – like those of Stallone's violent Rambo – rife with the possibility of one human body hurting the other. These ponderings soon led me to conceptualise what I call *caring self-protection*.

Caring self-protection[5] in dementia care consists of tactics and techniques that carers utilise to defend themselves from the care-recipient's aggression, while simultaneously trying to make sure they do not hurt the care-recipients *and* that adequate care is provided. In caring self-protection, care engenders corporeal choreographies (cf. Puumala and Pehkonen 2010; Väyrynen et al. 2016), where conflict, relations and use of power, violence, and care are balanced against one another, so that care takes place as well as possible. It is a direct response to the mundane situations where different entanglements of violence *become with* care, and hence the concept helps us to think further the paradoxes of care/violence that Kelly and Simplican discuss.

During my fieldwork, I discussed the concept explicitly with the nurses in two focus group discussions, inviting them to reflect upon the particular techniques and tactics they use. In the first meeting (9 October 2018, with thirteen nurses, twelve women and one man), I read the nurses my notes on Maija's shower day, while introducing my observations of caring self-protection as the most central finding of my study. At the time of this meeting, I still called the practices *caring self-defence* (*hoivaava itsepuolustus*).[6] While the nurses said they were never taught such skills as part of their training in dementia care, many embraced my terms (both 'caring self-defence' and, later, 'caring self-protection') as suitably expressing their methods of responding to mundane violence at work. Some did recall techniques of self-defence being briefly taught in the nursing school, but these were methods relevant to situations where one works in a hospital reception, for instance, and someone attacks, or behaves in threatening ways. They remembered the advice to call security personnel, and leave their desk – useless advice when facing violence in intimate dementia care.

The nurses also recalled a trade union campaign from some years ago, with posters saying 'Don't break your caregiver' on the walls of hospitals and health centres (Focus Group Discussion, 9 October 2018). While the campaign – recently renewed with the hashtag #älärikohoitajaasi [#dontbreakyournurse] (The Union of Social and Health Care Professionals in Finland 2018) – had a good intention, and it managed to raise consciousness in relation to some violence experienced by health workers in Finland (The Union of Social and Health Care Professionals in Finland 2011), it failed to address the violence particular to dementia care. Indeed, a poster in a dementia care home, telling the residents not to break their nurses, would be an absurd idea at best, hurtful and stigmatising at worst. Rational talk of zero tolerance of violence at work, or recommendations to give aggressive clients a 'clear message that violent behaviour has its consequences' (The Union of Social and Health Care Professionals in Finland 2011), would not be of use in situations where the violence is caused by severe cognitive disabilities. My nurse interlocutors pointed out that what they would rather need is a public discussion that does not seek culprits for the violence, and would thus be destigmatising for people living with dementia, their carers, as well as the care homes. As one of the nurses put it, what is needed is a 'dementia nurses' #metoo-campaign, carried out in a positive fashion' (Focus Group Discussion, 9 October 2018, my translation from Finnish).

Short of such a campaign, in their everyday work, the nurses develop subtle forms of protecting themselves, while protecting the violently behaving other, caringly. In the second focus group discussion (4 December 2019, with nine nurses; eight women and one man), I asked the nurses to write down the particular techniques of caring self-protection they use. The findings can only be considered as tentative, and further research is required to systematically map the best practices of caring self-protection. The list of skills that this small group of nurses in a single care home listed and discussed during the hour-long meeting is, however, eye-opening in regard to the high skills of violence-prevention and management that professional dementia-carers possess. The nurses discussed, for instance, the importance of preparing oneself properly for each particular care encounter, mentally as well as physically, well before going to the resident's room. This means managing one's fear, so that the resident does not sense it and become anxious; and working in pairs where necessary, but having only one nurse to take the main responsibility for speaking, so the care-recipient has space to participate in the interaction, rather than just being worked upon by a team of people. If there are issues in personal chemistry between the carers and the care-recipient, changing the nurse in the lead may tame aggressions before or once they erupt. Sometimes, the right kind of joking and humour works, or simply stepping back, silently, while letting the care-recipient curse, shout, spit, and swing their fists in the air, to get their aggression out.

Similarly, if the person has no words to express their frustration, the nurse can try and verbalise their anxiety, while giving it adequate time to develop – and pass. The nurses emphasised how with persons living with dementia, it is always crucially important to account for the entire sensual experience of the situation from the viewpoint of the care-recipient: Does the room echo, can something be done about the acoustics? Do reflections from the mirror appear threatening, can they be covered? Is the room cold, or too warm? Would music or singing help to calm down this person in this particular moment of time? Can something be done about the smells, or 'taste' of the situation (as in the case of the 'magic chocolate')? Sometimes adjusting one's tone of voice and speed of speaking may calm down the care-recipient – also and in particular when they no longer understand the words being spoken. Other times, a particular *manner* of speaking may turn the situation from threatening to jolly, and the key is to 'respond [to the resident] in the ways their self-expressions invite you to respond' (Nurse, Female, 4 December 2018). One of the nurses pointed out that such interactional skills are at the heart of the profession: they are the most demanding skills, on the top of which 'you build everything else' (Nurse, Female, 4 December 2018, my translation from Finnish).

Similarly, whether or not to touch the care-recipient, when to touch, where and how, matters. An intricate modification in the position of one's thumb may change the touch on the care-recipient's shoulder from threatening to caring: the thumb evenly pressed next to the other fingers may feel gentle, whereas if the thumb is separated from the other fingers it may feel as if someone is grabbing the shoulder in a threatening manner. Or it is the other way around, depending on the person's history, and then you adjust accordingly. Similarly, standing next to (and above) the person sitting on the toilet may appear dominant, whereas squatting so the carer's face is on an even level with that of the care-recipient, may appear friendly. In all situations, one needs to have adequate time to adjust one's actions to those of the care-recipient, and let them do independently as much as they can do. As many of the aggressions derive from past experiences, one would need also to know the history of the resident well. Since 'the body remembers', one of the nurses explained, the carers need to try and comprehend,

> whether the aggression derives from . . . experiences of abuse, war traumas, being subjugated or dominated, anything like that. . . . Are there questions of religion, shame? Because everyone hits for a reason, but the reason is always an image of the hitter. (Nurse, Female, Focus Group Discussion 4 December 2018, my translation from Finnish)

The nurses' methods of caring self-protection thus involve a whole range of corporeal choreographies, where one adjusts one's body and mind to the kind of inter-corporeal interaction that the care-recipient's embodied being invites them to, in the particular situation. Caring self-protection also requires adjusting the material realities of the environment: removing or covering mirrors in the bathroom; covering one's own arms with long sleeves; avoiding scratching, bleeding, and scars; and covering the care-recipients hands with soft mittens, so they cannot hurt the nurses by scratching them. Or, if the care-recipient is very reserved, it may help to partly cover them with towels while showering, so the person does not feel naked and exposed. In the following section, I argue that all these discursive-material methods of caring self-protection are best understood as conflict transformation.

CARING SELF-PROTECTION AS CONFLICT TRANSFORMATION

Developed by John Paul Lederach (2003, 2014), conflict transformation is a particular 'strategy for approaching conflict' (Lederach 2003). Instead of seeing a conflict as a problem to be solved, the conflict transformation approach orients itself positively to conflicts, understanding them as normal part of human relationships, and as dynamic openings for change. Conflict transformation does not seek to do away with conflicts, or their causes, but instead seeks to transform them constructively. It operates through three 'lenses', seeking (i) to see the immediate situation in which the conflict emerges; (ii) understand the 'deeper relationship patterns that form the context of the conflict'; and (iii) envisage a framework that links the immediate situation together with the deeper patterns of the relationship, so that peaceful ways of responding to the conflict can be found (Lederach 2003; also 2014, Ch. 2). In this understanding, conflicts do not necessarily include violence, although they may escalate to violence, and peaceful transformation of conflicts requires addressing the underlying factors, such as structural or other forms of violence. Conflict transformation thus always involves not only practices of reducing violence but also the promotion of justice, for example, by ensuring that people can influence the processes that shape their lives. In dementia care, this means, for instance, reducing the structural violence of working conditions, so that the care-participants have adequate space and time to mutually and inter-corporeally negotiate the epistemic boundaries, in the particular situation where the potentially threatening situation of care takes place.

Lederach's understanding of conflict transformation goes well together with this chapter's aims to first understand care as inclusive of violence, and then to develop constructive ways of speaking about that violence in a destigmatising manner. For instance, what my research participants' reflections on caring self-protection indicate is that, while they explicitly embraced the concept as describing the ways they protect themselves from violence, their techniques and tactics of protection are never aimed at violence per se, or even the violent person (cf. Åkeström 2002). Rather, *their actions are aimed at the conflicts emerging in the relationship* as differentially vulnerable bodies engage in practices of care. Through a range of techniques and tactics of caring self-protection, the nurses *together with* the care-receivers seek to transform this relationship in ways that the mutual experiences of threatening violence turn to peaceful – or at least less violent – coexistence. Often, these inter-corporeal practices of caring self-protection transform the conflict in ways that direct violence is avoided altogether.

The methods of caring self-protection can be read through Lederach's three-lens approach to conflict transformation. First, the nurses seek to understand the immediate conflict, and how it emerges through an epistemic friction between two conflicting perceptions of reality. Second, the disease and its symptoms in the particular structural conditions of the care encounter provide the 'deeper relationship pattern', forming a disjointedly emergent context for the encounter, and its sometimes forced, yet necessary, disgust-materialist embraces. Then, third, applying the different methods of caring self-protection, the nurses improvise a situated framework of action, where they seek to connect this particular deeper structure of relatedness with the immediate conflict at hand. Placing the opaque agency of the person who lives with dementia in the centre of action, they provide space for the seemingly unintelligible, epistemic realities of the demented mind, in ways that the person's frustration would not result in aggression. In this way, even when a conflict in care turns violent, the skills of caring self-protection allow the nurses to transform it into *a more peaceful and less violent* relationship of being with the other.

In this regard, the nurses' skills of caring self-protection have the potential to teach us something about the possibilities of seeking epistemic peace – that is, the absence of epistemic violence. Namely, what the nurses do once care starts to emerge with and include violence – be it about adjusting the environment or their embodied being with the care-recipient – is aimed at *transforming a conflict between two epistemic realities* equally true to the care-participants: the reality of the nurse and that of the person living with dementia. The nurses understand that, while they are exposed to physical violence, the other's violence derives from the experience of being/feeling threatened, too – as well as from the persistent epistemic violence where the knowledge of the demented mind never quite fits in, and the person living with/in that mind cannot speak.

Caring self-protection is thus not only about engaging with the entanglements of care and violence, but doing so in ways that seek to disentangle the different forms of violence (including potential violence) that make care threatening. When the violences are disentangled, it is possible to work with them in more nuanced ways, so that some of the experienced threats are diluted, and peaceful coexistence stands a chance in the midst of the violent situation. Here, of course, the structural conditions of care work always intertwine with the situation, and they can do so both in peaceful and violent ways. As described earlier in the chapter, structural violence such as inadequate staffing increases the risks of other types of violence, too, and indeed caring self-protection is only possible with adequate time provided for the care encounter – that is, in the absence of grave forms of structural violence.

In the second focus group discussion (4 December 2019), my research participants, for instance, could not think of a situation of intimate care, where they would not have adequate *time to work together with* the care-receiver. This implies that the structures in which these nurses work are rather peaceful, enabling practices of caring self-protection – and hence transformation of conflicts over epistemic realities. This does not mean that the nurses who participated in my study would not have structural pressures of time, that they would not have to continuously make choices between competing care needs, or that structural violence would be completely absent in this care home. Rather, it means that the structural conditions are *peaceful enough* for the nurses to take time and disentangle the intertwinements of epistemic, structural, and direct violence, as they emerge with/in particular inter-corporeal situations of intimate care. In the following, concluding section, I move to consider what caring self-protection as conflict transformation can contribute to our thinking about global health.

FEMINIST GLOBAL HEALTH AS CONFLICT TRANSFORMATION

Drawing on feminist ethics of care, feminist peace researchers have for a long time argued that practices of care give rise to alternative ways of knowing, and to situated, relational ethics of living with others. Heavily influenced by this tradition (see Vaittinen 2015, 2017; Vaittinen et al. 2019), and drawing on my ethnography of everyday peace and conflict in residential dementia care, I have developed in this chapter an empirically grounded concept of caring self-protection, best understood as mundane, inter-corporeal work of conflict transformation. The concept draws attention not only to the uncomfortable truth that care sometimes includes violence, but also to peaceful methods of working with such violence(s). Focusing on cognitive disabilities, dementia in particular, the analysis brought me to consider the role of epistemic violence in practices of care, which, in turn, led me to briefly address the possibilities of epistemic peace.

Many of the chapters in this book deal with the failure of global health to address the needs of differentially gendered marginalised groups – indeed, the failure to respond to *silenced care needs*. This is a question of epistemic violence in global health, where – as I have elaborated elsewhere (Vaittinen 2017) – the care needs of some cannot speak, because they are written out of the gendered and sexualised material-discursive orders in which care is provided. By way of conclusion – and as an opening for a new discussion on the nature of global health – I want to suggest that thinking about global health as caring self-protection and as conflict transformation may help us to better address such epistemic violences.

I have argued that caring self-protection involves techniques and tactics of protecting the self from violence, while seeking to protect the violent other *and* simultaneously seeking to provide good care. This, as shown throughout the chapter, demands adequately peaceful structural conditions, so that carers can seek to negotiate over conflicting epistemic realities, also in difficult circumstances. This applies to the need to listen to the particular needs of *waria* in Indonesia (Nuño, this volume), for instance, the experiences of women with breast cancer in Uganda (Ikhile et al., this volume), and the expertise of the volunteer counsellors of HIV patients in South Africa (Oinas, this volume). In all these contexts of gendered global health and violence, various feminised skills of caring self-protection already play a role. Yet, they should be increasingly made visible, valorised, and enabled by peaceful structures that allow adequate inter-corporeal time for care, and caring – also in difficult circumstances.

Understanding feminist global health as caring self-protection would also require a feminist orientation to conflict transformation that follows what Confortini and Ruane (2014) have conceptualised as 'weaving epistemology'. This is a 'flexible way of knowing *positioned to reduce dehumanization*'. This epistemology is a 'gut-level commitment' to practices (i) of '*living with dissonance*'; (ii) of '*creatively overcoming disconnects* between the interests of the self and the other'; and (iii) of 'bridging practical goals for surviving the present with more idealistic goals for "best practices" in the future' (Confortini and Ruane 2014, 73, emphasis mine). Following such a three-pronged approach in policies and practices of global health would turn global health into ongoing, situated, and inter-corporeal field of conflict transformation. It would mean an epistemological stance that respects the situated knowledges of the care-recipients – however irrational they might seem from the perspective of predominant biomedical knowledges – and a commitment to live with this dissonance, while seeking the best practices for the future.

Like the search for peace as an absence of all kinds of violence, the feminist search for global health is an endless task. It requires a recognition that care includes conflicts – and those conflicts can get violent. Yet, conceptualising feminist global health as conflict transformation would make us better equipped to recognise these gendered violences as they *emerge with* global health policies, practices, and discourses. What is more, it might help us to work with these violences, erase or at least erode them, and thus bring global health closer to the feminist ideals of peace as social justice.

NOTES

1. The research was part of a wider project, entitled *Mundane Practices of Peace*, funded by the Academy of Finland (project #297053). Ethical clearance to the research design was received from the Ethics Committee of the Tampere Region.

2. I acknowledge that elderly abuse in dementia care is also a serious problem, and that carers can treat their vulnerable care-recipients violently, too. In this chapter, however, I do not discuss the violence experienced by care-recipients, since my empirical data do not allow or call for such analysis.

3. Going to the sauna is generally a mundane part of people's lives in Finland, regardless of class or wealth. In care homes, there is always a sauna in the premises, and residents are regularly provided bathing in the sauna, assisted by the nurses.

4. Nurses working in mental health and psychiatry may be taught techniques such as Management of Mutual and Potential Aggression, MAPA®. Such skills, however, are not included in the training for elderly care – a feminised, low-skilled job in the professional hierarchies of healthcare professions.

5. Originally in Finnish: *hoivaava itsesuojelu*.

6. I want to thank the participants of the Cardiff Ethnography, Culture and Interpretive Analysis Research group, and Tampere University Social and Health Care Politics SOTEPO seminar for the valuable comments that helped me to develop the term from caring self-defence to self-protection.

REFERENCES

Åkeström, Malin. 2002. 'Slaps, Punches, Pinches – But Not Violence: Boundary-Work in Nursing Homes for the Elderly'. *Symbolic Interaction* 25, no. 4: 515–536.

Baines, Donna. 2006. 'Staying with People Who Slap Us Around: Gender, Juggling Responsibilities and Violence in Paid (and Unpaid) Care Work'. *Gender, Work and Organization* 13, no. 2: 129–151.

Banerjee, Albert, Tamara Daly, Hugh Armstrong, Pat Armstrong, Stirling Lafrance and Marta Szebehely. 2008. *'Out of Control': Violence against Personal Support Workers in Long-Term Care*. York University and Carleton University. https://www.longwoods.com/articles/images/Violence_LTC_022408_Final.pdf. Accessed 7 September 2019.

Banerjee, Albert, Tamara Daly, Pat Armstrong, Martha Szebehely, Hugh Armstrong and Stirling Lafrance. 2012. 'Structural Violence in Long-Term, Residential Care for Older People: Comparing Canada and Scandinavia'. *Social Science and Medicine* 74, no. 3: 390–398.

Butler, Judith. 2004. *Precarious Life: The Powers of Mourning and Violence*. London and New York: Verso.

Butler, Judith. 2005. *Giving an Account of Oneself*. New York: Fordham University Press.

Carroll, Berenice A. 1972. 'Peace Research: The Cult of Power'. *The Journal of Conflict Resolution* 16, no. 4: 585–616.

Confortini, Catia C. and Abigail Ruane. 2014. 'Sara Ruddick's *Maternal Thinking* as Weaving Epistemology for *Justpeace*'. *Journal of International Political Theory* 10, no 1: 70–93.

Confortini Catia C. and Tiina Vaittinen. 2019. 'Introduction: Analysing Violences in Gendered Global Health'. In *Gender, Global Health and Violence: Feminist Perspectives on Peace and Disease*, edited by Tiina Vaittinen and Catia Confortini. London and New York: Rowman & Littlefield.

Connors, Joanna. 2009. 'Kent State Professor Trudy Steuernagel's Fierce Protection of Her Autistic Son, Sky Walker, Costs Her Life: Sheltering Sky'. Accessed 18 April 2019. http://blog.cleveland.com/metro/2009/12/kent_state_professor_trudy_ste.html.

Erkkilä, Sari, Sara Simberg and Merja Hyvärinen. 2016. *'Jos minä nyt kuitenkin jaksan'. Suomen lähi-ja perushoitajaliitto SuPerin selvitys lähi- ja perushoitajien kokemasta työkuormasta 2016*. Helsinki: SuPer. Accessed 29 April 2019. https://www.superliitto.fi/site/assets/files/64616/tyohyvinvointiselvitys_verkko_07062016.pdf.

Featherstone, Katie, Andy Northcott and Jackie Bridges. 2019. 'Routines of Resistance: An Ethnography of the Care of People Living with Dementia in Acute Hospital Wards and Its Consequences'. *International Journal of Nursing Studies*. Accessed 7 September 2019. https://doi.org/10.1016/j.ijnurstu.2018.12.009.

Finley, Laura. 2019. 'Domestic Violence and Public Health: Beginning Steps for Creating More Just and Effective Community Responses'. In *Gender, Global Health and Violence: Feminist Perspectives on Peace and Disease*, edited by Tiina Vaittinen and Catia Confortini. London and New York: Rowman & Littlefield.

Galtung, Johan. 1969. 'Violence, Peace and Peace Research'. *Journal of Peace Research* 6: 167–191.

Harman, Sophie. 2019. 'Violence and the Paradox of Global Health'. In *Gender, Global Health and Violence: Feminist Perspectives on Peace and Disease*, edited by Tiina Vaittinen and Catia Confortini. London and New York: Rowman & Littlefield.

Hoppania, Hanna-Kaisa and Tiina Vaittinen. 2015. 'A Household Full of Bodies: Neoliberalism, Care and "the Political"'. *Global Society* 29, no. 1: 70–88.

Ikhile, Deborah, Gibson Linda and Azrini Wahidin. 2019. '"I Cannot Know That Now I Have Cancer!" A Structural Violence Perspective on Breast Cancer Detection in Uganda'. In *Gender, Global Health and Violence: Feminist Perspectives on Peace and Disease*, edited by Tiina Vaittinen and Catia Confortini. London & New York: Rowman & Littlefield.

Isaksen, Lise W. 2002. 'Toward a Sociology of (Gendered) Disgust: Images of Bodily Decay and the Social Organization of Care Work'. *Journal of Family Issues* 23, no. 7: 791–811.

Karsio, Olli and Anneli Anttonen. 2013. 'Marketisation of Eldercare in Finland: Legal Frames, Outsourcing Practices and the Rapid Growth of For-Profit Services'. In Gabrielle Meagher and Marta Szebehely (eds.) *Marketisation in Nordic eldercare: A research report on legislation, oversight, extent and consequences.* Stockholm: Stockholm University.

Kelly, Christine. 2017. 'Care and Violence through the Lens of Personal Support Workers'. *International Journal of Care and Caring* 1, no. 1: 97–113.

Kelly, Fiona. 2010. 'Abusive Interactions: Research in Locked Wards for People with Dementia'. *Social Policy & Society* 9, no. 2: 267–277.

Kittay, Eva F. 1999. *Love's Labour: Essays on Women, Equality and Dependency.* New York: Routledge.

Kröger, Teppo, Lina van Aerschott and Jiby M. Puthenparambil. 2018. *Hoivatyö muutoksessa. Suomalainen vanhustyö pohjoismaisessa vertailussa.* YFI Publications 6. Jyväskylä: University of Jyväskylä.

Lederach, John Paul. 2003. 'Conflict Tranformation'. An abridged version of Lederach's *The Little Book of Conflict Transformation*, shortened and edited by Michelle Maiese. Accessed 9 September 2019. https://www.beyondintractability.org/essay/transformation.

Lederach, John Paul. 2014. *The Little Book of Conflict Transformation.* New York: Good Books.

Lindholm, Camilla. 2015. 'Parallel Realities: The Interactional Management of Confabulation in Dementia Care Encounters'. *Research on Language and Social Interaction* 48, no. 2: 176–199.

Lukić, Dragana. 2019. 'Multiple Ontologies of Alzheimer's Disease in *Still Alice* and *A Song for Martin*: A Feminist Visual Studies of Technoscience Perspective'. *European Journal of Women's Studies*. Accessed 7 September 2019. https://doi.org/10.1177/1350506819831718.

Lukić, Dragana and Ann Therese Lotherington. 2019. 'Fighting Symbolic Violence through Artistic Encounters: Searching for Feminist Answers to the Question of Life and Death with Dementia'. In *Gender, Global Health and Violence: Feminist Perspectives on Peace and Disease*, edited by Tiina Vaittinen and Catia Confortini. London and New York: Rowman & Littlefield.

Molinier, Pascale. 2011. 'Care as Work: Mutual Vulnerabilities and Discrete Knowledge'. In *New Philosophies of Labour: Work and the Social Bond*, edited by Nicholas Smith and Jean-Philippe Deranty, 251–270. Leiden and Boston: Brill.

Nolan, Mike R., Sue Davies, Jayne Brown, Keady John and Janet Nolan. 2004. 'Beyond "Person-Centred" Care: A New Vision for Gerontological Nursing'. *International Journal of Older People Nursing* in association with *Journal of Clinical Nursing* 13, 3a: 45–53.

Nuño, Néstor M. 2019. 'Rethinking Global Health Priorities from the Margins: Health Access and Medical Care Claims among Indonesia's *Waria*'. In *Gender, Global Health and Violence: Feminist Perspectives on Peace and Disease*, edited by Tiina Vaittinen and Catia Confortini. London and New York: Rowman & Littlefield.

Oinas, Elina. 2019. 'HIV Politics and Structural Violence: Access to Treatment and Knowledge'. In *Gender, Global Health and Violence: Feminist Perspectives on Peace and Disease*, edited by Tiina Vaittinen and Catia Confortini. London and New York: Rowman & Littlefield.

Puumala, Eeva and Samu Pehkonen. 2010. 'Corporeal Choreographies between Politics and the Political: Failed Asylum Seekers Moving from Body Politics to Bodyspaces'. *International Political Sociology* 4: 50–65.

Reuterswärd, Camilla. 2019. '¡Malas Madres, Malas Mujeres, Malas Todas! The Incarceration of Women for Abortion-Related Crimes in Mexico'. In *Gender, Global Health and Violence: Feminist Perspectives on Peace and Disease*, edited by Tiina Vaittinen and Catia Confortini. London and New York: Rowman & Littlefield.

Robinson, Fiona. 1999. *Globalizing Care: Ethics, Feminist Theory and International Relations*. Westview Press: Boulder.

Robinson, Fiona. 2011. *The Ethics of Care: A Feminist Approach to Human Security*. Philadelphia: Temple University Press.

Robinson, Fiona and Catia Confortini. 2014. 'Symposium: Maternal Thinking for International Relations? Papers in Honor of Sara Ruddick'. *Journal of International Political Theory* 10, no. 1: 38–45.

Ruddick, Sara. 1990. *Maternal Thinking: Towards a Politics of Peace*. New York: Ballantine Books.

Rytkönen, Arja. 2018. *Hoivatyöntekijöiden työn kuormittavuus ja teknologian käyttö vanhustyössä*. PhD diss. (published). Tampere University Press. Accessed 7 September 2019. http://urn.fi/URN:ISBN:978-952-03-0829-2.

Simplican, Stacy C. 2015. 'Care, Disability and Violence: Theorizing Complex Dependency in Eva Kittay and Judith Butler'. *Hypatia* 30, no. 1: 217–233.

Sointu, Liina. 2018. 'Slipping into "That Nurses Dress": Caring as Affective Practice in Mixed-Sex Couples' Relationships'. In *Affective Inequalities in Intimate Relationships*, edited by Tuula Juvonen and Marjo Kolehmainen, 95–107. London: Routledge.

Tedre, Silva. 2004. 'Tukisukkahousut sosiaalipolitiikkaan: Inhomaterialistinen hoivatutkimusote'. In *Ruumis töihin! Käsite ja käytäntö*, edited by Eeva Jokinen, Marja Kaskisaari and Marita Husso, 41–64. Tampere: Vastapaino.

Tronto, Joan C. 1993. *Moral Boundaries: A Political Argument for an Ethic of Care*. New York/London: Routledge.

Twigg, Julia. 2000. *Bathing: The Body and Community Care*. London and New York: Routledge.

The Union of Social and Health Care Professionals in Finland. 2011. 'Tehy: älä riko hoitajaasi'. Press release, 14 March. Accessed 7 September 2019. https://www.tehy.fi/fi/mediatiedote/tehy-ala-riko-hoitajaasi.

The Union of Social and Health Care Professionals in Finland. 2018. 'Älä riko hoitajaasi – seminaari väkivallan teemoista'. Seminar announcement, 14 August 2018. Accessed 7 September 2019. https://www.tehy.fi/fi/ajankohtaista/ala-riko-hoitajaasi-seminaari-vakivallan-teemoista.

Vaittinen, Tiina. 2017. *The Global Biopolitical Economy of Needs: Transnational Entanglements between Ageing Finland and the Global Nurse Reserve of the Philippines*. PhD diss. (published). Tampere Peace Research Institute and Tampere University Press. Accessed 7 September 2019. http://urn.fi/URN:ISBN:978-952-03-0505-5.

Vaittinen, Tiina, Amanda Donahoe, Rahel Kunz, Silja B. Ómarsdóttir and Sanam Roohi. 2019. 'Care as Everyday Peacebuilding'. *Peacebuilding* 7, no. 2: 194–209.

Vaittinen, Tiina, Hoppania Hanna-Kaisa and Olli Karsio. 2018. 'Marketization, Commodification and Privatization of Care Services'. In *Handbook of the International Political Economy of Gender*, edited by Juanita Elias and Adrienne Roberts, 379–391. Cheltenham and Norhampton: Edward Elgar.

Väyrynen, Tarja, Eeva Puumala, Samu Pehkonen, Anitta Kynsilehto and Tiina Vaittinen. 2017. *Choreographies of Resistance: Mobile Bodies and Relational Politics*. London and New York: Rowman & Littlefield.

Chapter 12

Conclusion: Violence and the Paradox of Global Health

Sophie Harman

Global health is underpinned by violence and this violence is gendered. To draw together the main conclusions of the book, I revisited two important bodies of work that came to mind when reading and thinking about the collected chapters. The first, familiar to feminists working on the everyday, violence, gender, and global health (see, for example, Anderson 2015): Nancy Scheper-Hughes' (1992) ground-breaking *Death without Weeping: The Violence of Everyday Life in Brazil*. The second, common to people working in global health but perhaps less familiar to feminists working on violence: Paul Farmer's work on Haiti and the relationship between structural violence, HIV/AIDS, and human rights in *AIDS and Accusation* (1992) and later *Pathologies of Power* (2005). Both published in 1992, these bodies of work engage with the main themes of this book: the intersecting nature of violence, health, and gender; the importance of context in understanding how such violence occurs and is reproduced; the social and political structures that embed violent practice; and the routinisation of violence, either in the case of Scheper-Hughes with regard to child mortality or Farmer, HIV/AIDS. Reading the chapters in this volume, I was struck by the nagging thought, what has changed in our understanding and practices of violence, gender, and global health in the twenty-five years since *Death without Weeping* and *AIDS and Accusation* were first published? Are the relationships, intersections, and routinisation the same?

The chapters in this book suggest little has changed with regard to structural violence and health outcomes: stigma, routinised death, and state neglect all persist and impact on health outcomes. What has changed is the globalised nature of healthcare delivery and the upsurge in attention towards global health, new sources and increases in global health financing, the creation of multiple types of public and private global health actors, and investment in global health research. The health problems and patterns of structural violence explored in Farmer and Scheper-Hughes' work were included as key targets in both the United Nations Millennium Development Goals (Goal 4 Reduce Child Mortality and Goal 5 Improve Maternal Health) and the Sustainable Development Goals (Goal 3 Good Health and Well-Being).

This upsurge in global health has led to tangible outcomes: global mortality of older children has dropped by 50 per cent since 1990, and by 2016 the rate of under-five child mortality was one in twenty-six in comparison to one in eleven in 1990 (UNICEF 2018); new infection rates of children with HIV have declined by 70 per cent since 2001 (UNAIDS 2016); and by June 2017, 20.9 million people living with HIV were able to access treatment in comparison to 685,000 people in 2000 (UNAIDS 2017). In addition, over the last twenty years, a new range of social welfare strategies such as conditional cash transfer programmes have been introduced, with the specific aim of targeting the health and education outcomes of the most poor and marginalised in society. Conditional cash transfer programmes such as *Bolsa Familia* were established in Brazil, with the specific intent of helping women such as those from the Alto do Cruzeiro in Scheper-Hughes' book. The impact of these initiatives, financing strategies, and goals are not without criticism, particularly by feminist scholars (see, for example, Bradshaw 2008; Chant 2006). However, what is important here is to note the intense and significant change in the scale of response to global health challenges. The question thus becomes not only what has changed in the last twenty-five years in our understanding of global health, gender, and violence, but also how the significant changes in global health have furthered or challenged our understanding of this relationship.

Confortini and Vaittinen argue at the outset of this book that we have not done enough to further our understanding of this relationship. Peace Research has not kept pace with the rapid changes in global health, global health scholarship rarely engages with Peace Research, and gender – while central to understanding this relationship – tends to be side-lined or an add-on to the analysis of both fields of study. For Confortini and Vaittinen, we need to see global health as less of a case study in which to explore the impact and outcomes of violence but recognise how global health interventions, institutions, and actors may be reproducing the very violence they seek to address. The relationship between global health and violence is more than just structural violence: it involves intersecting symbolic, everyday, and epistemic forms of violence. What Confortini and Vaittinen point to, and the chapters in this book demonstrate, is a central paradox to the relationship between global health and violence: violence is embedded and reproduced within the very structures and practices of global health governance that seek to ameliorate its negative effects.

This is not surprising or new to anyone with a basic understanding of violence and how it is embedded within society. However, what is revealing here is the paradox of global health governance: it is a system of governance based on care, born of a need to address, mitigate, and ameliorate the consequences of structural and other forms of violence to deliver the highest attainability of physical and mental health for all. Yet, the findings of this book suggest that rather than ameliorating violence, such systems of governance reproduce it. The paradox of global health governance is thus the tension between a normative commitment to treat, prevent, care, and heal, and how the very structures that deliver on such normative commitments enact and reproduce forms of violence.

The notion of global health as violence is somewhat distasteful or contrary to the normative aims and intent of global health governance to provide health for all. However, as this book demonstrates, conceptualising global health as violence generates new questions as to where violent practices, assumptions, and constructions exist; how they are reproduced and resisted; how they exclude; and how they act as barriers in the realisation of the healthy lives for all in the world. This conclusion explores the paradox of global health governance by focusing on four specific themes that arose from the chapters: context, stigma, hierarchy, and the violence of health professionals.

CONTEXT AND GENDER

Context matters when understanding violence. This is a common concern for studies of individual, state, institutional, structural, symbolic, epistemic, or everyday violence. There is no general theory of violence or the practice of violence (Lawrence and Karim 2007, 7). Thus, we need detailed theories and empirical work in which to understand different types of violence, its effects, and the processes within which it is reproduced. Context is particularly relevant for scholars looking to understand everyday, symbolic, epistemic, and structural violence because of the ways in which social orders intersect and have differing consequences and impact on people's lives. Without context, violence risks becoming a redundant concept: catch all in application, or a throw away word ascribed to a range of activities without either empirical or theoretical grounding. Violence loses meaning and value without context and as such can be ignored or used rhetorically with limited commitment to redress or change.

Context and empirical research do not just provide material for peace researchers to evidence their claims but are about the very nature of violence itself. As Kleinman (1997) argues, structural violence is about social orders and 'the study of the violences of everyday life is significant, because it offers an alternative view of human conditions that may give access to fundamental, if deeply disturbing, processes of social organization' (Kleinman 1997, 238). Violence is located within everyday practices and, as Arendt (1969) argues, 'power and violence, though they are distinct phenomena, usually appear together'. What is crucial therefore for understanding structural violence, or the many other forms of indirect violence the chapters expose in global health, is how they operate within specific social orders or systems of governance. If a core component of structural violence is the impact it has on the health and wellbeing of people around the world, and most acutely to the poorest and most marginalised in society, we need to understand what these structures are, how they exert power and enact violence, and how structures and orders of global health reproduce such violence.

Global health is not an add-on to understanding violence: it provides specific context and understanding to how violence is reproduced and routinised. Global health pertains to a specific form of governance, dependent on how states organise their health systems; the financial aid commitments of international donors and institutions; and social norms as to behaviour, stigma, and healthcare access and delivery. I have argued previously that global health governance refers to 'trans-border agreements or initiatives between states and/or non-state actors to the control of public health and infectious disease and the protection of people from health risks or threats' (Harman 2011, 2). What is particular about global health, and how it differs from other social forms of violence, is its primary emphasis on care and amelioration of suffering, death, and illness. Global health, in principle, is normatively committed to care, treatment, and healing: the opposite of violence. However, global health governance also has the capacity to help 'normalise' forms of violence, for example, that it is not uncommon for a woman to die in childbirth of preventable causes, health care is expensive and unaffordable, or a woman living with HIV brought the disease on herself. It, therefore, provides an extreme context to our understanding of structural violence as a sphere of governance where violence is to be addressed, avoided, and healed rather than enacted.

As scholars such as Anderson (2015) and the chapters in this book argue, forms of governance and social orders, specifically global health, are gendered. Gender is always present when considering the relationship between global health and violence (Anderson 2005; Farmer 1992; Scheper-Hughes 1992). Examining the contexts in which violence takes place and is embedded, challenged, and reproduced by social orders and forms of governance requires a gender lens. A gender lens not only looks at how men and women (trans and cis) and non-binary people are affected differently by health interventions or lack thereof; it considers how the systems aimed to ameliorate such difference in providing health for all can reproduce gender and difference. Difference can be positive – identifying groups at risk of violence, poor health, or both to target and tailor interventions; recognising that not everyone in the world is a white cis male and therefore may have different concerns and be subjected to different forms of structural violence. It can also be negative for example, assuming that women will provide care for free, that women's health can be reduced to maternal mortality and that people should fit into gendered categories.

One of the key contributions of a gender lens to understanding the relationship between global health and violence is to shine light on the silenced, marginalised, and unseen relationships and entanglements between health and different forms of violence. This is not necessarily just identifying where the women are, but also the issues, assumptions, and machinations of violence that happen in informal settings are known but taken for granted, or strategically ignored. It is often those issues and people that are hidden in plain sight or 'conspicuously invisible' (Harman 2016) that lead to, or are subject to, different forms of violence. This is a theme that runs through the chapters of this book. It is, for instance, clearly the case with regard to Reuterswärd's work on abortion in Mexico, Finley's depiction of intimate partner violence, Féron's chapter on sexual violence against men, and Vaittinen's chapter on nurses' exposure to violence in dementia care: the epistemic violence enacted through global health that governs whose voice and knowledge counts, and how knowledge can be used as power over rather than power to care and heal.

The second key contribution of a gendered lens to understanding global health and violence is to enact change. DeLaet, Golden, and Laveta make this point clearly in their chapter on survivors of human rights violations, global health, and therapeutic justice. For the authors, a gender lens on the issue of human rights violations and forms of therapeutic justice offer a framework for redress, change, and improvement in the lives of survivors. At the core of their work is the need to understand the relationship between human rights violations and global health as a basis for improvement in individual lives and as a means of sustaining peace in post-conflict situations. The basis for such understanding is to challenge the epistemic violence of justice systems to change how survivors are involved in justice and how their needs can be met through an emphasis on therapeutic justice. Underpinned by feminist theory and feminist activism, a gender lens should not only shine light on the unseen but do so in a way that becomes a basis for change and redress to the improvement of people's lives and progress towards gender equality. It is not enough to understand different forms of violence: the point of understanding is to change.

Global health is thus important for understanding gendered violence for three reasons. First, it provides a distinct case study and context in which to explore violence. What makes global health distinct is its emphasis on care, treatment, and healing seeming to exist, in principle at least, in direct opposition to violence. Second, gendered aspects of violence are reproduced in forms of global health governance in specific ways. Gendered forms of indirect violence are conspicuously invisible in global health: violence occurs in everyday ways and is dominant across different aspects of global health, yet is deliberately invisible in how we understand and address global health concerns. Third, this volume demonstrates that global health is relevant to more than just understanding structural violence: it is also a crucial space in which to explore and critically engage with symbolic, epistemic, and everyday violence; and how these different forms of violence overlap, reproduce, and sustain each other.

STIGMA

Stigma, in many respects, is the ordering principle of the relationship between violence and global health. Stigma is present in how people access health care, whether they are dealing with diseases known to be associated with stigma such as HIV/AIDS (Nuño; Oinas, this volume) or concerns that have not been considered in terms of stigma such as Breast Cancer (Ikhile et al., this volume). Such stigma is driven by individualised self-stigma, community based-stigma, and stigma drawn from social norms and conduct such as women's position in society. Stigma is also present in how people deliver health services. What is perhaps most concerning in some of the chapters is how health professionals stigmatise specific health concerns, particularly health concerns specific to women, such as abortion rights and the people accessing treatment for a variety of health issues. In the case of Reuterswärd's chapter on access to abortion rights in Mexico, it is clear that it is both the act of abortion and the women who seek abortions who were stigmatised by medical professionals.

If stigma is the ordering principle of the relationship between global health and violence, it is exacerbated, reproduced, and embedded within society by gender. Women's health needs, such as reproductive health and access to safe abortion, are stigmatised in specific contexts as a means to control women's bodies (Tanyag, this volume; Reuterswärd, this volume). Such control comes from stigma as a social norm, internalised self-stigma that acts as a limit or control to an individual's behaviour, and stigma that becomes a part of both formal domestic law and customary international law. Stigma as a social norm is clear in prejudicial attitudes to people living with HIV as being promiscuous, somehow remiss in not preventing transmission, or a potential threat to others. Social stigma not only is about societal prejudice but also occurs through everyday assumptions and fears as identified in Ikhile et al.'s chapter that prevent women from seeking medical attention, and consequently early detection of breast cancer. Internalised stigma can similarly be seen when someone living with HIV is aware of such social norms and thus changes or adapts their behaviour and starts to internalise feelings of shame to the detriment of both their mental and physical wellbeing (Nuño, this volume). Féron's chapter demonstrated the extreme consequences the combination of social stigma and individual self-stigma can have on the ability of people, in this case, men, to have healthy lives. Finally, stigma can become entrenched in legal attitudes towards people living with specific diseases or health concerns through targeted interventions in extreme cases, such as quarantine, and everyday legal norms throughout the world such as the notion that reproductive health is something to be curtailed rather than a right (Harman and Davies 2019).

Violence is personal in how the individual internalises such violence through stigma or shame (e.g. in the case of sexual violence), or uses such violence as a force for change (e.g. mobilisation of people and communities living with HIV/AIDS, see Oinas, this volume). As Lukić and Lotherington suggest in their chapter, individual internalisation of violence and symbolic violence can lead to violence against self, rendering suicide an option preferable to living with the disease. Violence is mediated and reproduced by both structures of global health governance, and as Foucault would argue, through human consciousness (Lawrence and Karim 2007, 6). In global health, violence is mutually constituted between human consciousness and the individual and structures that create and reproduce stigma, isolation, and neglect.

Stigma and how stigma is gendered is a core component of Farmer and Scheper-Hughes' work on global health and structural violence. While gendered stigma has been latent in understandings of structural violence and how it pertains to health, both are now a prominent feature and lens for analysis. Simply put you cannot understand structural violence in the context of global health without understanding gender and its relationship to stigma. The chapters in this volume demonstrate that social stigma, individual self-stigma, and customary legal stigma are united in how they are all gendered. Structural and epistemic violence are mediated through gendered stigma that controls the services available to women (reproductive health and abortion), stops women from accessing health services (breast cancer), perpetuates female self-stigma as to what is appropriate behaviour or health concerns for a differentially gendered individuals to have (HIV/AIDS and breast cancer), orders which knowledge is relevant and what knowledge is silenced and shamed, and ignores categories of gender beyond male or female, thus rendering large populations invisible or redundant from global health service delivery. Increasingly gendered stigma is the ordering principle of violence and global health that limits the delivery of health for all.

HIERARCHY OF HEALTH

In 1992, HIV/AIDS exceptionalism was not related to the attention and money it received but the stigma that was associated with it. What has changed twenty-five years on is how HIV/AIDS is seen as exceptional within global health governance because of the donor support, global attention, and political commitment mobilised to address the care, treatment, and prevention of the disease. For some, including authors in this book, this has led to a distortion in funding and attitudes towards specific populations and states where access to resources for health expenditure has required claims to HIV/AIDS funding and attention (Nuño, this volume). Such distortion and HIV/AIDS financing points to a significant issue in understanding global health, gender, and violence: hierarchies of health.

Different health issues and diseases exist in a global hierarchy of importance, interest, and value. Hierarchy exists as to which health concerns take precedence and which ones are of less concern to health policy-makers and practitioners. Such hierarchies are embedded in forms of epistemic violence as to who knows best and whose knowledge matters more for prioritising specific issues over others (cf. Oinas, this volume). This takes on a form of violence that sidelines or neglects health concerns that are not topical, a security threat, or of political and social significance to key actors in health (see Harman 2016). What the chapters demonstrate here is that hierarchy is both an everyday factor in what health concerns are privileged or ignored, and a prominent factor in the complex entanglements of violence that can occur in the context of emergencies.

HIV/AIDS has come to dominate debates on exceptionalism (Benton 2015; Lisk 2009) and hierarchy in global health. The chapters in this collection contribute directly to such debate. As Oinas suggests, access to anti-retroviral treatment (ART) for HIV/AIDS has always been political and HIV/AIDS occupies its specialised status on account of political and civic activism and mobilisation. The hierarchical position of HIV/AIDS in global health can potentially be mediated within communities to their own ends. It is the everyday engagement with these health hierarchies that reproduces forms of structural, symbolic, and epistemic violence wherein individuals have to mould their health needs and position themselves along a continuum of health priorities that are shaped by global political interests. Nuño contributes to understanding the violence of HIV/AIDS exceptionalism, by showing how the *waria* have to distinguish themselves from the omnipresence of HIV/AIDS interventions in their lives and create space for their health needs to be identified and recognised.

The need to order global health through categories – male/female, children under five, people living with HIV, high risk populations – all serve to identify, manage, and target health interventions to help those in need. Categories and labels order preferences and priorities within global health, measure indicators of success, provide coherence to strategy, and identify those who are overlooked or ignored in wider health policy. The basics of epidemiology and public health – contact tracing, mapping vulnerable populations, ratios, and prevalence rates – all require and include a specific level of categorisation. However such categories can also overlook populations that do not fit within specific models, mis-label, or make certain populations fit into certain boxes, it can also lead to hierarchies between categories. As Nuño argues, the *waria* have not only to navigate categories of gender based on two genders of male and female in Indonesian society, but their categorisation within a health system. This points to a duality of violence within the health system: the *waria* do not fit within two categories of gender within wider society, and in addition, they are then wrongly categorised when it comes to their health needs. This exacerbates issues of stigma and neglects the complex and differing health needs of a diverse group of people. To address their needs, the *waria*, like many stigmatised groups before them, have to collectively organise and engage in activism to have their health needs recognised and met within wider structures of symbolic and epistemic violence.

The need to fit within categories or boxes to assist with the overall management of global health is a form of violence. As Féron's chapter suggests, this is particularly problematic for male survivors of sexual violence and their ability to access the physical and mental health care they need. Labelling of male rape in war as torture and female rape as sexual violence, according to Féron, feeds wider narratives of women as vulnerable and men as having agency. This has obvious practical limitations for the health services men and women can access and how they access such services. Fundamentally, it reproduces the violent practice inherent in sexual violence: to have power over people, shame, stigma, and a lack of agency.

Hierarchy of health is further exacerbated when thinking how needs are met in times of crisis. Triage is a standard mechanism for addressing health needs and concerns in global emergencies. What Tanyag's chapter shows is how sexual and reproductive health rights are commonly ignored or sidelined through such emergency processes. Everyday needs of women such as access to contraception or sanitary products are a low priority on the hierarchy of emergency health concerns. Global health emergencies present extreme evidence of the everyday structural, symbolic, and epistemic violence of ordering women's health concerns as a low priority.

If a hierarchy of health exists within global health, the chapters in this volume suggest the health needs of women and gender non-conforming people are at the bottom of this hierarchy. Women's health needs, for instance, exist at the top of the hierarchy when their function in reproducing and sustaining child health and wellbeing, or managing their own HIV status, is concerned. Otherwise, women's health needs are sidelined as less important than other health concerns, or such needs are afforded attention but come up against the ordering principle of violence and global health: gendered stigma.

VIOLENCE OF HEALTH PROFESSIONALS

Structures of governance that control, mitigate, and address global health challenges have historically been born of a need to ameliorate the consequences of such violence either to protect the self, other, or state. What is, therefore, controversial is the notion that such structures could somehow be complicit in or create violence. We know that health outcomes are socially determined (Wilkinson and Marmot 2003), 'diseases and premature death are unjustly distributed; institutions protect some while exposing others to the brutal vectors of economic and political power' (Kleinman 1997, 226). The aforementioned section demonstrated how hierarchy of health and disease and the need to categorise and label all reproduce forms of structural and internalised individual violence based on stigma, neglect, and isolation. In the present volume, the chapters broaden our understanding of violence by considering the paradox of global health: a form of governance concerned with care, treatment, and healing that can enact and reproduce violence through its practice. What is different and revealing within this volume is the role of individual health professionals in enacting different forms of violence.

The act of violence by health professionals can be first seen in the process of triage. As Finley argues in her chapter, the global systems we have to address physical and sexual intimate partner violence rest on a shelter triage model that is just about coping. While not critical of this system, such a model forces individuals working within the system to undertake everyday acts of violence as they prioritise need and case work of different individuals. This is compounded by criminal justice systems around the world that do not serve the needs of women. Triage is not just particular to the case of intimate partner violence, as Finley explores, but is a model of crisis and health management that transfers the burden of structural violence on to individual health professionals. These individual caregivers, nurses, social workers, doctors, and administrators of health have to mitigate the direct impact of such violence while minimising the violence they enact themselves – and while perhaps protecting themselves from violence the structures expose them to, as in Vaittinen's chapter. This puts individual health workers in an impossible position (that also impacts on their own wellbeing): to know they are acting to mitigate and address the outcomes of violence while aware that such action means depriving someone else of care. What is, therefore, revealing about the relationship between violence and global health is the responsibility and individualised nature of mitigating and addressing such violence.

An uncomfortable truth to some of the chapters in this collection is that health professionals do not necessarily seek to mitigate the consequences of structural or other forms of violence but directly reproduce or exacerbate such violence through choice. As Reuterswärd's chapter on abortion in Mexico explores, in some instances, medical professionals are reporting women who seek abortion as a means of protecting themselves and the potential repercussions they face. On the one hand, these cases suggest a clear example of a structure of violence conditioning individuals into complicity or hard choices within such structures. The structural element of this is important: health professionals have to make a number of moral questions about their role in reporting within the structural limitations in their own lives – whether failure to report results in their loss of employment, dependents on their employment, and the community they serve. The wider structures in which they operate condition the choices that they have in whether to report or not.

An emphasis on structure and the societal conditions in which medical professionals and other health professionals operate should not substitute for the agency and political interests of such individuals. Compounding their decision could be ideological concerns based on religious or political positions. Decision-making is also based on a power imbalance based on knowledge and access to treatment. Doctors, for example, may deduce from their years of medical training and expertise that they have better knowledge for what is best for the patient than the patient themselves. This is where a feminist lens becomes crucial to understanding this relationship. As Reuterswärd's chapter suggests, the judgement on identifying and reporting cases is not universal: with the case on abortion in Mexico, it is with regard to the most marginalised. One interpretation of this is that medical professionals working in complex contexts and more impoverished sectors have greater demands and pressures on triage and the factors that shape their decision-making. Another interpretation is that such marginalised groups are more susceptible to the gross imbalance of power between medical health professionals (educated, well paid, high standing in the community) and the patients and people in which they serve (less educated, living on the poverty line, often marginalised from the wider community).

Marginalised groups clearly show how forms of violence intersect in global health. First, structural violence can drive health outcomes and how the poor and marginalised are able to access health care. Second, the category of poor or marginalised enacts a symbolic violence as to perceptions of their ability to know what is best for themselves, that they need or depend on external assistance or expertise. This, in turn, third, produces a form of epistemic violence as to how their knowledge, awareness of their bodies, or concerns at best are seen as secondary to other forms of knowledge or, at worst, ignored altogether. In both interpretations, the more marginalised and susceptible to interlocking forms of violence the patients are, the greater the imbalance in relations between medical professionals and the patients, and the agency afforded to health professionals to enact or resist practices of violence. Decision-making and the types of violence mediated through health interventions are therefore not only determined by structures, with individual choice curtailed or determined by these structures, but the individual choice is also based on religious, political, or knowledge-based agency and power relations.

The privileged position of medical professionals and healthcare workers throughout local and global governance structures puts them in a position of power as providers of health care that have the ability to mediate, embed, or resist forms of structural violence. This points to a fundamental issue with violence and global health: the power relations between the knower and the known. This, in itself, is a form of epistemic violence, as it curtails the agency of the sick person or patient when they are dependent on physicians or other health professionals for treatment (see also Oinas, this volume).

GLOBAL HEALTH GOVERNANCE AS VIOLENCE

Structural violence, entangled with various forms of direct and indirect violence, has a long history of association with global health. Global health outcomes and the susceptibility of the poorest and most marginalised in society have long been held up as evidence of the devastating impact such violence has on everyday lives. Global health has attended to its relationship with structural violence by considering the social determinants of health, globalisation and health inequalities, and the everyday violence of living in poverty and managing complex health needs. The position of gender within this relationship is in evidence in the pioneering work of Scheper-Hughes and Farmer nearly twenty-five years ago. Such work is now being revisited and advanced by a range of scholars and feminist activists such as Emma Louise Anderson (2015) and the contributors to this volume.

Some aspects of this work are similar and draw a direct line from groundbreaking texts such as *Death without Weeping*. Stigma and shame are ever-present factors that feed structural violence, its reproduction, and the internalisation of violence within individuals. Unequal relations of power still persist, between the holder of medical knowledge, and resources, and those that need them, and the mediators that use such access as power over people and within the communities in which they operate. What this volume demonstrates is that global health is not just a case study in which violence and its outcomes can be explored. Global health cuts to the core of structural violence – it is both the end point, what stops people from dying or suffering when they do not have to – and it is that which drives the inequalities underpinning such violence – who can afford to stay alive and who cannot.

Beyond the focus on structural violence in global health, this book makes several advancements in understanding the relationship between gender, global health, and complex entanglements of violence. The first is that stigma is the first principle of understanding violence and global health, and that this stigma is gendered. The second is the paradox of global health: it is a social order that emphasises care and health for all as its fundamental principles, yet reproduces practices of different forms of violence that limits this. These practices include hierarchy of health concerns, diseases, and issues that are often dependent on donor preferences and political strategic choices; categorisation and labelling of populations that while necessary for targeted interventions can also exclude, discriminate, and overlook; and emphasise a form of triage that puts the onus on individual decision-making.

Central to understanding the paradox of global health and the relationship between violence, global health, and gender is the role of agency and individuals within this. Individual internalisation of stigma – self-stigma and stigma to others – perpetuates and fuels different forms of violence. Medical professionals seeking to ameliorate, mediate, or embed practices of these violences operate within personal and social constraints. Such constraints can lead to impossible and difficult choices. However, these choices can also be highly subjective and dependent on individual political, epistemic, and social preferences. The greater the inequality between the medical professional and the patient in terms of both finance and knowledge, the greater autonomy and agency the medical professional has in reproducing forms of violence.

The purpose of this book is to highlight the relationship between gender, global health, and different forms of violence: to evidence this relationship, to expand our knowledge and understanding; and to show the value of Global Health and gender to Peace Research, and vice versa. However, at its core is the feminist principle to use knowledge and research to enact change. As outlined in the introduction to this final chapter, a lot of progress has been made since the work of Scheper-Hughes and Farmer. Yet, as these chapters suggest, a lot of progress still needs to be made. Making the links, showing the evidence, identifying different and intersecting forms of violence – epistemic, symbolic; not just structural, sexual, and everyday – and calling out the paradox of global health – are the basis from which we can advance in the next twenty-five years, to seek out and address violence and its gendered impact.

REFERENCES

Anderson, Emma Louise. 2015. *Gender, HIV and Risk: Navigating Structural Violence*. London: Palgrave Macmillan.

Arendt, Hannah. 1969. 'Reflections on violence'. *Journal of International Affairs* 23, no. 1: 1–35.

Benton, Adia. 2015. *HIV Exceptionalism: Development through Disease in Sierra Leone*, Minneapolis: University of Minnesota Press.

Bradshaw, S. 2008. 'From Structural Adjustment to Social Adjustment'. *Global Social Policy* 8, no. 2: 188–207.

Chant, S. 2006. 'Re-Thinking the "Feminisation of Poverty" in Relation to Aggregate Gender Indices'. *Journal of International Development* 7, no. 2: 201–220.

Confortini, Catia C. and Tiina Vaittinen. 2019. 'Introduction: Analysing Violences in Gendered Global Health'. In *Gender, Global Health and Violence: Feminist Perspectives on Peace and Disease*, edited by Tiina Vaittinen and Catia Confortini. London and New York: Rowman & Littlefield.

D'Cruze, Shani and Anupama Rao. 2005. 'Violence and the Vulnerabilities of Gender'. In *Violence, Vulnerability and Embodiment: Gender and History*, edited by Shani D'Cruze and Anupama Rao, 1–18. Oxford: Blackwell.

DeLaet, Debra L., Shannon Golden and Veronica Laveta. 2019. 'Therapeutic Justice for Survivors of Human Rights Violations and Wartime Violence'. In *Gender, Global Health and Violence: Feminist Perspectives on Peace and Disease*, edited by Tiina Vaittinen and Catia Confortini. London and New York: Rowman & Littlefield.

Farmer, Paul. 1992. *AIDS and Accusation: Haiti and the Geography of Blame*. Berkeley: University of California Press.

Farmer, Paul. 2005. *Pathologies of Power: Health, Human Rights, and the New War on the Poor*. Berkeley: University of California Press.

Féron, Élise. 2019. 'When Is It Torture? When Is It Rape? Discourses on Wartime Sexual Violence'. In *Gender, Global Health and Violence: Feminist Perspectives on Peace and Disease*, edited by Tiina Vaittinen and Catia Confortini. London and New York: Rowman & Littlefield.

Finley, Laura. 2019. 'Domestic Violence and Public Health: Beginning Steps for Creating More Just and Effective Community Responses'. In *Gender, Global Health and Violence: Feminist Perspectives on Peace and Disease*, edited by Tiina Vaittinen and Catia Confortini. London and New York: Rowman & Littlefield.

Harman, Sophie. 2011. *Global Health Governance*. London: Routledge.

Harman, Sophie. 2016. 'Ebola, Gender and Conspicuously Invisible Women in Global Health Governance'. *Third World Quarterly* 37, no. 3: 524–541.

Harman, Sophie. 2016. 'Norms Won't Save You'. *Global Health Governance* X, no. 1: 11–16.

Harman, Sophie. 2019. 'Violence and the Paradox of Global Health'. In *Gender, Global Health and Violence: Feminist Perspectives on Peace and Disease*, edited by Tiina Vaittinen and Catia Confortini. London and New York: Rowman & Littlefield.

Harman, Sophie and Sara Davies. 2019. 'President Donald Trump as Global Health's Displacement Activity'. *Review of International Studies* (forthcoming).

Ikhile, Deborah, Gibson Linda and Azrini Wahidin. 2019. '"I Cannot Know That Now I Have Cancer!" A Structural Violence Perspective on Breast Cancer

Detection in Uganda'. In *Gender, Global Health and Violence: Feminist Perspectives on Peace and Disease*, edited by Tiina Vaittinen and Catia Confortini. London and New York: Rowman & Littlefield.

Kleinman, Arthur. 1997. 'The Violences of Everyday Life: The Multiple Forms and Dynamics of Social Violence'. In *Violence and Subjectivity*, edited by Veena Das, Arthur Kleinman, Mamphela Ramphele and Pamela Reynolds, 226–241. Berkeley: University of California Press.

Lawrence, Bruce B. and Aisha Karim. eds. 2007. *On Violence: A Reader*. Durham: Duke University Press.

Lisk, Franklyn. 2009. *Global Institutions and the HIV/AIDS Epidemic: Responding to an International Crisis*. Abingdon: Routledge.

Lukić, Dragana and Ann Therese Lotherington. 2019. 'Fighting Symbolic Violence through Artistic Encounters: Searching for Feminist Answers to the Question of Life and Death with Dementia'. In *Gender, Global Health and Violence: Feminist Perspectives on Peace and Disease*, edited by Tiina Vaittinen and Catia Confortini. London and New York: Rowman & Littlefield.

Nuño, Néstor M. 2019. 'Rethinking Global Health Priorities from the Margins: Health Access and Medical Care Claims among Indonesia's *Waria*'. In *Gender, Global Health and Violence: Feminist Perspectives on Peace and Disease*, edited by Tiina Vaittinen and Catia Confortini. London and New York: Rowman & Littlefield.

Oinas, Elina. 2019. 'HIV Politics and Structural Violence: Access to Treatment and Knowledge'. In *Gender, Global Health and Violence: Feminist Perspectives on Peace and Disease*, edited by Tiina Vaittinen and Catia Confortini. London and New York: Rowman & Littlefield.

Reuterswärd, Camilla. 2019. '¡Malas Madres, Malas Mujeres, Malas Todas! The Incarceration of Women for Abortion-Related Crimes in Mexico'. In *Gender, Global Health and Violence: Feminist Perspectives on Peace and Disease*, edited by Tiina Vaittinen and Catia Confortini. London and New York: Rowman & Littlefield.

Scheper-Hughes, Nancy. 1992. *Death without Weeping: The Violence of Everyday Life in Brazil*. Berkeley: University of California Press.

Tanyag, Maria. 2019. 'Replenishing Bodies and the Political Economy of SRHR in Crisis and Emergencies'. In *Gender, Global Health and Violence: Feminist Perspectives on Peace and Disease*, edited by Tiina Vaittinen and Catia Confortini. London and New York: Rowman & Littlefield.

UNAIDS. 2016. 'UNAIDS Warns That after Significant Reductions, Declines in New HIV Infections among Adults Have Stalled and Are Rising in Some Regions'. Accessed 1 October 2018. http://www.unaids.org/en/resources/presscentre/pressreleaseandstatementarchive/2016/july/20160712_prevention-gap.

UNAIDS. 2017. 'UNAIDS Announces Nearly 21 Million People Living with HIV Now on Treatment'. Accessed 1 October 2018. http://www.unaids.org/en/resources/presscentre/pressreleaseandstatementarchive/2017/november/20171121_righttohealth_report.

UNICEF. 2018. 'Under Five Mortality'. Accessed 1 October 2018. https://data.unicef.org/topic/child-survival/under-five-mortality/.

Vaittinen, Tiina. 2019. 'Exposed to Violence While Caring: From Caring Self-Protection to Global Health as Conflict Transformation'. In *Gender, Global Health and Violence: Feminist Perspectives on Peace and Disease*, edited by Tiina Vaittinen and Catia Confortini. London and New York: Rowman & Littlefield.

Wilkinson, Richard and Michael Marmot. 2003. *Social Determinants of Health: The Solid Facts*. 2nd edition. Geneva: World Health Organization Europe.

Index

Aberystwyth school of critical security studies, 11
abortion-related crimes, incarceration in Mexico for: in context, 16, 139–42, 155n7; gendered legal structures and reform with, 144–47; GIRE data on, 155n8; medical sphere with legal uncertainty and mandatory reporting with, 147–48; reports, trials and sentences per state, *146*; social expectations of motherhood and sexuality with, 150–53; state violence as gender-based structural, cultural and direct violence with, 153–54; structural violence and flawed legal processes with, 148–50; theorising state as perpetrator of gender violence and, 142–44
Abu Ghraib/Guantánamo, 175n2
abuser-victim model, 210
Academy of Finland, 109n1, 246n1
Acedo Ung, Leyla Guadalupe, 143
Acheson, Donald, 72
Achmat, Zackie, 97
activism: HIV/AIDS, 82, 89, 90, 97; TAC movement, 89–90, 92, 96–99, 107
AD. *See* Alzheimer's disease
ADD. *See* Alzheimer's disease or other dementias

adolescent birth rates, 37–38, 42n5
Afghanistan, 185, 206
African Americans, homicide rates for males, 218
ageing, 118, 128–31, 133
agential cuts, 125–29
AIDS and Accusation (Farmer), 251
'AIDS denialism', 94. *See also* HIV/AIDS
Akayesu rape case, 163
Alcock, Norman, 6
Alice Howland (fictional character), 119, 120, 122–30, 133, 134
Alzheimer's disease (AD), 118, 119. *See also* dementia, feminist answers to life-death question with
Alzheimer's disease or other dementias (ADD), 118
American Cancer Society, 72
analytical tool, violence as, 13
Anderson, Emma-Louise, 13, 254, 262
Antiretroviral Therapy (ART), 53, 55, 91, 92, 95, 102, 108–9, 258. *See also* HIV/AIDS
anti-torture advocacy, 188–90
anti-violence work, 92, 108
apartheid, 89, 93–94, 96, 104–5
Arendt, Hannah, 254
Argentina, 139, 153

ART. *See* Antiretroviral Therapy
artistic encounters, with dementia and art of life, 133–34
artistic entanglements, dementia and, 122–25
ASEAN. *See* Association of Southeast Asian Nations
assisted suicide, 118–22, 126, 135n1
Association of Southeast Asian Nations (ASEAN), 35–36, 40
Australia, domestic violence in, 212

Baines, Donna, 215
Baja California, abortion in, 145
Bali, 52, 59
Banerjee, Albert, 232, 233
Barad, Karen, 125–26, 127, 129, 132
Beattie, A., 83
Bedford, Kate, 155n4
Beijing Platform for Action (BfPA), 42n1
being alongside, dementia and enactments of, 131–33
Bejarano Celaya, Margarita, 143
Belfast/Good Friday Peace Agreement (1998), 161
Bem, Daryl, 121, 122, 129, 132
Bem, Emily, 121, 122
Bem, Jeremy, 121
Bem, Sandy, 118–22, 125–29, 132–33, 135n1
Berk, Richard, 213
Berns, Nancy, 216
BfPA. *See* Beijing Platform for Action
biomedicine: ADD and, 188; dementia and, 119, 129; epistemic violence of, 93, 104–7, 108
biopolitics, 50, 52, 84n7, 97
biopower, 50, 108
bissu, in Indonesia, 63n2
boda boda (motorcycle), 78, 84n9
bodies: 'body-political care manifesto', 231; menstruation and, 34; SRHR with security and replenishing, 37–40. *See also* breast cancer detection, structural violence in Uganda with; HIV/AIDS; wartime sexual violence

'body-political care manifesto', 231
Boellstorff, Tom, 48, 62n1, 63n2, 63n7
Bolivia, 139
Bolsa Familia, 252
Bosnia, 160, 161, 162–63
Boulding, Elise, 4
Bourdieu, Pierre, 30, 91, 119, 127, 129, 131
Brainard, Lori, 217
Brand-Jacobsen, Jai Frithjof, 6
Brazil, 139, 251, 252
breast awareness, 72, 78, 84n2
breast cancer detection, structural violence in Uganda with: addressing, 82–83; background, 71–73; barriers in Kajjansi town council, 75–82; as concept, 84n6; fears about, 76; with global health and development, 74–75; global health and new directions for, 83–84; with global health governance and international donors, 79–82; illustration of analysis of, *81*; incidence of, 84nn4–5; with primary health care infrastructure, poor, 77–78; with prioritisation for intervention, low, 78–79; risk and, 84n7; in social context, 15, 70–71; study methodology, 73–74; women and low knowledge of, *76*
Breast Health Global Initiative, 73
breast self-examination (BSE), 72–73, 82
Brunei, 42n3
BSE. *See* breast self-examination
Bumiller, Kristin, 216
Burton, Robert, 72
Burundi, 169, 172, 191
Buss, Doris, 168
Butler, Judith, 235

Caballero-Anthony, Mely, 36
Callahan, Sidney, 119
Cambodia, 37, 38, 42n3
Canada, 232, 234
cancer, 72; stages of, 84n2; WHO and, 79. *See also* breast cancer detection, structural violence in Uganda with
'Can the Subaltern Speak?' (Spivak), 8
capitalism, neoliberal, 7, 108

Index

care: epistemic violence and, 235–37, 243–45; medical, 56–61, 77–78; needs silenced, 245

care workers: interviews, 240–41; self-defence and, 239–40; with violence and dementia care, 230–32

caring self-protection: care workers with violence and dementia care, 230–32; as conflict transformation, 242–44; in context, 227–28; in empirical context, 229; with feminist global health as conflict transformation, 244–46; role of, 238–42; structural and direct violence with, 232–33; with violent refusals of care, 236–38; when care includes violence, 234–36

Carroll, Berenice, A., 227

Catholic Church, 150–51

CBE. *See* clinical breast examination

CEDAW. *See* UN Committee on the Elimination of Discrimination against Women

Center for Disease Control, US, 218

Center for Victims of Torture (CVT), 187–201; clinical model and right to rehabilitation, 190–92; role of, 182; from silos to integration, 192–201; survivor-centered documentation, 194–96; therapeutic documentation, 196–201; with trauma rehabilitation and anti-torture advocacy, 188–90; trauma-sensitive documentation, 193–94

Centro Las Libres, 144, 155n6

Chernobyl, 50–51

Chi, Primus Che, 26

children: adults with dementia as, 231–32; born of rape, 184; domestic violence influencing, 212, 215; marriage and, 38. *See also* youths

child soldiers, 38

Chile, 139

civil disobedience, with HIV, 96–99

clients, HIV counselling practice with, 102–4

climate: change, 5, 26, 36–37, 90; resilience, 35

clinical breast examination (CBE), 72–73, 82

clinical management, of rape, 39

clinics, HIV counselling practice and, 102–4

Cockburn, Cynthia, 28

cognitive decline, 121. *See also* dementia, feminist answers to life-death question with

cognitive disorders, stigma of, 235

Coker, Donna, 213

Colombia, 139

communicable diseases, 52, 71, 77–79

community: HIV counselling practice with client, clinic and, 102–4; Indonesian AIDS, 63n5

complex dependency, 234, 235, 236

conflict transformation: caring self-protection as, 242–44; feminist global health as, 244–46

Confortini, Catia C., 143, 245

Corbett, Kitty, 47

Corbex, Marilys, 72

costs: cancer control plan funding, 79; with crime, monetisation of, 211; of domestic violence, 211–13; medical care, 57, 77–78; war finances and, 210

counselling: practice, HIV and trajectories of, 102–4; VCT, 53

crime: HIV/AIDS, leadership and, 97; monetisation of, 211; wartime sexual violence as, 161–68. *See also* abortion-related crimes, incarceration in Mexico for

criminal justice approach, to domestic violence, 207, 213–17

crisis: as global governance technique, 32; Southeast Asia as prone to, 26–27

Cruz Sánchez, Verónica, 150, 152, 153

cultural violence: abortion and, 150–53; defined, 141; state violence as gender-based structural and, 153–54

CVT. *See* Center for Victims of Torture

D'Adesky, Anne-Christine, 97

Davies, Sara E., 2, 38–39

Davis, Kathy, 118

deaths: breast cancer mortality rate, 72; domestic violence, 206; genocide, 31, 96–99; HIV/AIDS, 89; homicide rates for African-American males, 218; maternal, 25, 26, 35, 42, 140; of police officers, 214; 'right to die' movement, 118, 119, 134; from structural violence, 7; suicide and, 120–22, 125–29, 211; of women, 7, 25, 26, 35, 42, 140, 206, 235. *See also* dementia, feminist answers to life-death question with

Death without Weeping (Scheper-Hughes), 251, 262

Declaration on the Elimination of Violence against All Women, 143

Declaration on the Elimination of Violence against Women (DEVAW), 40, 42n1

dementia: with adults as children, 231–32; care workers and violence with, 230–32. *See also* caring self-protection

dementia, feminist answers to life-death question with: artistic encounters and art of life with, 133–34; artistic entanglements, 122–25; biomedicine and, 119, 129; in context, 117–20; enactments of being alongside, 131–33; fears about, 121; neoliberal structures of symbolic violence and, 129–31; suicide and, 118, 120–22, 125–29

Democratic Republic of the Congo (DRC), 160, 169, 171, 191

Denmark, 232

Department of Injuries and Violence Prevention, WHO, 219

dependency: complex, 234, 235, 236; power and, 235–36, 239

depletion, 35, 37

determinants of health, 80–82, 262

DEVAW. *See* Declaration on the Elimination of Violence against Women

direct violence: state violence as gender-based structural, cultural and, 153–54; structural and, 232–33

disability studies, 128

disaster-induced displacement, populations, 36, 37

diseases: AD, 118, 119; communicable, 52, 71, 77–79; infectious, 9, 218; NCDs, 9, 71–72, 75, 79; sickle cell, 75; US Center for Disease Control, 218

displacement camps, 32, 34

Doctors without Borders, 95

Dolan, Chris, 162

domestic abuse: children and, 212, 215; poverty and, 214

domestic abusers, incarceration of, 213–14

domestic violence: costs of, 211–13; criminal justice approach to, 207, 213–17; deaths, 206; feminism and, 207; feminist public health approach to, 221–22; GBV and, 208–10, 212, 217, 221–22; incident rate of, 206; labour influenced by, 211–12; Minneapolis Domestic Violence Experiment, 213; police officers and, 214, 215; public health approach to, 218–19; as public health issue, 219–21; shelter-based approach to, 213–17

Dominguez, Silvia, 30

donors, global health governance and international, 79–82

DRC. *See* Democratic Republic of the Congo

dynamic peace, 4, 15

ebola, 75, 80

ecological model, domestic violence and, 219–20

education: domestic violence influencing, 212; illiteracy rates, 37

ejido commissioner, 152, 155n1

elderly abuse, 246n2

electric shock, 167

El Salvador, 139, 151

Elson, Diane, 35
emasculation, 167
empiricism, with caring self-protection, 229
empowerment, feminism and, 216
enactments, being alongside dementia, 131–33
England, domestic violence in, 211–12
Enloe, Cynthia, 142
entanglements of violence, 3, 13–14, 161, 233, 236, 239, 258, 263
epidemic, global AIDS, 79, 93–96
epistemic peace, 243, 245
epistemic violence, 7, 10, 127, 161, 174; of biomedicine, 93, 104–7, 108; care and, 235–37, 243–45; with context and gender, 255; defined, 15; with health hierarchy, 258–59; health professionals and, 261–62; sexual and, 169; stigma and, 257; structural and, 92; subaltern and, 8, 91, 101, 236; survivors, 168–73
Epstein, Steven, 90
Eritrea, 191
Erwin, Alec, 96
Ethiopia, 188, 191
euthanasia, 118, 126
Excelsior (newspaper), 150

fa'afafine, in Samoa, 63n2
families: *Bolsa Familia*, 252; with health of women, 32; PKBI, 51–53, 55–58, 63n5; World Congress of Families, 29; youth, 37–38, 42n5, 184, 212, 215, 231–32. *See also* dementia, feminist answers to life-death question with
Farmer, Paul, 12, 48, 74–75, 251–52
fears: about breast cancer, 76; about dementia, 121; shame and, 55
Feldman, Allen, 167
feminisation, 169–70
feminism: domestic violence and, 207; empowerment and, 216; with GBV, analyses of, 183; postcolonial, 7; with public health and domestic violence, 221–22; with research and IR, 32; 'right to die' movement and, 118, 119, 134; with violence, analysis of, 15–16. *See also* dementia, feminist answers to life-death question with
Feminism and Psychology (journal), 118
feminist global health, conflict transformation and, 244–46
feminist peace research, 4, 10, 13, 15, 188, 234
feminist peace researchers, 4, 227, 244
Ferraro, Kathleen, 216
film, dementia in, 122–24
Finland, 109n1, 228, 231, 232–33, 239, 240, 246n1, 246n3
Fonn, Sharon, 31
forced marriages, 32, 159
Foucault, Michel, 50, 91
Fourie, Pieter, 3
France, 50–51
Fraser, Nancy, 217
The Free (*Las Libres*), 139–40, 144–45, 149, 151
Fulda, Isabel, 150
funding, for cancer control plan, 79

Gag Rule, 29
Galtung, Johan, 6, 7, 12, 74, 140–41, 143, 150, 153
GBV. *See* gender-based violence
gender: with internal displacements in Southeast Asia, 35–37; as ordering principle, 1; SGBV, 32; Southeast Asia and expressions of, 62n2; transgender, 13, 15, 62n1, 82; violence with context and, 253–56. *See also waria*, in Indonesia
gender-based violence (GBV), 26, 29, 154; domestic violence and, 208–10, 212, 217, 221–22; feminist analyses of, 183; SGBV, 32, 38–39, 171; transitional justice with invisibility and silence with, 183–84. *See also* domestic violence

gendered global health: ordering principle and, 1; peace research and, 2–11; with violence, 12–16
gendered legal structures, abortion policy reform and, 144–47
gender responsive policies, 71, 82–83
gender violence, 140–44, 153
Geneva Convention, 166
genocide: civil disobedience with HIV, politicised jar of pills and, 96–99; HIV/AIDS and, 97; rape as, 31
Genova, Lisa, 119, 122–24
Gilligan, James, 6
GIRE. *See Grupode Información en Reproducción Elegida*
Glatzer, Richard, 122
Global Climate Risk Index, 36
global governance, 1, 32, 79–80, 262
global health: caring and, 227; conflict transformation and feminist, 244–46; gendered, 1, 2–16; IR and, 3; new directions for cancer and, 83–84; priorities on HIV, 47–48; securitised, 9–11; structural violence with development and, 74–75; with violence, approaches to, 12–16; *waria* in Indonesia with neoliberalisation of, 49–52
global health, paradox of: in context, 251–53; with governance as violence, 262–63; with health, hierarchy of, 258–60; stigma with violence and, 256–57; with violence of health professionals, 260–62; violence with context, gender and, 253–56
global health governance, international donors and, 79–82
Globalization and Health (journal), 84n3
global military-industrial complex, 5
Global Politics of Medicine, 10
Gonzales, Simon, 215
governmentality, 50
grassroots interventions, within medical practice and HIV, 99–101
Great Lakes Region of Africa (2009–2014), 160

Grey, Rosemary, 170
Grupode Información en Reproducción Elegida (Information Group on Chosen Reproduction, GIRE), 147, 155n1, 155n8
Guantánamo/Abu Ghraib, 175n2
Guardado Bautista, Jose Santos, 151
Guatemala, 206
Gullette, M. Margaret, 129

Haglund, Jilliene, 213
Haiti, 251
Harman, Sophie, 14
Harrington, Mona, 155n3
healing: CVT with justice and, 192–201; therapeutic justice, trauma and, 185–87
health: access and medical care problems among *waria*, 56–58; determinants of, 80–82, 262; *Globalization and Health*, 84n3; hierarchy of, 258–60; peace research and, 4–5; professionals, violence of, 260–62; promotion, 71, 82–83, 98; public, 218–22; services for mental, 197, 212; as social construct, 81–82; UN Special Rapporteur on the Right to Health, 33; WHO, 1, 39, 73, 79, 81–82, 160, 168, 206, 219; of women, 32. *See also* breast cancer detection, structural violence in Uganda with; global health; HIV/AIDS
health care: costs with domestic violence, 212; primary, 73, 77–78, 80–81; *waria* claiming access to medical and, 58–61
Henig, Robin M., 120
hijras, in India Nanda, 63n2
'hir', as pronoun, 60, 63n7
HIV/AIDS, 6, 245, 251, 252; activism, 82, 89, 90, 97; ART of, 53, 55, 91, 92, 95, 102, 108–9, 258; deaths, 89; genocide and, 97; global health priorities on, 47–48; Indonesian AIDS community, 63n5; interviews, 100–103, 109n2; leadership, crime

and, 97; in media, 93, 96; resilience versus structural responses to, 61–62; stigma and structural violence against *waria*, 49, 52–56; subaltern with women and, 101; syndemic factors and, 54, 63n6; women and, 13–14
HIV politics, structural violence and: civil disobedience, genocide and politicised jar of pills, 96–99; with client, clinic and community, 102–4; with cyborg embodiment and structural material violence in treatment, 107–9; with epistemic violence of biomedicine, 104–7; with global AIDS epidemic as context, 79, 93–96; grassroots interventions within medical practice and, 99–101; in social context, 89–93
homicide rates, for African-American males, 218
Honduras, 139
Hoppania, Hanna-Kaisa, 233
Hoskyns, Catherine, 35
Howard, Natasha, 12
Howell, Alison, 9–10
human rights, 163, 215. *See also* therapeutic justice, for human rights violations and wartime violence
Hunt, Paul, 25

IACHR. *See* Inter-American Commission on Human Rights
ICC. *See* International Criminal Court
ICCPR. *See* International Covenant on Civil and Political Rights
ICC Prosecutor v. Kenyatta, 164
ICESCR. *See* International Covenant on Economic, Social and Cultural Rights
ICPD. *See* International Conference on Population and Development
ICTR. *See* International Criminal Tribunal for Rwanda
ICTY. *See* International Criminal Tribunal for the former Yugoslavia
IDMC data. *See* Internal Displacement Monitoring Centre

Ikatan Waria Jogjakarta (*waria* bonds Jogjakarta, IWAYO), 63n5
Ilaboya, Deborah Evho, 73, 74, 75
illiteracy rates, 37
IMF. *See* International Monetary Fund
incarceration: of domestic abusers, 213–14; sexual torture with, 175n2. *See also* abortion-related crimes, incarceration in Mexico for
incidence, of breast cancer, 84nn4–5
Incite! Women of Color against Violence, 215–16
India, domestic violence in, 212
India Nanda, *hijras* in, 63n2
indirect violence, 5, 11, 13, 143, 219, 254, 256, 262
individualism, 50, 61, 130
Indonesia, 42n3; adolescent birth rates in, 38; *bissu* and *tomboi* in, 63n2; PKBI, 51–53, 55–58, 63n5. *See also waria*, in Indonesia
Indonesian AIDS community (*Komunitas AIDS Indonesia*), 63n5
Indonesian Family Planning Association. *See Perkumpulan Keluarga Berencana Indonesia*
infectious diseases, 9, 218
Information Group on Chosen Reproduction. *See Grupo de Información en Reproducción Elegida*
infrastructures, primary health care, 77–78
Inter-American Commission of Women of the Organization of American States, 209
Inter-American Commission on Human Rights (IACHR), 215
Internal Displacement Monitoring Centre (IDMC) data, 36
International Conference on Population and Development (ICPD), 25; Program of Action, 42n1
International Covenant on Civil and Political Rights (ICCPR), 42n1
International Covenant on Economic, Social and Cultural Rights (ICESCR), 42n1

International Criminal Court (ICC), 163–64, 183
International Criminal Law, 163
International Criminal Tribunal for Rwanda (ICTR), 163–64, 183
International Criminal Tribunal for the former Yugoslavia (ICTY), 163–65, 183
international donors, 77, 79–82, 254
international human rights, 33, 42n1
International Human Rights Law, 163, 213
International Monetary Fund (IMF), 47
International Physicians for the Prevention of Nuclear War (IPPNW), 5
International Relations (IR), 2, 3, 8, 32
interviews: care workers, 240–41; HIV/AIDS, 100–103, 109n2; sexual violence, 167, 172; with *waria* in Indonesia, 63n4
intimate partner violence (IPV), 206, 212, 255, 260
intra-actions, 125, 129, 131
invisibility: transitional justice with silence and, 183–84; women and, 14–15, 34
IPPNW. *See* International Physicians for the Prevention of Nuclear War
IPV. *See* intimate partner violence
IR. *See* International Relations
Iraq, 175n2, 185, 191, 195, 206
Iraqi prisoners, sexual torture of, 175n2
IWAYO. *See* Ikatan Waria Jogjakarta

Jamkesmas health insurance, 56–57, 59
Janes, Craig, 47
Jennings, K. Patricia, 126
Jogjakarta, population of, 52. *See also waria*, in Indonesia
Jordan, 188, 193, 198, 200
Jungar, Katarina, 92, 107
justice: CVT with healing and, 192–201; domestic violence and criminal, 207, 213–17; social, 49, 51, 90, 107–8, 209, 216, 234, 246. *See also* therapeutic justice, for human rights violations and wartime violence; transitional justice

Kajjansi town council, with breast cancer detection barriers, 75–82
kathoey, in Thailand, 62n2
KEBAYA. *See Keluarga Besar Waria Yogyakarta*
Kelly, Christine, 227, 234
Keluarga Besar Waria Yogyakarta (KEBAYA), 53, 55–58
Kenya, 188
Khmer Rouge, 37
Kittay Feder, Eva, 235
Kitzinger, Celia, 118–19
Kivel, Paul, 217
Klawiter, Maren, 84n7
Kleinman, Arthur, 253–54
Köhler, Gernot, 6
Komunitas AIDS Indonesia (Indonesian AIDS community), 63n5

Labonté, Ronald, 31–32
labour: care workers and, 228; division of, 210; domestic violence influencing, 211–12; unions, 240
Lambourne, Wendy, 186
Lamont, Gary, 97
Laos, 42n3
Latimer, J. Elizabeth, 119, 128, 132
law, abortion and: with medical sphere, legal uncertainty and related crimes, 147–48; reform and gendered legal structures, 144–47; with structural violence and flawed legal processes, 148–50
leadership, crime with HIV/AIDS and, 97
Lederach, John Paul, 242, 243
Lee, Bandy X., 6–7, 12
Lee, Kelley, 34
Leiby, Michele, 162
Lenahan-Gonzales, Jessica, 215
Lewis, Clear, 128–29
liberalism, 50, 217
Las Libres (The Free), 139–40, 144–45, 149, 151
life: adolescent birth rates, 37–38, 42n5; dementia with artistic encounters and

art of, 133–34; right-to-life, 140, 145–48. *See also* deaths; dementia, feminist answers to life-death question with
Lindroth, Marjo, 51
literature, dementia in, 122–24
López de la Cruz, Hilda, 149, 151

MacKinnon, Catherine, 207
Makerere University, 73
Makerere University School of Public Health, Uganda, 84n3
malaria, 47, 78, 79
Malawi, 13
Malaysia, 42n3
male aggression, state violence and, 210
males, homicide rates for African-American, 218
mammography screenings, 72, 79, 82
Management of Mutual and Potential Aggression (MAPA)®, 246n4
Mandela, Nelson, 94
Manzanares Calletano, Adriana, 150, 152
MAPA®. *See* Management of Mutual and Potential Aggression
MAPW. *See* Medical Association for the Prevention of War
Marcus, Sharon, 166
marriages, 121, 152, 153; children and, 38; forced, 32, 159
Masculine Domination (Bourdieu), 127
masculinities, 3, 170
material violence, 91–92, 99, 102–4, 107–9
maternal deaths, 25, 26, 35, 42, 140
Mbeki, Thabo, 89, 94, 99, 108
MCANW. *See* Medical Campaign against Nuclear Weapons
McInnes, Colin, 34
McPherson, Dafne, 139, 151
MDGs. *See* Millennium Development Goals
Medact, 5
media: HIV/AIDS in, 93, 96; women incarcerated for abortion in, 144–45, 151

Medical Anthropology, 2
Medical Association for the Prevention of War (MAPW), 5
Medical Campaign against Nuclear Weapons (MCANW), 5
medical care: costs, 57, 77–78; problems and health access among *waria*, 56–58; *waria* claiming access to health and, 58–61
medical norm, 130
medical practice, HIV and grassroots interventions within, 99–101
medical sphere, with abortion, 147–48
Medicine, Conflict and Survival (journal), 12
Melber, Henning, 90
men: as domestic violence victims, 206; homicide rates for African-American males, 218. *See also* wartime sexual violence
Menjivar, Cecilia, 30
menstruation, 34
mental health services, 197, 212
#MeToo movement, 222
Mexico. *See* abortion-related crimes, incarceration in Mexico for
militarism, 28, 32, 210, 221
military, 33, 166, 173; global industrial complex, 5; paramilitary groups, 160–61, 167; role of, 142, 143; spending, 39
Millennium Development Goals (MDGs), 40, 208, 252
Mills, Elizabeth, 13–14, 75
Minić et al. case, 163
Ministry of Health, Uganda, 73
Minneapolis Domestic Violence Experiment, 213
Moeketsi, Kebareng, 89
Mohindra, K. S., 31–32
Mol, Annemarie, 131
monetisation, of crime, 211
Moro Islamic rebels, 37, 38–39
mortality. *See* deaths
motherhood, 142, 149, 154; politics of, 31; social expectations of sexuality and, 150–53

276　Index

motorcycle (*boda boda*), 78, 84n9
Mundane Practices of Peace, 246n1
muscular dystrophy, 50–51
Myanmar, 36–37, 42n3

narrative exposure therapy, 186
National Census of Domestic Violence Services, 215
NCDs. *See* non-communicable diseases
negative peace, 4, 5
neoliberal capitalism, 7, 108
neoliberalisation, of global health with *waria*, 49–52
neoliberalism, 50, 217
neoliberal structures, of symbolic violence with dementia, 129–31
New York Times Magazine, 120
NGOs. *See* non-governmental organizations
Nicaragua, 139
non-communicable diseases (NCDs), 9, 71–72, 75, 79
non-governmental organizations (NGOs), 29, 50–51, 61, 63n5, 80, 170
non-profit industrial complex, 216
Northern Ireland, 160–61, 167
Norway, 232
Nottingham Trent University School of Social Sciences, UK, 84n3
Novartis, 78
Nunes, João, 9, 10–11, 13
Nurse-Rambos, 239
nursing homes, 117, 124, 129–30, 133
Nwoma, Chatinka, 97

Oetomo, Dédé, 63n2
O'Manique, Colleen, 3
opacity, vulnerability and, 235
ordering principles, 1, 28, 169, 256–57, 260
Oregon, assisted suicide in, 122, 135n1
the Other, 8

Pacific Ring of Fire, 36, 42n4
paramilitary groups, 160–61, 167
Parks, A. Jennifer, 118–19
Pathologies of Power (Famer), 251

patriarchal violence, 173–74
peace, 34, 40, 161, 246n1; SRHR in continuum of, 41–42; types of, 4, 5, 15, 234, 245
peaceful transformation, 7, 242
peace research, 13, 15, 188, 227, 234, 244; gendered global health and, 2–11; health and, 4–5; with securitised global health, 9–11; TAPRI, 2; violence in, 6–11
pentobarbital, 121–22
Perkumpulan Keluarga Berencana Indonesia (Indonesian Family Planning Association, PKBI), 51–53, 55–58, 63n5
Peru, 162
Petchesky, R., 27
phenomena, defined, 125–26
Philippines, 42n3; adolescent birth rates in, 38; climate change and, 36; conflict intensity in, 38–39; Moro Islamic rebels in, 37
physical violence, 27, 30, 41, 54, 159, 161, 165, 228–30
physician-assisted dying. *See* suicide, with dementia
PKBI. *See Perkumpulan Keluarga Berencana Indonesia*
Pleck, Emily, 216
police officers: domestic violence and, 214, 215; resources for, 33
political will, 77, 81, 84, 96
politics: biopolitics, 50, 52, 84n7, 97; 'body-political care manifesto', 231; of motherhood, 31. *See also* HIV politics, structural violence and
populations: control, 28–29; disaster-induced displacement, 36, 37; of Jogjakarta, 52; Southeast Asia and youth, 38; UNFPA, 29, 37; of *waria*, 63n5
positive peace, 4, 234
postcolonial feminism, 7
poverty: abortion-related crime and, 147–50, 154; breast cancer detection and, 74; domestic abuse and,

214; eradication of, 47; rates, 37; reduction, 208; stigma of, 54, 94
power, 251; biopower, 50, 108; dependency and, 235–36, 239; with empowerment and feminism, 216; structural violence and, 48
primary health care, 73, 77–78, 80–81
primary health care infrastructure, 77–78
privatisation, 31, 47
Prosecutor v. Bagosora, 164
Prosecutor v. Muhimana, 164
Prosecutor v. Sesay, Kallon and Gbao, 163–64
protector-protected model, 210
public health: domestic violence and, 218–19; domestic violence and feminist, 221–22; domestic violence as issue of, 219–21
pulmonary docimasia technique, 149–50
Purandare, Nitin, 128

racism, 6, 7, 94, 96, 232
Rai, Shirin, 35
rape: cases, 163; children born of, 184; clinical management of, 39; as genocide, 31. *See also* wartime sexual violence
RavenLight, 82
Ravindran, Sundari, 31
reform: abortion policy, 144–47; right-to-life, 140, 145–48
rehabilitation, right to, 188–92
reporting: abortion-related crimes and mandatory, 147–48; wartime sexual violence and under-, 159–60, 168–69
resilience, 37, 52, 53, 174; climate, 35; governmentality and, 50; HIV with structural responses versus, 61–62; logics, 51, 60
Resolution WHA49.25, 218
Richards, David, 213
Richmond, Julius B., 218
rights: human, 163, 215; IACHR, 215; ICCPR, 42n1; to life reforms, 140, 145–48; UN Special Rapporteur on the Right to Health, 33; for *waria*

in Indonesia, 57–58, 60, 259. *See also* Sexual and Reproductive Health and Rights; therapeutic justice, for human rights violations and wartime violence
'right to die' movement, feminists and, 118, 119, 134
right to rehabilitation, 188–92
risk, breast cancer and, 84n7
risk group, 93
Robinson, Fiona, 35
Rohingya minority ethnic group, 37, 38
Rojas, Clarissa, 221
Rooney, Phyllis, 126
Ross, Marlon B., 167
Ruane, Abigail, 245
Ruddick, Sara, 228
Ruttenberg, Maria, 213
Rwanda, 163, 183, 191

Samoa, *fa'afafine* in, 63n2
Sancho-Garnier, Hélène, 72
San Francisco Lesbian-Gay-Bisexual-Transgender Pride Parade (1993), 82
saunas, 229, 246n3
Scheper-Hughes, Nancy, 12, 251–52, 262
securitisation theory, 8–10
securitised global health, 9–11
security, SRHR with replenishing bodies and, 37–40
self-defence, care workers and, 239–40
senior citizens, 246n2. *See also* dementia, feminist answers to life-death question with
sexual abuse, 165, 232, 233
sexual and gender-based violence (SGBV), 32, 38–39, 171
Sexual and Reproductive Health and Rights (SRHR): defined, 25; with gender and internal displacements, 35–37; in peace, continuum of, 41–42; promotion of, 26–27; security and replenishing bodies with, 37–40; with violences, different, 27–35
sexual intimate partner violence (IPV), 206, 260

sexuality, social expectations of motherhood and, 150–53
sexual torture, 160–62, 167, 175n2
sexual violence: in conflict, ending, 40; defined, 160; epistemic and, 169; interviews, 167, 172; against women with wartime sexual violence, 165–68. *See also* wartime sexual violence
sex workers, *waria* as, 49, 52, 54
SGBV. *See* sexual and gender-based violence
shame, 55, 58, 99, 127, 165, 168–69, 183–84, 257
shelter-based approach, to domestic violence, 213–17
Shepherd, Laura J., 143, 170
Sherman, Lawrence, 213
sickle cell disease, 75
Sierra Leone, 75, 163–64
silence: around care needs, 245; IR and, 8; the Other and, 8; sexual violence and, 172; transitional justice with invisibility and, 183–84; violence and, 13, 183
Simplican, Stacy Clifford, 227, 234, 235
Sinevaara-Niskanen, Heidi, 51
Singapore, 42n3
Siplon, Patricia, 217
situated practices, 131
Smith-Oka, Vania, 150–51, 152
social construct, 71, 73, 81–82
social expectations, of motherhood and sexuality, 150–53
social justice, 49, 51, 90, 107–8, 209, 216, 234, 246
Somalia, 191
Sondorp, Egbert, 12
South Africa, 14, 245; apartheid in, 89, 93–94, 96, 104–5; domestic violence in, 212; with HIV politics and structural violence, 90–102, 108–9; TAC movement in, 89–90, 92, 96–99
Southeast Asia: adolescent birth rates in, 37–38; ASEAN, 35–36, 40; climate change and, 36; countries in, 42n3; as crisis-prone, 26–27; with gender, expressions of, 62n2; regional cooperation in, 39–40; SRHR with gender and internal displacements in, 35–37; youth population in, 38
South Sudan, 191
space-time-matters, 125–26, 131, 133
Spain, domestic violence in, 212
Special Court for Sierra Leone, 163–64
Spitzer, Denise, 31–32
Spivak, Gayatri, 7–8, 91
SRHR. *See* Sexual and Reproductive Health and Rights
SSA. *See* sub-Saharan Africa
Stallone, Sylvester, 239
state violence: gender and, 142–44; as gender-based structural, cultural and direct violence, 153–54; male aggression and, 210
Steinbock, Bonnie, 128
Steurnagel, Trudy, 235
stigma: abortion and, 152; of cognitive disorders, 235; of poverty, 54, 94; role of, 263; with violence and paradox of global health, 256–57; *waria* in Indonesia with structural violence and HIV, 49, 52–56
Still Alice (film), 122–24
Still Alice (Genova), 119, 122–24
storytelling, 186
structural racism, 6, 7
structural violence: abortion and flawed legal processes with, 148–50; as complicated to observe, 48–49; deaths from, 7; defined, 30, 75; direct and, 232–33; epistemic and, 92; with global health and development, 74–75; with HIV stigma against *waria*, 49, 52–56; power and, 48; roots of, 141; state violence as gender-based direct, cultural and, 153–54. *See also* breast cancer detection, structural violence in Uganda with; HIV politics, structural violence and

subaltern: cyborg embodiment and HIV treatment, 107–9; epistemic violence and, 8, 91, 101, 236; with women and HIV/AIDS, 101
subjectivity, 91–92, 108, 127
sub-Saharan Africa (SSA), 71–72, 79, 84
suicide, with dementia: agential cuts, 125–29; assisted suicide or, 118–22, 126, 135n1
Suicide and Assisted Dying: Reflections on Sandra Bem's Death (Wilkinson), 118
suicide rates, 211
survivor-centered documentation, CVT and, 194–96
Sustainable Development Goals, 34, 208, 252
Sweden, 232
symbolic violence, 107; defined, 30, 91; dementia and neoliberal structures of, 129–31; masculine domination and, 127; youth and, 38
syndemic factors, HIV/AIDS and, 54, 63n6
Syria, 191, 198, 200

TAC movement. *See* Treatment Action Campaign movement
Tadić, Duško, 163
Talley, Clarence R., 126
Tampere Peace Research Institute (TAPRI), 2
Tanyag, Maria, 38–39, 42n2
TAPRI. *See* Tampere Peace Research Institute
technoscience, 119
Tedre, Silva, 231, 238
Ter Veen, Annemarie, 12
testimony therapy, 186
Thailand, 36, 42n3, 62n2
therapeutic documentation, CVT and, 196–201
therapeutic justice, for human rights violations and wartime violence: in context, 181–82; CVT and, 187–201; key principles of, 182; role of, 201–2; transitional justice and trauma with, 183–87

Thomas, Dania, 35
Thompson, Charis, 107
Thunder Hawk, Madonna, 217
Tickner, Ann, 142
tomboi, in Indonesia, 63n2
torture: anti-torture advocacy, 188–90; sexual, 160–62, 167, 175n2; UNCAT, 191. *See also* Center for Victims of Torture; wartime sexual violence
toxoplasmosis, 63n8
transgender, 13, 15, 62n1, 82
transitional justice: with invisibility and silence with GBV, 183–84; with trauma, healing and therapeutic justice, 185–87; trauma and, 183–87; vulnerability and, 184–85
trauma: rehabilitation and anti-torture advocacy with CVT, 188–90; therapeutic justice, healing and, 185–87; therapy, 186; transitional justice and, 183–87
trauma-sensitive documentation, CVT and, 193–94
Treatment Action Campaign (TAC) movement, 89–90, 92, 96–99, 107
True, Jacqui, 38–39, 42n2, 208, 210, 211–12, 221
Trump, Donald, 29, 221
Truth and Reconciliation Commission, Peru, 162
Tshabalala-Msimang, Manto, 96
Tulloch, Gail, 119

Uganda, 73, 77–78, 188, 191, 212. *See also* breast cancer detection, structural violence in Uganda with
Uganda Cancer Institute, 73, 77–78
Uganda Women's Cancer Support Organisation, 73
ultrasounds, 72
UN. *See* United Nations
UNAIDS, 90, 95
UNCAT. *See* United Nations Convention against Torture

UN Committee on the Elimination of Discrimination against Women (CEDAW), 40, 42n1, 163, 213
UN Declaration of Commitment to End Sexual Violence in Conflict, 40
UN Declaration on the Elimination of All Forms of Violence against Women, 208
UNFPA. *See* UN Population Fund
United Nations (UN), 1
United Nations Convention against Torture (UNCAT), 191
United States (US): Center for Disease Control, 218; population assistance from, 28; VAWA, 206–7
UN Population Fund (UNFPA), 29, 37
UN Security Council Resolutions, 159, 166
UN Special Rapporteur on the Right to Health, 33
Urdal, Henrik, 26
Uruguay, 139
US. *See* United States
USAID, 28, 52
US Christian Right, 29

Valentine, David, 62n1
VAWA. *See* Violence against Women Act
VCT. *See* Voluntary Counselling and Testing
Vellacott, Jo, 4
victims. *See* Center for Victims of Torture
Vietnam, 36, 42n3
violence: as analytical tool, 13; anti-violence work, 92, 108; care including, 234–36; care workers with dementia care and, 230–32; cultural, 141, 150–53; *Declaration on the Elimination of Violence against All Women*, 143; defined, 6; entanglements of, 3, 13–14, 161, 233, 236, 239, 258, 263; feminism analysis of, 15–16; forms of, 29–32; gender, 140–44, 153; gender and context with, 253–56; gendered global health with, 12–16; global health approaches to, 12–16; global health governance as, 262–63; of health professionals, 260–62; Incite! Women of Color against Violence, 215–16; indirect, 5, 11, 13, 143, 219, 254, 256, 262; IPV, 206, 212, 255, 260; layers of, 28–29; material, 91–92, 99, 102–4, 107–9; patriarchal, 173–74; in peace research, 6–11; phases of, 32–35; physical, 27, 30, 41, 54, 159, 161, 165, 228–30; public health approach to, 218–19; with refusals of care, 236–38; silence and, 13, 183; SRHR and accumulation of different, 27–35; state, 142–44, 153–54, 210; stigma with global health paradox and, 256–57; symbolic, 129–31; UN Declaration on the Elimination of All Forms of Violence against Women, 208. *See also* direct violence; domestic violence; epistemic violence; gender-based violence; sexual violence; structural violence; symbolic violence; therapeutic justice, for human rights violations and wartime violence; wartime sexual violence
Violence against Women Act (VAWA), 206–7
Viterna, Jocelyn, 151
Voluntary Counselling and Testing (VCT), 53
vulnerability: opacity and, 235; transitional justice and, 184–85

Walby, Sylvia, 211–12
Wales, domestic violence in, 211–12
Wallstrom, Margot, 160
waria, in Indonesia: defined, 48, 62n1; etymology of, 63n2; health access and medical care problems among, 56–58; health and medical care access claimed by, 58–61; with 'hir' as pronoun, 60, 63n7; HIV stigma and structural violence

against, 49, 52–56; interviews with, 63n4; medical care costs for, 57; neoliberalisation of global health and, 49–52; population of, 63n5; with resilience versus structural responses to HIV, 61–62; rights for, 57–58, 60, 259; as sex workers, 49, 52, 54; in social context, 47–49
waria bonds Jogjakarta. *See Ikatan Waria Jogjakarta*
wars: child soldiers and, 38; costs and finances, 210; fatalities compared to domestic violence deaths, 206; IPPNW, 5; MAPW, 5; MCANW, 5
wartime sexual violence: in context, 159–61, 175n1; with depoliticisation of sexual violence against women, 165–68; with male survivors, support programmes for, 168–73; against men as coded and prosecuted, 161–68; against men as patriarchal violence, 173–74; underreporting of, 159–60, 168–69
wartime violence. *See* therapeutic justice, for human rights violations and wartime violence
Watts, Charlotte, 166
Waylen, Georgina, 155n4
'weaving epistemology', 245
Weber, Max, 141
Westmoreland, Wash, 122
WHO. *See* World Health Organization
WHO Commission on the Social Determinants of Health Report (2008), 81–82
Whyte, S. R., 80
Wilkinson, Sue, 118
women: with AD, 119; with breast cancer, low knowledge of, 76; CEDAW, 40, 42n1, 163, 213; deaths of, 7, 25, 26, 35, 42, 140, 206, 235; *Declaration on the Elimination of Violence against All Women*, 143; depoliticisation of sexual violence against, 165–68; DEVAW, 42n1; families with health of, 32; HIV and, 13–14; Incite! Women of Color against Violence, 215–16; invisibility and, 14–15, 34; subaltern with HIV/AIDS and, 101; suicide and, 118–29; UN Declaration on the Elimination of All Forms of Violence against Women, 208; VAWA, 206–7. *See also* abortion-related crimes, incarceration in Mexico for; breast cancer detection, structural violence in Uganda with; domestic violence
Women, Peace and Security (WPS) agenda, 34, 40
World Bank, 7, 28, 47
World Congress of Families, 29
World Health Assembly, 218
World Health Organization (WHO), 39, 73; Department of Injuries and Violence Prevention, 219; gender and, 1; on health as social construct, 81–82; on IPV, 206; national cancer control plan and, 79; on sexual violence, 160, 168
World Report on Violence (WHO), 219
WPS agenda. *See* Women, Peace and Security (WPS) agenda

youths: adolescent birth rates, 37–38, 42n5; children, 38, 184, 212, 215, 231–32; population in Southeast Asia, 38; symbolic violence and, 38
Yugoslavia, 163–64, 183

Zimmerman, Cathy, 166

About the Authors

Catia C. Confortini is Associate Professor in the Peace & Justice Studies Programme at Wellesley College in Massachusetts (US). Her research and publications explore the contributions of women's peace activism to peace studies as an academic field and as a practice, as well as feminist theorising of peace and violence. She is the author of *Intelligent Compassion: Feminist Critical Methodology in the Women's International League for Peace and Freedom* (OUP 2012); co-editor (with Tarja Väyrynen, Élise Féron, Peace Meadie, and Swati Parashar) of *The Handbook of Feminist Peace Research* (forthcoming, Routledge 2020); and co-editor (with Tiina Vaittinen and Shweta Singh) of the book series *Feminist Studies on Peace, Justice, and Violence* (Rowman & Littlefield International). Her current interests lie at the intersection of feminist peace research and global health. As a feminist peace activist, she has served as Vice President of WILPF from 2015 to 2018.

Debra L. DeLaet is professor of Political Science at Drake University in Des Moines, Iowa, where she serves as the David E. Maxwell Distinguished Professor of International Affairs. Her major research interests are in the area of human rights, global health, and gender issues in world politics. She has published three books: *U.S. Immigration Policy in an Age of Rights* (Praeger 2000), *The Global Struggle for Human Rights* (Wadsworth 2006), and (co-authored with David E. DeLaet) *Global Health in the 21st Century: The Globalization of Disease and Wellness* (Paradigm Publishers 2012). In addition to these books, she has published numerous articles and book chapters in her areas of interest. In her current scholarly work, Professor DeLaet is particularly interested in questions related to human rights in everyday politics, and in investigating how to build capacity in civil society to translate abstract global norms into concrete human rights practices within communities.

Élise Féron is a senior researcher at the Tampere Peace Research Institute, Tampere University. She is an invited professor at the Université Catholique de Louvain (Belgium), the University of Turin (Italy), Sciences Po Lille (France), and the Université Lumière de Bujumbura (Burundi) where she co-convenes a Gender Studies Master Programme. She holds an Accreditation to Supervise Research (Docent 2003) and a PhD in Political Science (1999). Her main research interests include gender and peace negotiations, sexual violence in conflict settings, as well as conflict-generated diaspora politics. Her latest book is *Wartime Sexual Violence against Men: Masculinities and Power in Conflict Zones* (Rowman & Littlefield 2018).

Laura Finley is associate professor of Sociology and Criminology at Barry University in Miami, Florida. She is author, co-author, or editor of eighteen books and numerous book chapters and journal articles. Dr Finley is also a syndicated columnist with PeaceVoice and a contributing author with New Clear Vision. In addition, Dr Finley is actively involved with a number of state, local, national, and international peace, justice, and human rights groups.

Linda Gibson is an associate professor of Public Health. Her current roles include student supervision, research, and consultancy. She is passionate about the promotion of health and upstream interventions at individual, community, and global levels. She is involved in several research projects in Europe, Uganda, Burkina Faso, Nigeria, and the UK. Her research focus is on health promotion and health systems/services and community development/engagement, as well as patient safety to explore non-communicable diseases (CVD, Breast Cancer, Diabetes) – all through the lens of the social determinants of health, using a socio-ecological model. Dr Gibson's current research work is funded by the DfID (through the Tropical Health Education Trust [THET]), the British Academy, and the EU Commission (Horizon 2020).

Shannon Golden is research associate at the Center for Victims of Torture (CVT), where she provides research and programme evaluation support for CVT's work with survivors of torture and other human rights violations in Africa and the Middle East. Her current research interests include efficacy of trauma rehabilitation interventions; representative surveys of mental health symptoms and needs in humanitarian contexts; and survivor-centred approaches to transitional justice. She is the co-author (with James Ron, David Crow, and Archana Pandya) of *Taking Root: Human Rights and Public Opinion in the Global South* (Oxford 2017). She received her PhD in Sociology and Human Rights from the University of Minnesota.

Sophie Harman is professor in International Politics at Queen Mary University of London where she teaches and conducts research into Global Health Politics, Africa and International Relations, and Global Governance. She has published six books on these topics, most notably *Global Health Governance*, and has written for *The Guardian*, *The Huffington Post*, and *The Independent*, and on Ebola and HIV/AIDS. Sophie is the trustee of Tanzanian HIV/AIDS charity 'TransTanz' and in 2016 she co-wrote and produced her first narrative feature film *Pili*, which was nominated for a BAFTA for outstanding debut for a British writer, producer, or director in 2019.

Deborah Ikhile is currently undertaking her doctoral study at Nottingham Trent University, UK. Her research focuses on exploring approaches to promote early detection of breast cancer in women in developing countries, with a focus on a semirural region in Uganda. Prior to this, she completed an extensive research on perceived barriers to early detection of breast cancer among women in Central Uganda, using a multilevel approach. She also works as a research assistant at Nottingham Trent University where she provides project management and research support to the Public Health department on international health projects across Europe, Eastern and Western parts of Africa, and South Africa. Deborah has a strong multidisciplinary background in community development and health. Over the years, she has developed an interest in a multi-level approach to women's health and how this is positioned and influenced by global health and development discourses. She holds an MA in Public Health from Nottingham Trent University and an MSc in Sustainable Planning and Environmental Management from the University of Hertfordshire.

Veronica Laveta is an international clinical advisor for mental health at the Center for Victims of Torture (CVT). She provides clinical supervision and programme oversight to CVT's mental health rehabilitation programmes for survivors of torture and war trauma, as well as capacity building for torture treatment centres around the world. She has worked in the Middle East, South Africa, and Uganda. In addition to her clinical degree (LCSW), Veronica has an MA in Conflict Transformation and is particularly interested in the intersection of trauma healing and peacebuilding. She has written a chapter titled 'Preventing Violence through a Trauma Healing Approach' for an edited volume.

Dragana Lukić is a PhD candidate in Gender Research at the Centre for Women's and Gender Research, HSL-Faculty, UiT the Arctic University of Norway. Her PhD research explores transformative powers of the creative arts for creating different understandings of lives with dementias. Her PhD project Artistic Entanglements: Multiple ontologies of Alzheimer's disease and other dementias is a part of Artful Dementia Research Lab at the Centre for Women's and Gender Research. Lukić's research interests include material feminisms, the politics of care, science and technology studies, health care practices, and fine arts. Her most recent publication is 'Multiple Ontologies of Alzheimer's Disease in Still Alice and A Song For Martin: A Feminist Visual Studies of Technoscience Perspective' in European Journal of Women's Studies.

Ann Therese Lotherington, PhD, is professor of Sociology and Vice Dean for Research, HSL-Faculty, UiT The Arctic University of Norway. She has a long-term commitment to gender and feminist research within different empirical fields. Currently she explores, together with an interdisciplinary research team, The Artful Dementia Research Lab, the potentials of art interventions for the development of an ethically sustainable qualitative research method for inquiring into living a gracious everyday life with dementia. This endeavour also demands a new theoretical framework combining relational aesthetics and feminist materialist theory. Lotherington has published widely within the field of health and social care.

Néstor Nuño Martínez is PhD candidate in Epidemiology at the Swiss Tropical and Public Health Institute. He is a graduate in Social Anthropology at the Universidad Complutense of Madrid and holds a master of science degree in Medical Anthropology and Sociology from the University of Amsterdam. He is specialised in the fields of religion, gender studies, and global health with research experience in Spain, Indonesia, and Peru. His recent publications include 'The Use of "Life-Enabling" Practices among Waria. Vulnerability, Subsistence and Paradoxes in Contemporary Jogjakarta', in *Intimate Economies: Bodies, Emotions and Sexualities on the Global Market*, edited by S. Hofmann and A. Moreno (Palgrave 2016); and 'El acceso y la atención sanitaria como reivindicaciones socio-políticas. Reconstruyendo la salud global desde los márgenes', *Revista de Antropologia Social* 26, no. 1: 73–91.

Elina Oinas is professor of Sociology at the Swedish School of Social Science at the University of Helsinki. Her work deals with gender, girls, and the body in various contexts. Her recent projects have been about youth and politics in contemporary Africa, and about academia as a site of contestation, with a focus on Development Studies, Gender Studies, and Biomedicine. They include an ethnographic study on a diarrhoea vaccine trial in Benin, West Africa, and a study on the epistemic practices of Gender Studies in Ethiopia, Finland, and South Africa. Elina acts as the chair of the council of the Nordic Africa Institute and is a board member of a number of academic societies, including the International Sociological Association.

Camilla Reuterswärd received her PhD from the Department of Political Science, University of Wisconsin-Madison, in 2019. Her work focuses on gender and politics in Latin America with a particular emphasis on abortion and LGBTQ+ policy, as well as party politics, religious institutions, and social movements in the region. She also holds broader interests in issues related to violence against women, especially feminicide. Camilla has a bachelor degree in Development studies from the Department of Government at Uppsala University and a master's degree from the University of Wisconsin-Madison. Her work has appeared in *Development and Change*. She is currently a postdoctoral fellow at the Freie Universität Berlin.

Maria Tanyag is a lecturer in International Relations at the Australian National University, Coral Bell School of Asia Pacific Affairs. Previously, she was a postdoctoral research fellow at the Gender, Peace and Security (GPS) Centre at Monash University, Australia, where she was also awarded her PhD in 2018. She is a recipient of the Australian Institute of International Affairs (AIIA) Early Career Research Impact Award; and the 2018 Australian International Political Economy Network (AIPEN) paper prize for her article 'Invisible Labor, Invisible Bodies: How the Global Political Economy Affects Reproductive Freedom in the Philippines' in the *International Feminist Journal of Politics* (2017).

Tiina Vaittinen is Academy of Finland Postdoctoral Research Fellow at Tampere University, Finland. She holds a PhD in Peace and Conflict Research. Drawing broadly on feminist theories of peace, ethics of care, new materialisms, science and technology studies, her work focuses on deconstructing the global politics of care and care needs. Her most recent project deals with peace and conflict in residential dementia care, and she is just commencing a new project on the global political economies of the adult incontinence pad. She has published in journals such as *International Feminist journal of Politics, Women's Studies International Forum, Peacebuilding*, and *Global Society*, and is a co-editor of the book series Feminist Studies on Peace, Justice and Violence (with Shweta Singh and Catia C. Confortini, Rowman & Littlefield International).

Azrini Wahidin is professor of Criminology and Sociology and the co-director of the Centre for Study of Women and Gender Studies at the University of Warwick. She has held the position of associate dean for research and innovation and head of department. She researches on the issues of imprisonment, youth justice, violence against women, women in the criminal justice system, the engendering of punishment, the experiences of elders in prison in the UK and US, as well as feminist research methods and ethics. Her book, *Ex-Combatants, Gender and Peace in Northern Ireland: Women, Political Protest and the Prison Experience* (Palgrave 2016), focuses on female political prisoners and the role of transitional justice in post-conflict societies. She is the co-editor (with Linda Moore Phil Scraton) of *Women's Imprisonment and the Case for Abolition: Critical Reflections on Corston Ten Years On* (Routledge 2018) and (with Malcolm Cowburn and Loraine Gelsthorpe) of *Research Ethics in Criminology – Dilemmas, Issues and Solutions* (Routledge 2017). She is a visiting professor at the University of Malaya in the faculty of law and a visiting Professor in the KANITA (Gender Studies) Department in the School of Social Sciences, Universiti Sains Malaysia.

www.ingramcontent.com/pod-product-compliance
Ingram Content Group UK Ltd.
Pitfield, Milton Keynes, MK11 3LW, UK
UKHW041832220426
470268UK00001B/24